Atlas of Laparoscopic Gastrectomy for Gastric Cancer

Chang-Ming Huang
Chao-Hui Zheng • Ping Li
Jian-Wei Xie

Atlas of Laparoscopic Gastrectomy for Gastric Cancer

High Resolution Image for New Surgical Technique

PMPH PEOPLE'S MEDICAL PUBLISHING HOUSE Springer

Chang-Ming Huang
Department of Gastric Surgery
Fujian Medical University
Union Hospital
Fuzhou
China

Chao-Hui Zheng
Department of Gastric Surgery
Fujian Medical University
Union Hospital
Fuzhou
China

Ping Li
Department of Gastric Surgery
Fujian Medical University
Union Hospital
Fuzhou
China

Jian-Wei Xie
Department of Gastric Surgery
Fujian Medical University
Union Hospital
Fuzhou
China

ISBN 978-981-13-2861-9 ISBN 978-981-13-2862-6 (eBook)
https://doi.org/10.1007/978-981-13-2862-6

Library of Congress Control Number: 2018962493

This Springer imprint is published by the registered company Springer Nature Singapore Pte Ltd.
The registered company address is: 152 Beach Road, #21-01/04 Gateway East, Singapore 189721, Singapore

This book commemorates the 10th anniversary of performing laparoscopic radical gastrectomies for gastric cancer and a total of over 5000 such cases treated at the Department of Gastric Surgery, Fujian Medical University Union Hospital (Fujian, China).

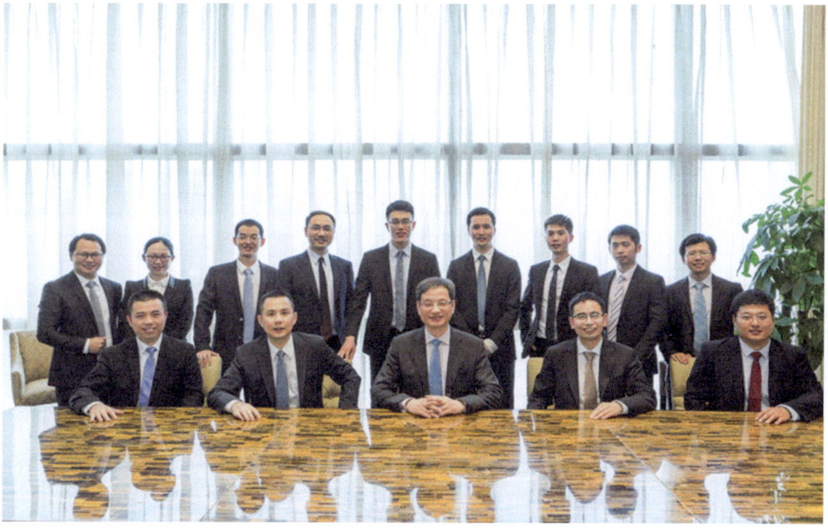

Our team: Department of Gastric Surgery, Fujian Medical University Union Hospital, China

Left→Right (row one): Jian-Wei Xie, Chao-Hui Zheng, Chang-Ming Huang, Ping Li, Jia-Bin Wang

Left→Right (row two): Jian-Xian Lin, Mi Lin, Ru-Hong Tu, Jun Lu, Ze-Ning Huang, Qi-Yue Chen, Hua-Long Zheng, Ju-Li Lin, Long-Long Cao

Preface

Laparoscopic technology has achieved satisfactory clinical effects in the treatment of early gastric cancer and has also been applied to the treatment of locally advanced gastric cancer. The success of laparoscopic radical gastrectomy for gastric cancer not only requires proficient surgical techniques but also high-level, standardized, and programmed surgical procedures. Accordingly, we decided to publish this atlas, which is based on *Laparoscopic Gastrectomy for Gastric Cancer: Surgical Technique and Lymphadenectomy*, published in 2015. All ultra-high-definition surgical images in the book were collected by the Highlights Storz IMAGE1 S™ Platform and are of an excellent quality that enhances the descriptions.

In this book, we introduce procedures and precautions associated with lymph node dissection of laparoscopic radical gastrectomy for gastric cancer, ranging from preoperative preparation to regional lymph node dissection, and digestive tract reconstruction. The content is pragmatic and comprehensive and relevant to clinical practical applications.

As the first specialized department in a large-scale Chinese general hospital devoted to the treatment of gastric cancer, the Department of Gastric Surgery, Fujian Medical University Union Hospital, performs more than 1000 gastric cancer surgeries each year. Since the first case of laparoscopic radical gastrectomy in May 6, 2007, ten years of unremitting efforts have enabled our department to become one of the most respected centers for laparoscopic gastric cancer surgery in the world.

During the past ten years, we have continuously evaluated the anatomic characteristics and variation of gastric vessels, which has laid solid foundations for the development of laparoscopic radical gastrectomy. We also optimized lymph node dissection, especially "Huang's three-step maneuver" in laparoscopic spleen-preserving splenic hilar lymphadenectomy, which simplifies the procedure, reduces its difficulty, and promotes popularization of the technique. We have regularly modified laparoscopic reconstruction of the digestive tract after radical gastrectomy and improved the safety of distal gastrectomy and total gastrectomy by first proposing the modified delta-shaped gastroduodenostomy technique, then later isoperistaltic later-cut Roux-en-Y anastomosis. At the same time, we have furthered high-level evidence-based medicine by conducting a number of multicenter prospective clinical trials associated with laparoscopic gastric cancer surgery. These included acting as principal investigator in the CLASS-04 test, and as the unit with the most effective cases in the CLASS-01 test and the CLASS-02 test.

Additionally, more than ten single-center prospective clinical trials are currently in progress.

Based on the spirit of an ancient Chinese poem from the Tang Dynasty which states that "ten years' hard working molds a sword," we have taken our valuable experience of laparoscopic gastric cancer surgery and compiled it into a book. We hope that it will inspire our colleagues who are committed to gastric cancer surgery and aspire to work together to promote the development of minimally invasive laparoscopic surgery for gastric cancer. This book is dedicated to the 10th anniversary of laparoscopic radical gastrectomies for gastric cancer and a total of over 5000 such cases at the Department of Gastric Surgery, Fujian Medical University Union Hospital.

The editors of this book are doctors at the clinical front line of this department. Besides their heavy clinical workload, they have sacrificed much of their precious spare time to help publish this book, for which we are immensely grateful. We would also like to express our appreciation to the related departments of People's Medical Publishing House and Springer for their encouragement and support. Meanwhile, we hope that all experts, fellows, and readers will feel free to enlighten us with suggestions to further improve this book and its later editions; together, we can make it extraordinary.

Fuzhou, China
December 2017

Chang-Ming Huang

Contents

Contributors and Editors

About the Authors

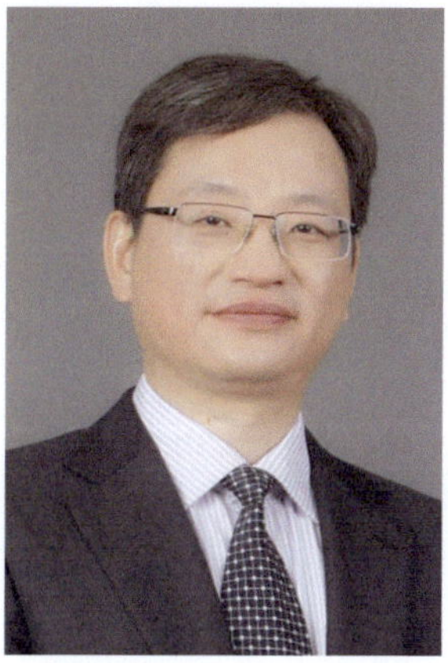

Chang-Ming Huang is a secondary level professor, chief physician, doctoral supervisor, recipient of a Government Special Allowance, a science and technology innovation talent from Fujian Province, and Director of the Department of Gastric Surgery of Fujian Medical University Union Hospital, China. He is a member of the Gastric Cancer Profession standing committee of the Chinese Anti-Cancer Association, the vice chairman of the Surgical Oncology Committee of the surgical branch of the Chinese Medical Doctor Association, a member of the gastrointestinal surgical branch of the Chinese Medical Association, and a member of the Minimally Invasive Surgery Committee of the surgical branch of the Chinese Medical Doctor Association. He is also an editorial board member of the *Chinese Journal of Gastrointestinal Surgery*, *Chinese Journal of Digestive Surgery*, and *Journal of Laparoscopic Surgery*, and a corresponding editor of the *Chinese Journal of Surgery*; he has also acted as a reviewer for more than ten core journals including *Annals of Surgical Oncology*, *Surgical Endoscopy*, *World Journal of Gastroenterology*, and *the Chinese Medical Journal*. He has published more than 200 articles, including more than 100 in SCI journals, as well as in Chinese medicine magazines, and other professional journals. As an editor-in-chief, he published

Laparoscopic Gastrectomy for Gastric Cancer: Surgical Technique and Lymphadenectomy in English (Springer, 2015) and two books in Chinese (People's Medical Publishing House, 2011 and 2015). Moreover, he has been awarded the Fujian Provincial Science and Technology Achievement Award many times and is currently undertaking a number of national and provincial scientific research projects.

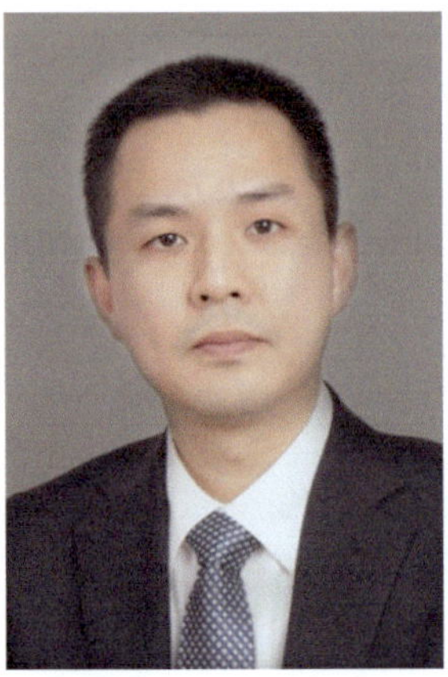

Chao-Hui Zheng is an associate professor, chief physician, and master's supervisor who currently works in the Department of Gastric Surgery of Fujian Medical University Union Hospital, China. He is a member of the Laparo-Endoscopic Surgery of the surgical branch of the Chinese Medical Association, a member of the Gastric Cancer Association of the Chinese Anti-Cancer Association, a member of the Surgical Oncology Physicians Committee of the surgical branch of the Chinese Medical Doctor Association, a member of the Obesity and Diabetes Surgeons Committee of the surgical branch of the Chinese Medical Doctor Association, a member of the Obesity and Diabetes Surgical Committee of the Chinese Research Hospital Association, and a member of the First Laparoscopic Subcommittee of the Endoscopic Physicians Committee of the Chinese Medical Doctor Association. He is also corresponding editor of the *Chinese Journal of Digestive Surgery* and on the editorial board of the *Chinese Journal of Obesity and Metabolic Diseases*. He has published more than 50 articles, including more than 40 in SCI journals, as well as in Chinese medicine magazines, and other professional journals. As an editor-in-chief, he published *Laparoscopic Gastrectomy for Gastric Cancer: Surgical Technique and Lymphadenectomy* in English (Springer, 2015) and two books in Chinese (People's Medical Publishing House, 2011 and 2015). Moreover, he has been awarded the Fujian Provincial Science and Technology Achievement Award many times and is currently undertaking a number of national and provincial scientific research projects.

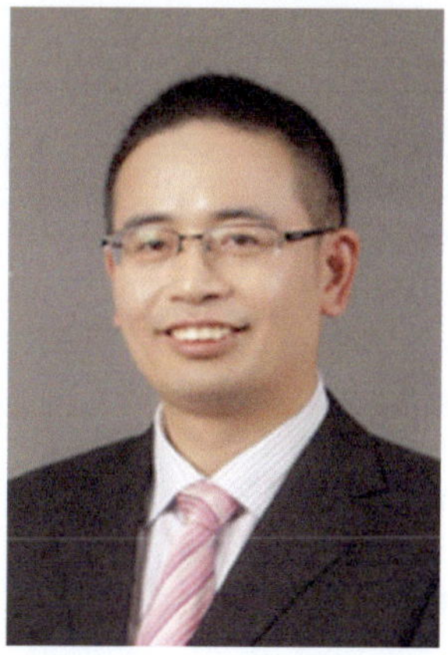

Ping Li is an associate professor, associate chief physician, master's supervisor, and medical postdoctoral fellow of the Memorial Sloan Kettering Cancer Center, New York (NY, USA). He is a member of the Bariatric and Metabolic Committee of the surgical branch of the Chinese Medical Association, a member of the Upper Gastrointestinal Surgical Committee and the Young Oncologists Committee of the Surgical Oncology Committee of the surgical branch of the Chinese Medical Doctor Association, a member of the Academic Instruction Rehabilitation Committee of the Chinese Anti-Cancer Association, and a health science member of the China International Exchange and Promotive Association for Medical and Healthcare. He has published 12 original articles in SCI journals, Chinese medicine magazines, and other professional journals as first author or co-corresponding author. He is also the deputy editor of *Laparoscopic Gastrectomy for Gastric Cancer: Surgical Technique and Lymphadenectomy* in English (Springer, 2015) and *Laparoscopic Radical Gastrectomy for Gastric Cancer: Technique of Lymphadenectomy* in Chinese (People's Medical Publishing House, 2015), as well as an editor of a previous version of this latter publication, published in 2011. Moreover, he won the César Roux Award in the Laparoscopic Gastric Cancer Surgery Group in the 2014 Gastric Cancer Surgery Video Contest for Young Chinese Physicians and was awarded the 2014 Award of National Scholarship for Doctoral Candidates, and the Fujian Provincial Science and Technology Progress Award many times. He is currently undertaking a number of national and provincial scientific research projects.

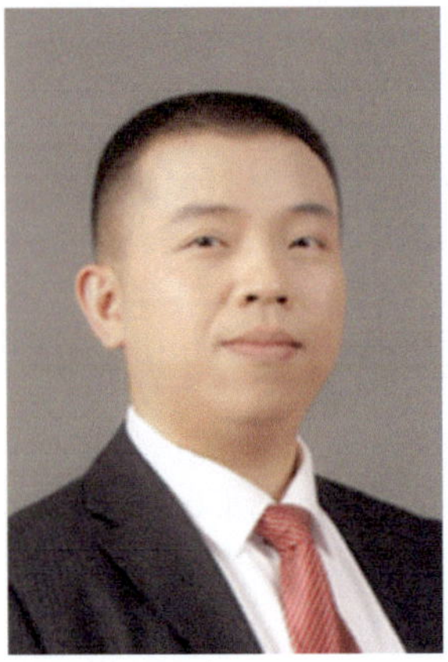

Jian-Wei Xie is a doctor of medicine and associate chief physician. He is a member of the Gastrointestinal Oncology Committee of the oncological branch of the Chinese Medical Association, a member of the neuroendocrine tumor branch of the China Science and Technology Industry Association, a young member of the surgical branch of the China Science and Technology Industry Association, a member of the Professional Committee of Gastrointestinal Stromal Tumor Diagnosis and Treatment of the Chinese Medical Doctor Association, and a member of the Robotic Surgery Committee of the surgical branch of the Chinese Medical Doctor Association. He has completed further study in renowned hospitals including the Mayo Clinic in the USA and the National Cancer Center, Japan. He has published more than 10 articles in SCI journals, Chinese medicine magazines, and other professional journals. He is also deputy editor of *Laparoscopic Gastrectomy for Gastric Cancer: Surgical Technique and Lymphadenectomy* in English (Springer, 2015) and *Laparoscopic Radical Gastrectomy for Gastric Cancer: Technique of Lymphadenectomy* in Chinese (People's Medical Publishing House, 2015), as well as an editor of a previous version of this latter publication, published in 2011. Moreover, he has been awarded the Fujian Provincial Science and Technology Achievement Award many times and is currently undertaking a number of national and provincial scientific research projects.

List of Contributors

Long-Long Cao Department of Gastric Surgery, Fujian Medical University Union Hospital, Fuzhou, China

Hai-Feng Chen Department of Gastric Surgery, Fujian Medical University Union Hospital, Fuzhou, China

Qi-Yue Chen Department of Gastric Surgery, Fujian Medical University Union Hospital, Fuzhou, China

Zhi-Jiang Chen Department of Gastric Surgery, Fujian Medical University Union Hospital, Fuzhou, China

Yun Dai Department of Gastric Surgery, Fujian Medical University Union Hospital, Fuzhou, China

Zhi-Liang Hong Department of Gastric Surgery, Fujian Medical University Union Hospital, Fuzhou, China

Chang-Ming Huang Department of Gastric Surgery, Fujian Medical University Union Hospital, Fuzhou, China

Ying-Qi Huang Department of Gastric Surgery, Fujian Medical University Union Hospital, Fuzhou, China

Ze-Ning Huang Department of Gastric Surgery, Fujian Medical University Union Hospital, Fuzhou, China

Ping Li Department of Gastric Surgery, Fujian Medical University Union Hospital, Fuzhou, China

Yang Liao Department of Gastric Surgery, Fujian Medical University Union Hospital, Fuzhou, China

Guang-Tan Lin Department of Gastric Surgery, Fujian Medical University Union Hospital, Fuzhou, China

Jian-Xian Lin Department of Gastric Surgery, Fujian Medical University Union Hospital, Fuzhou, China

Ju-Li Lin Department of Gastric Surgery, Fujian Medical University Union Hospital, Fuzhou, China

Jun-Peng Lin Department of Gastric Surgery, Fujian Medical University Union Hospital, Fuzhou, China

Mi Lin Department of Gastric Surgery, Fujian Medical University Union Hospital, Fuzhou, China

Zhi-Yu Liu Department of Gastric Surgery, Fujian Medical University Union Hospital, Fuzhou, China

Jun Lu Department of Gastric Surgery, Fujian Medical University Union Hospital, Fuzhou, China

Xin-Chang Shang-Guan Department of Gastric Surgery, Fujian Medical University Union Hospital, Fuzhou, China

Ru-Hong Tu Department of Gastric Surgery, Fujian Medical University Union Hospital, Fuzhou, China

Jia-Bin Wang Department of Gastric Surgery, Fujian Medical University Union Hospital, Fuzhou, China

Liang-Bin Wang Department of Gastric Surgery, Fujian Medical University Union Hospital, Fuzhou, China

Zu-Kai Wang Department of Gastric Surgery, Fujian Medical University Union Hospital, Fuzhou, China

Jian-Wei Xie Department of Gastric Surgery, Fujian Medical University Union Hospital, Fuzhou, China

Bin-Bin Xu Department of Gastric Surgery, Fujian Medical University Union Hospital, Fuzhou, China

Chao-Hui Zheng Department of Gastric Surgery, Fujian Medical University Union Hospital, Fuzhou, China

Hua-Long Zheng Department of Gastric Surgery, Fujian Medical University Union Hospital, Fuzhou, China

Zhi-Fang Zheng Department of Gastric Surgery, Fujian Medical University Union Hospital, Fuzhou, China

Qing Zhong Department of Gastric Surgery, Fujian Medical University Union Hospital, Fuzhou, China

1 Points for Attention Before Performing Laparoscopic Lymph Node Dissection for Gastric Cancer

1.1 Instrument Preparation

Routine laparoscopy equipment includes soft-acting gastric forceps, soft-acting intestinal forceps, aspirators, dissection forceps, scissors, needle holders, hemolock release clamps, vascular clamps, absorbable clip appliers, titanium clip appliers, small gauzes, 5 and 12 mm trocars, and ultrasonic scalpels (Figs. 1.1, 1.2, 1.3, 1.4, 1.5, 1.6, 1.7, 1.8, 1.9, 1.10, 1.11, and 1.12).

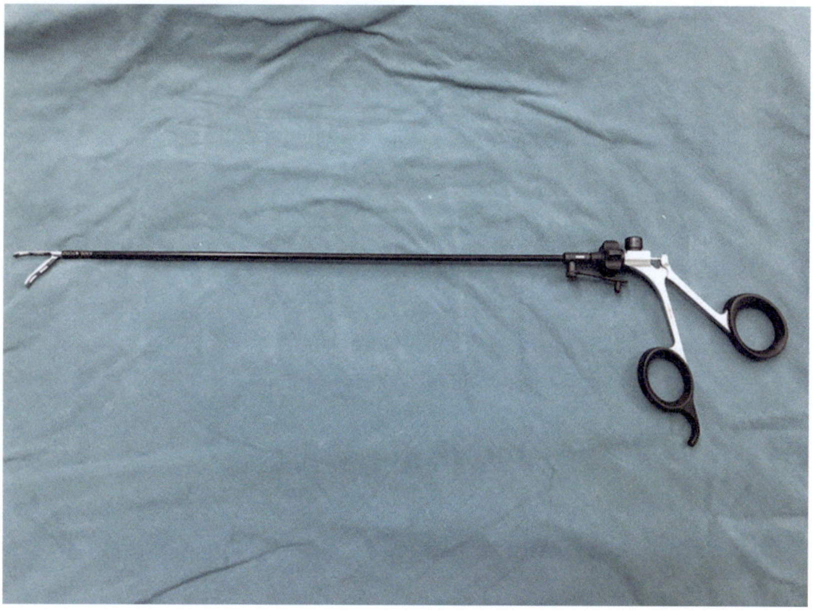

Fig. 1.1 Soft-acting gastric forceps

C.-M. Huang et al., *Atlas of Laparoscopic Gastrectomy for Gastric Cancer*,
https://doi.org/10.1007/978-981-13-2862-6_1

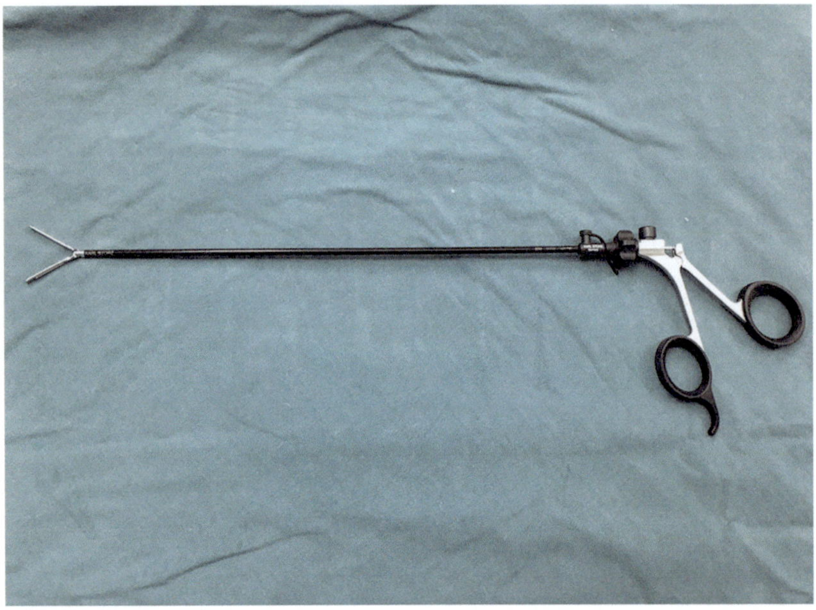

Fig. 1.2 Soft-acting intestinal forceps

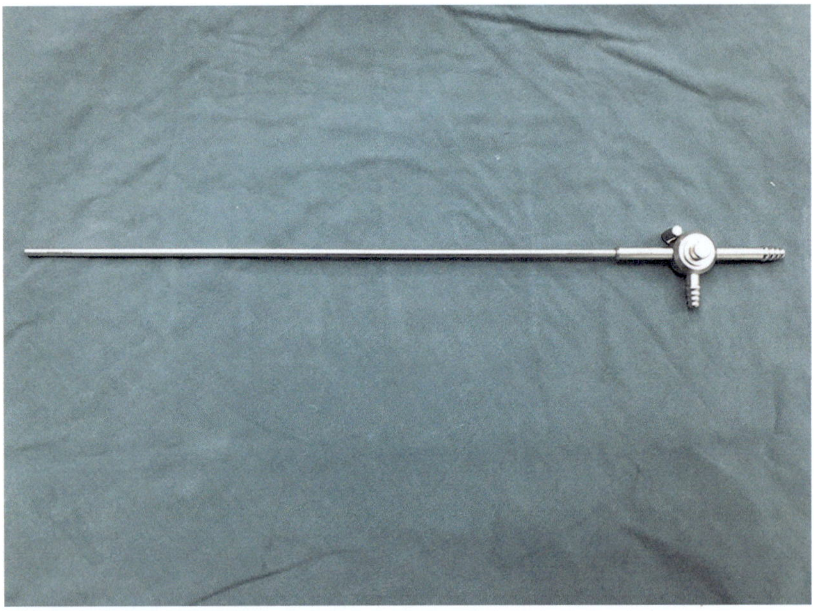

Fig. 1.3 Aspirator

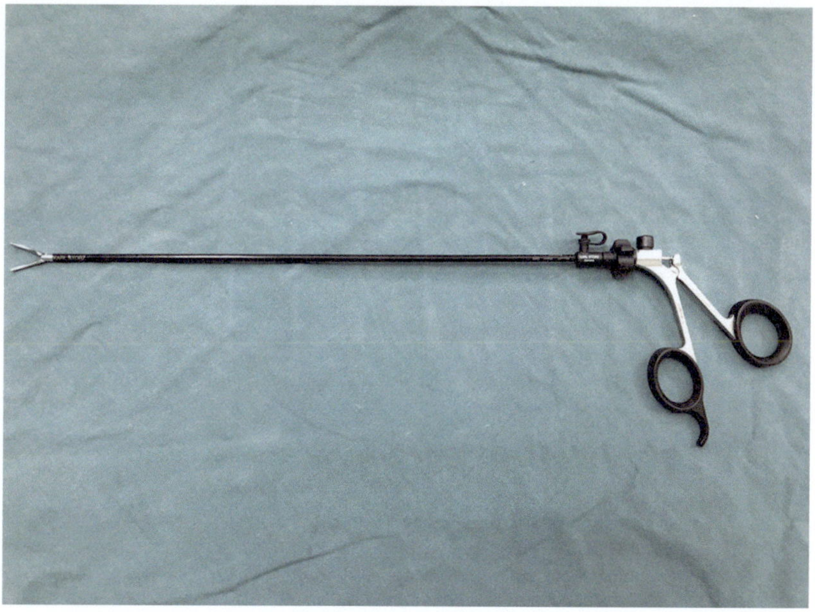

Fig. 1.4 Dissecting forceps

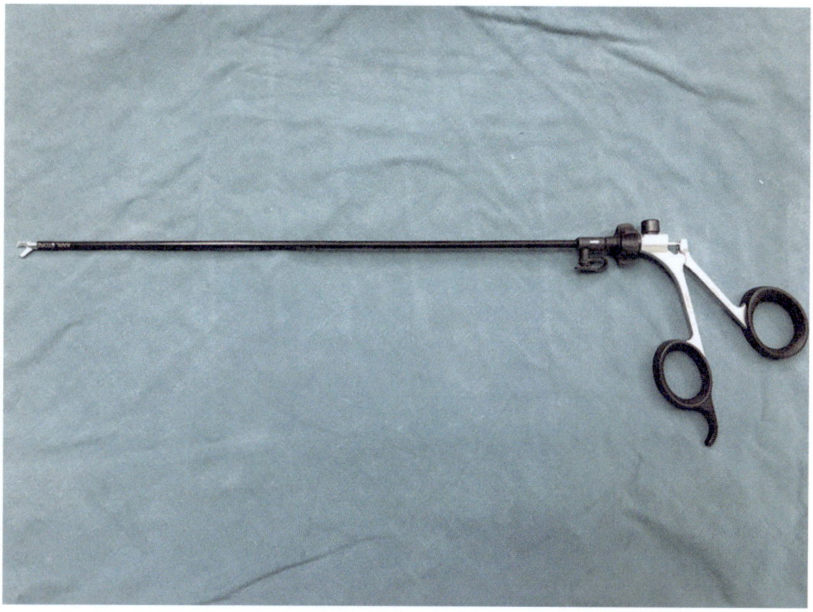

Fig. 1.5 Scissors

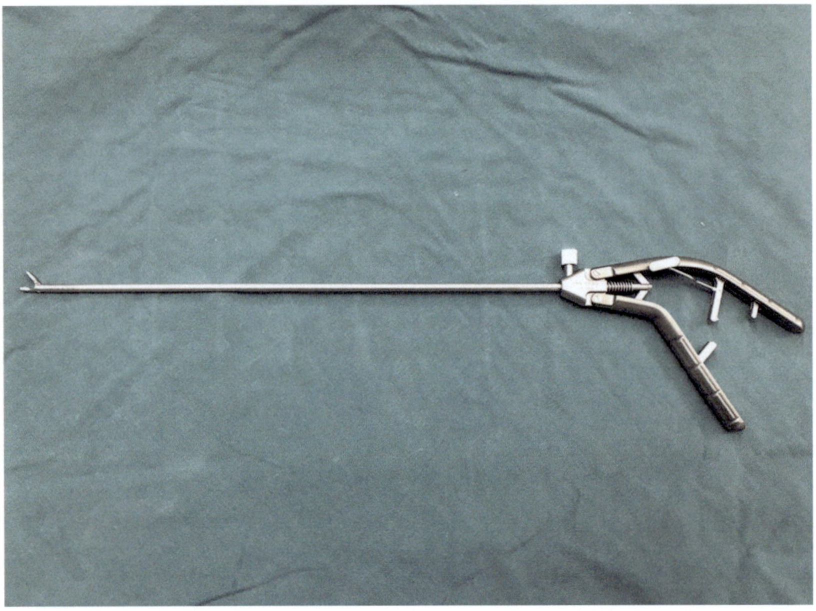

Fig. 1.6 Needle holder

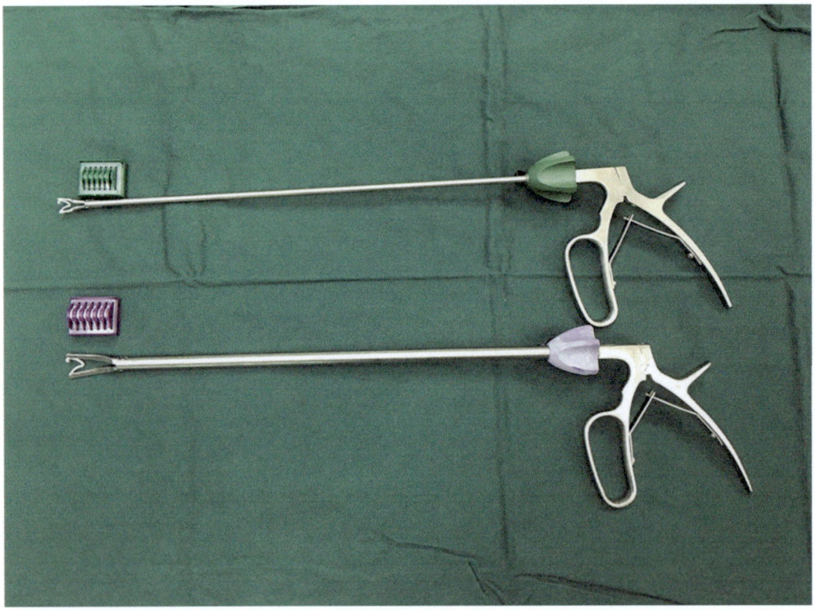

Fig. 1.7 Hemolock release clamp

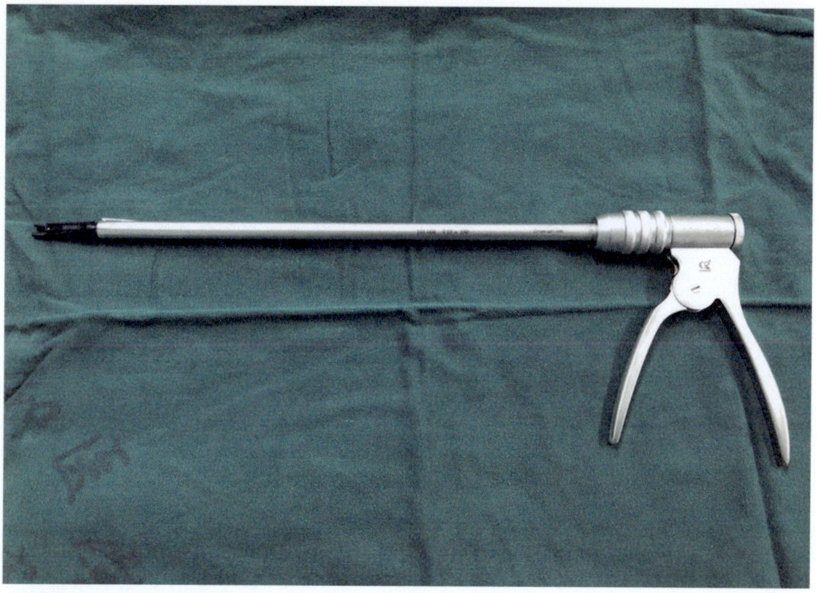

Fig. 1.8 Absorbable clip applier

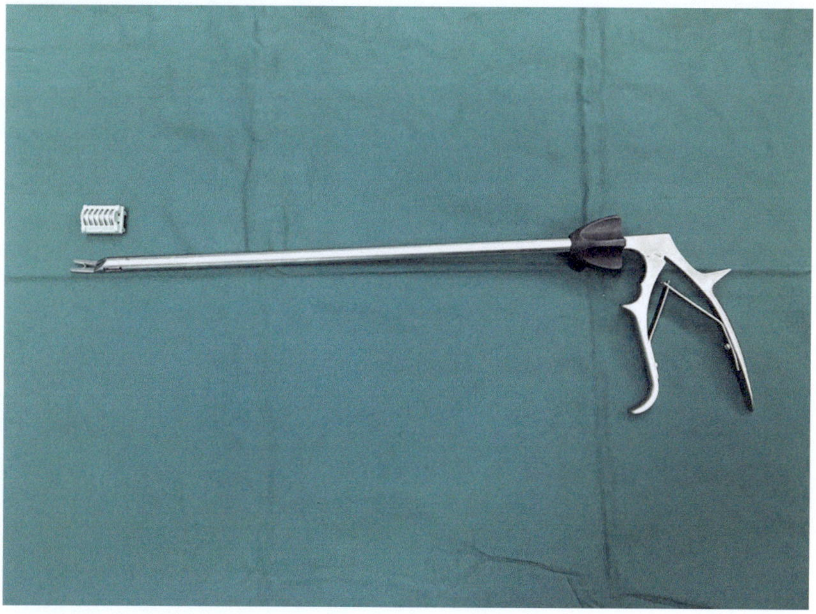

Fig. 1.9 Titanium clip applier

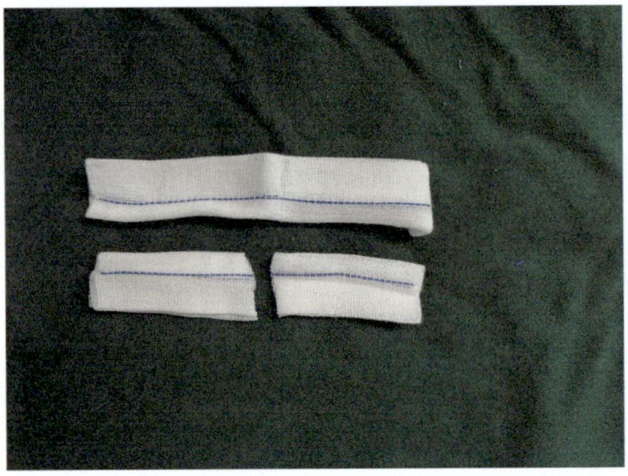

Fig. 1.10 Small gauze

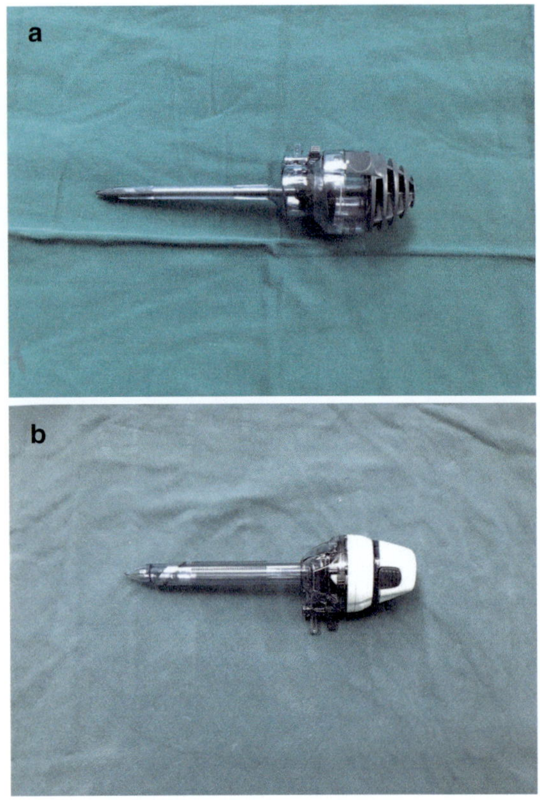

Fig. 1.11 (**a**) 5 mm trocar. (**b**) 12 mm trocar

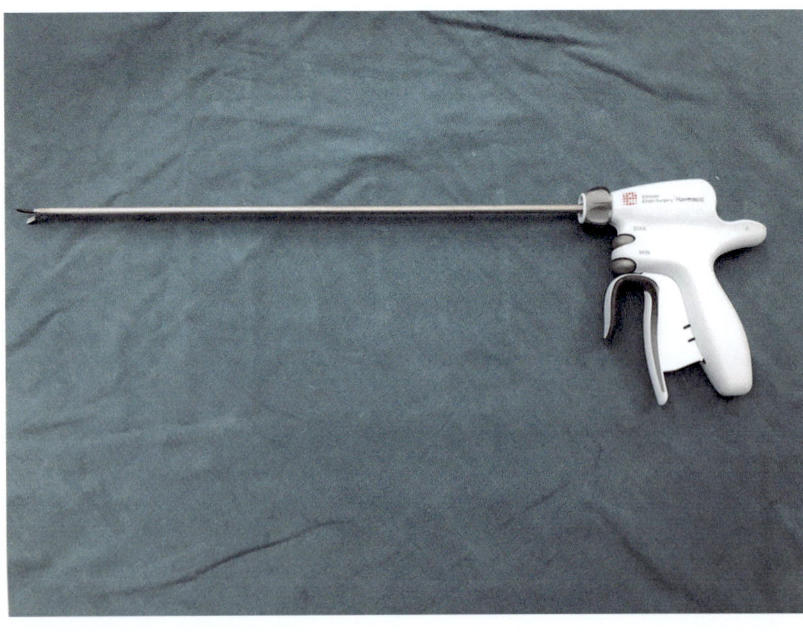

Fig. 1.12 Ultrasonic scalpel

1.2 Patient's Position

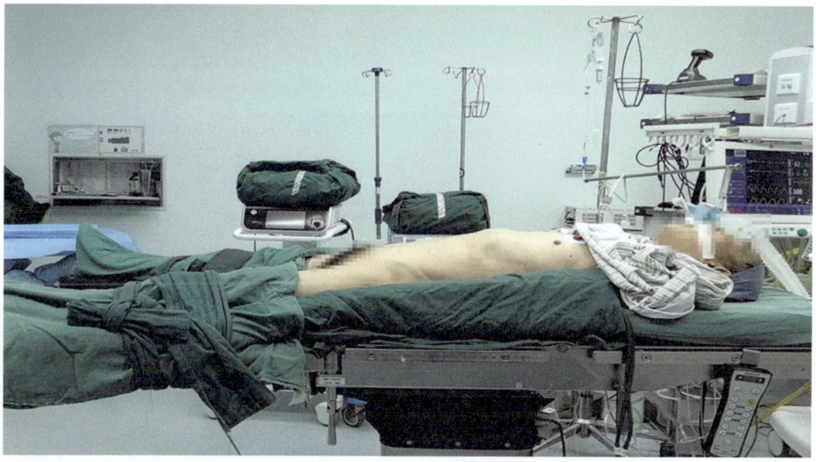

Fig. 1.13 Patient positioning: place in the supine and the reverse Trendelenburg position

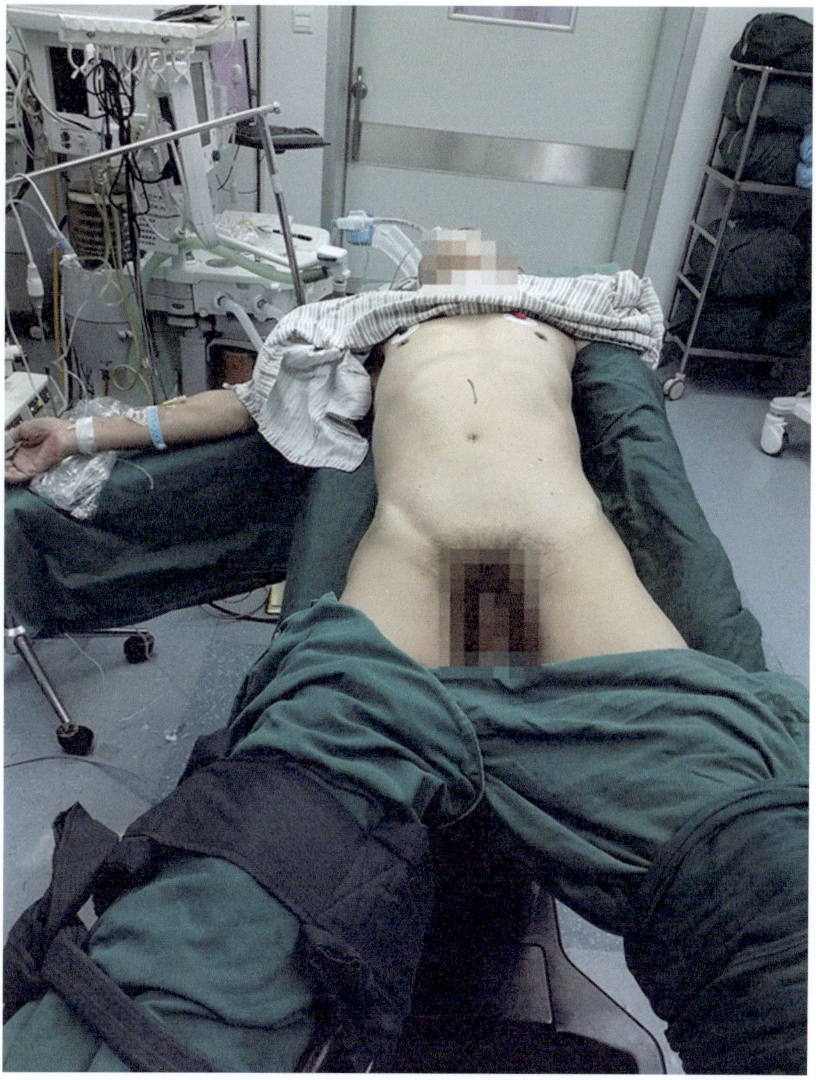

Fig. 1.14 Patient positioning for splenic hilar lymph node (LN) dissection: elevate the head of the bed by 10–20° and tilt it to the right by 20–30°

1.3 Surgeons' Positions

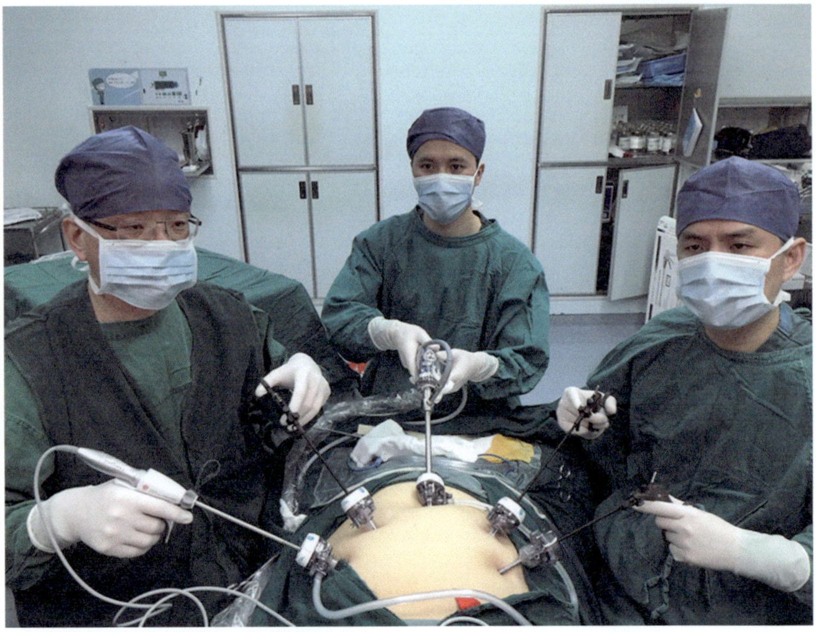

Fig. 1.15 General position of surgeons

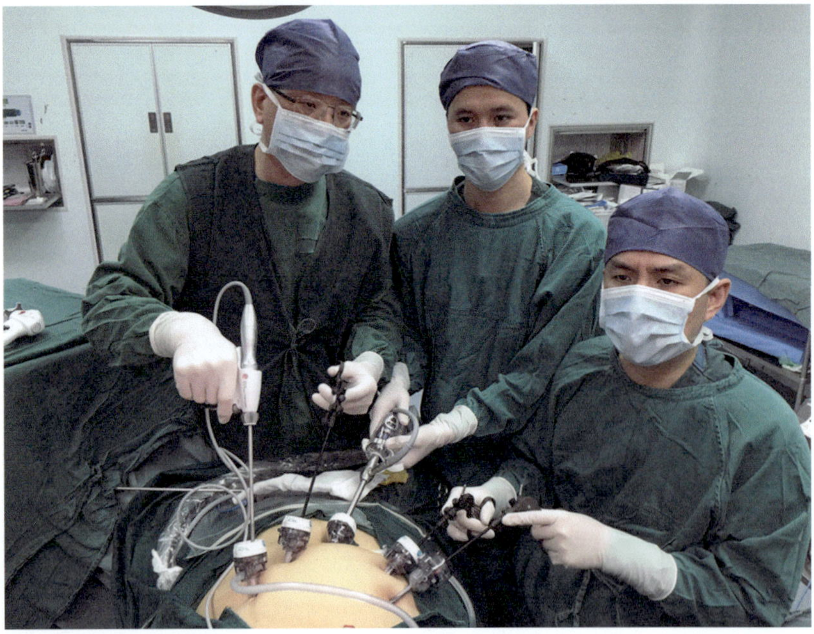

Fig. 1.16 Position of surgeons during splenic hilar LN dissection

1.4 Location of Trocars

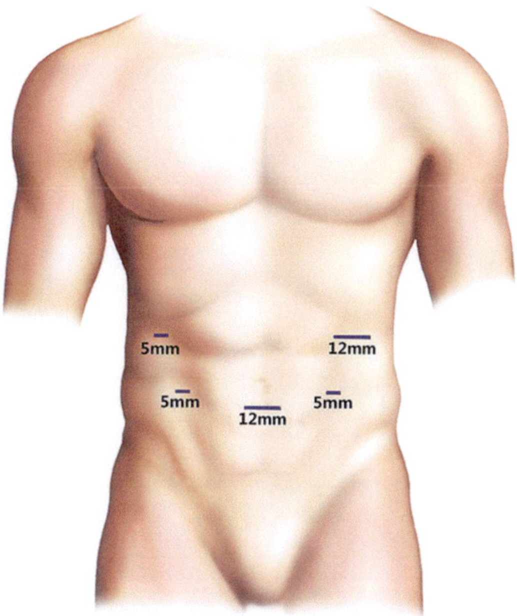

Fig. 1.17 Diagram of trocar locations

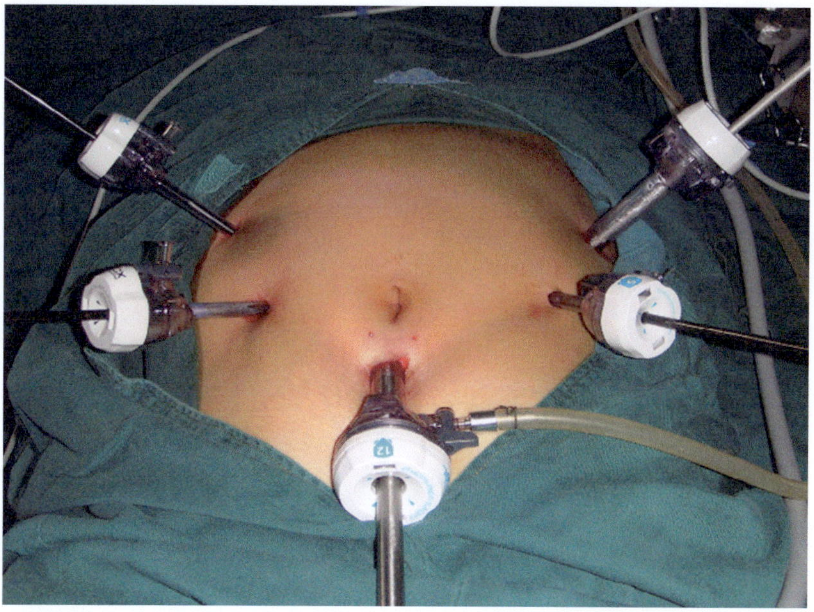

Fig. 1.18 Locations of the trocars (Reproduced with permission from [1])

1.5 Establishment of Pneumoperitoneum

SFVS (small flow vacuum suction).

To reduce the mist generated by the ultrasonic scalpel during the operation and help maintain a clear vision, a low vacuum suction set can be connected to the trocar in the major hand port (Fig. 1.19).

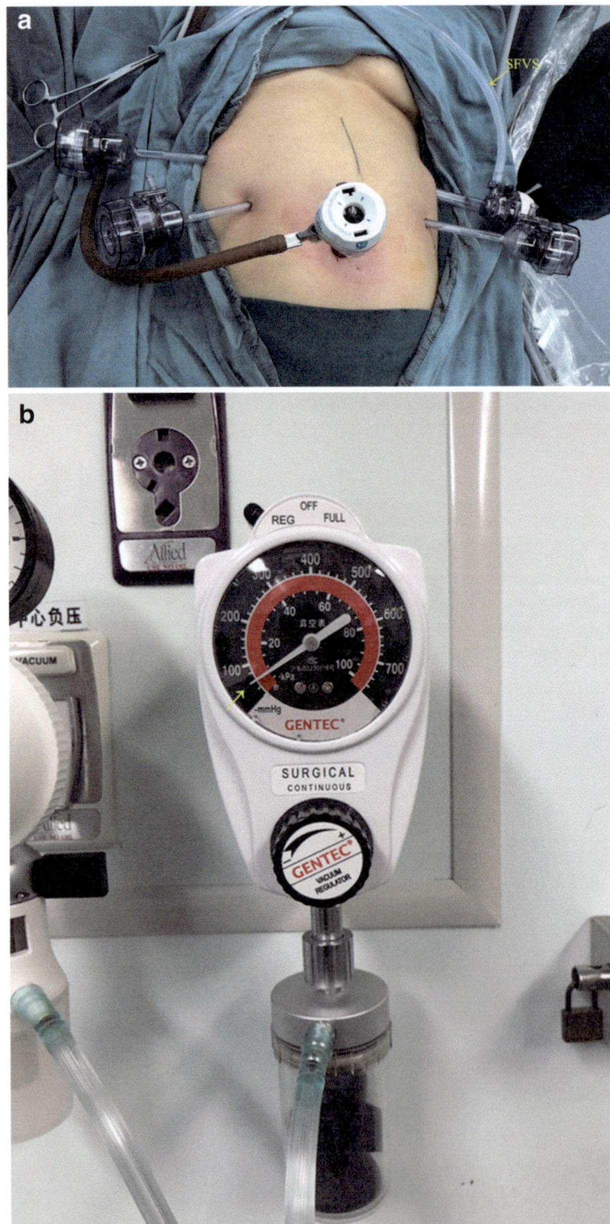

Fig. 1.19 (**a**) Major hand port connected with a small flow vacuum suction set. (**b**) Low vacuum suction

1.6 Preoperative Exploration

Preoperative diagnostic laparoscopic examination with a high-definition imaging system can effectively investigate the location, extent, and infiltration depth of the primary tumor, as well as the presence of lymph node metastasis (LNM), peritoneal implantation, ascites, and invasion of adjacent tissues (Figs. 1.20, 1.21, 1.22, and 1.23).

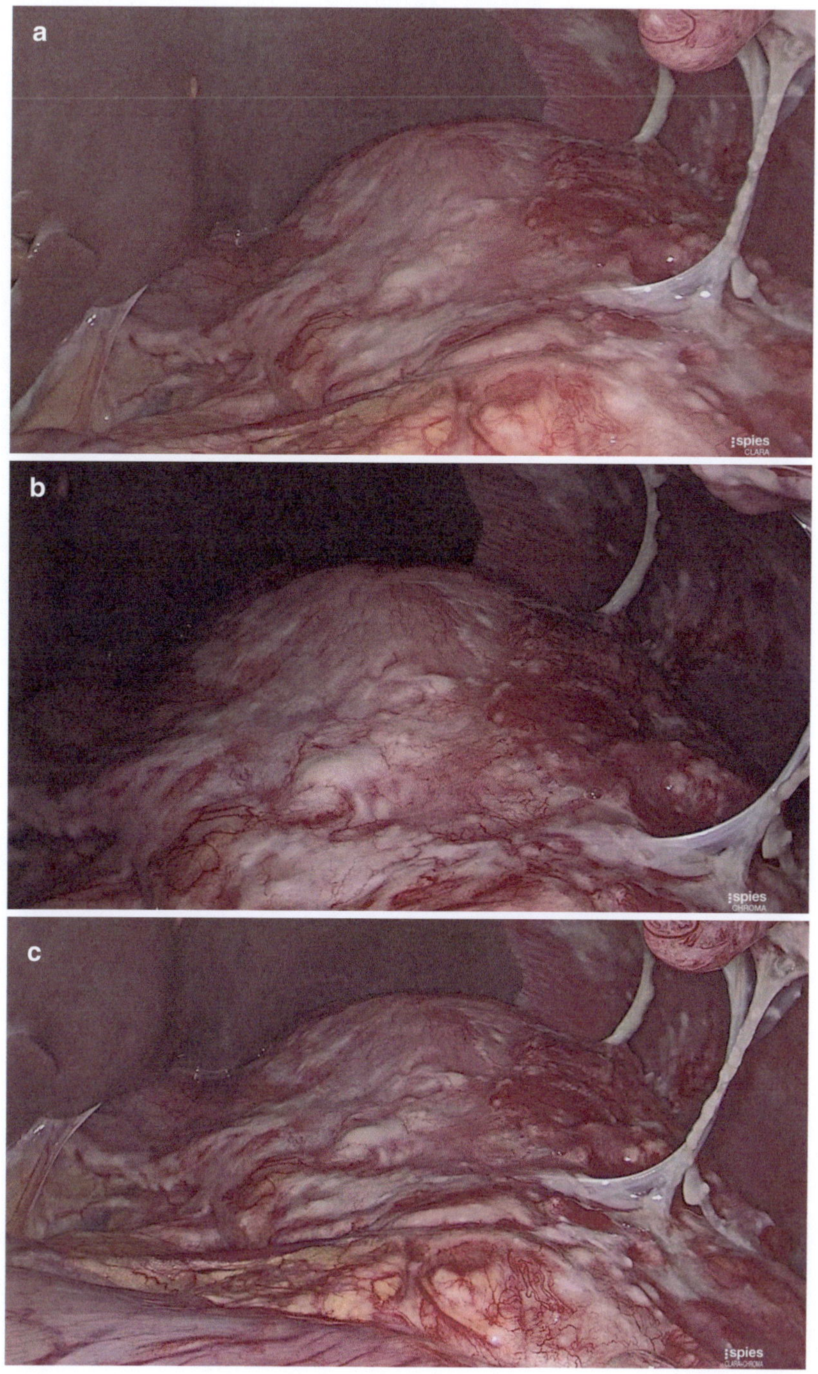

Fig. 1.20 (**a**) The tumor is located on the anterior gastric wall invading the serosa (model: CLARA), (**b**) The tumor is located on the anterior gastric wall invading the serosa (model: CHROMA), (**c**) The tumor is located on the anterior gastric wall invading the serosa (model: CLARA+CHROMA), (**d**) The tumor is located on the anterior gastric wall invading the serosa (model: SPECTRA A), (**e**) The tumor is located on the anterior gastric wall invading the serosa (model: SPECTRA B)

Fig. 1.20 (continued)

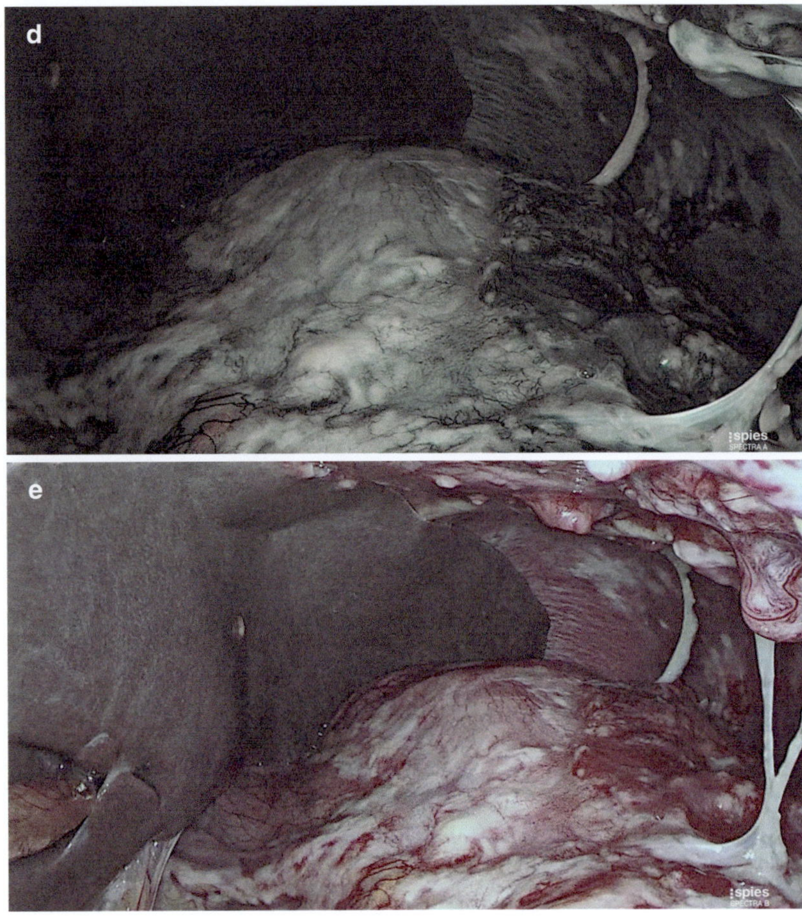

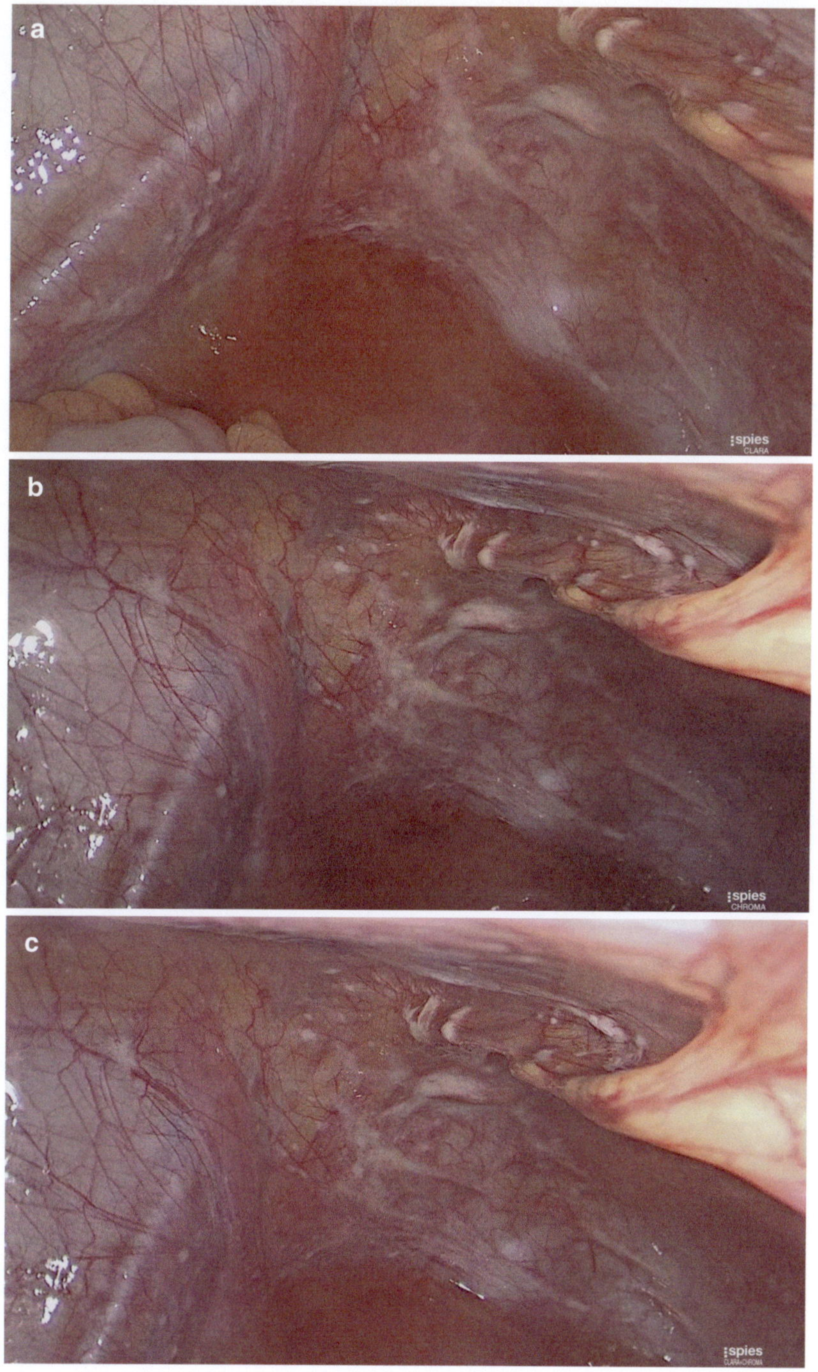

Fig. 1.21 (**a**) Gastric cancer with intraperitoneal metastasis and ascites (model: CLARA), (**b**) Gastric cancer with intraabdominal extensive metastasis and ascites (model: CHROMA), (**c**) Gastric cancer with intraperitoneal metastasis and ascites (model: CLARA+CHROMA), (**d**) Gastric cancer with intraperitoneal metastasis and ascites (model: SPECTA), (**e**) Gastric cancer with intraperitoneal metastasis and ascites (model: SPECTB)

Fig. 1.21 (continued)

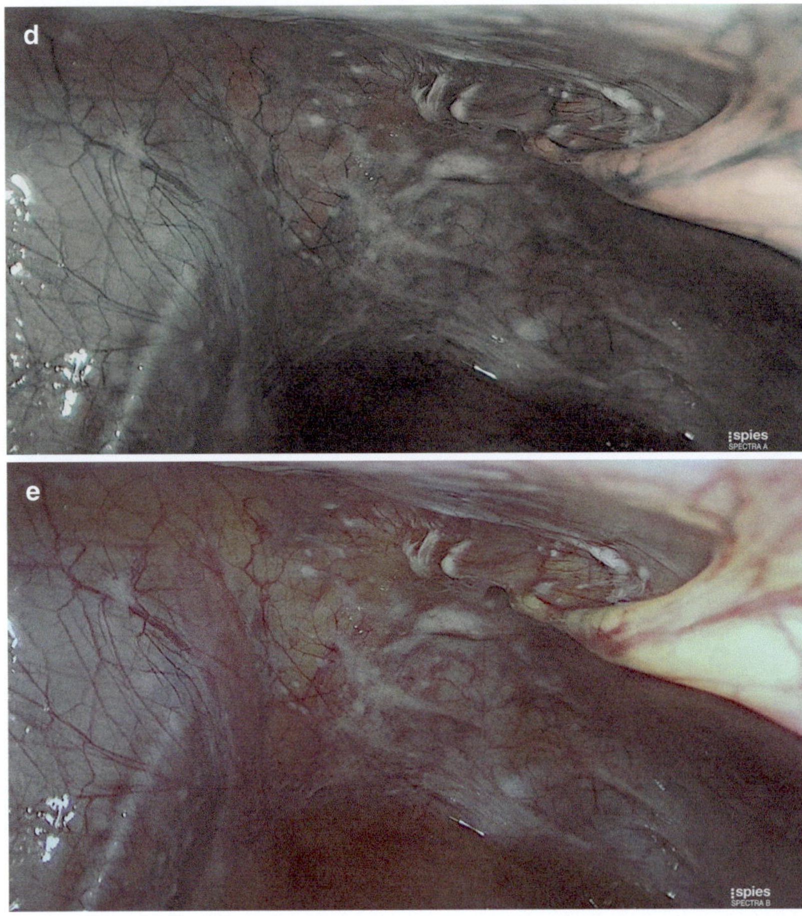

Fig. 1.22 Gastric cancer with liver metastasis (model: CLARA)

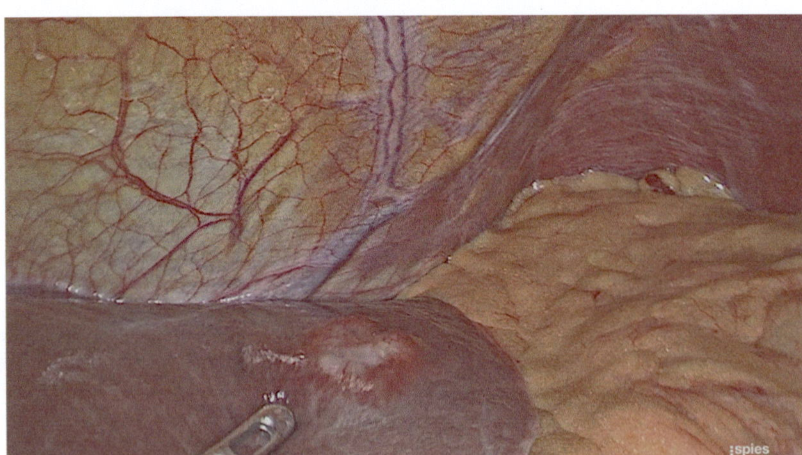

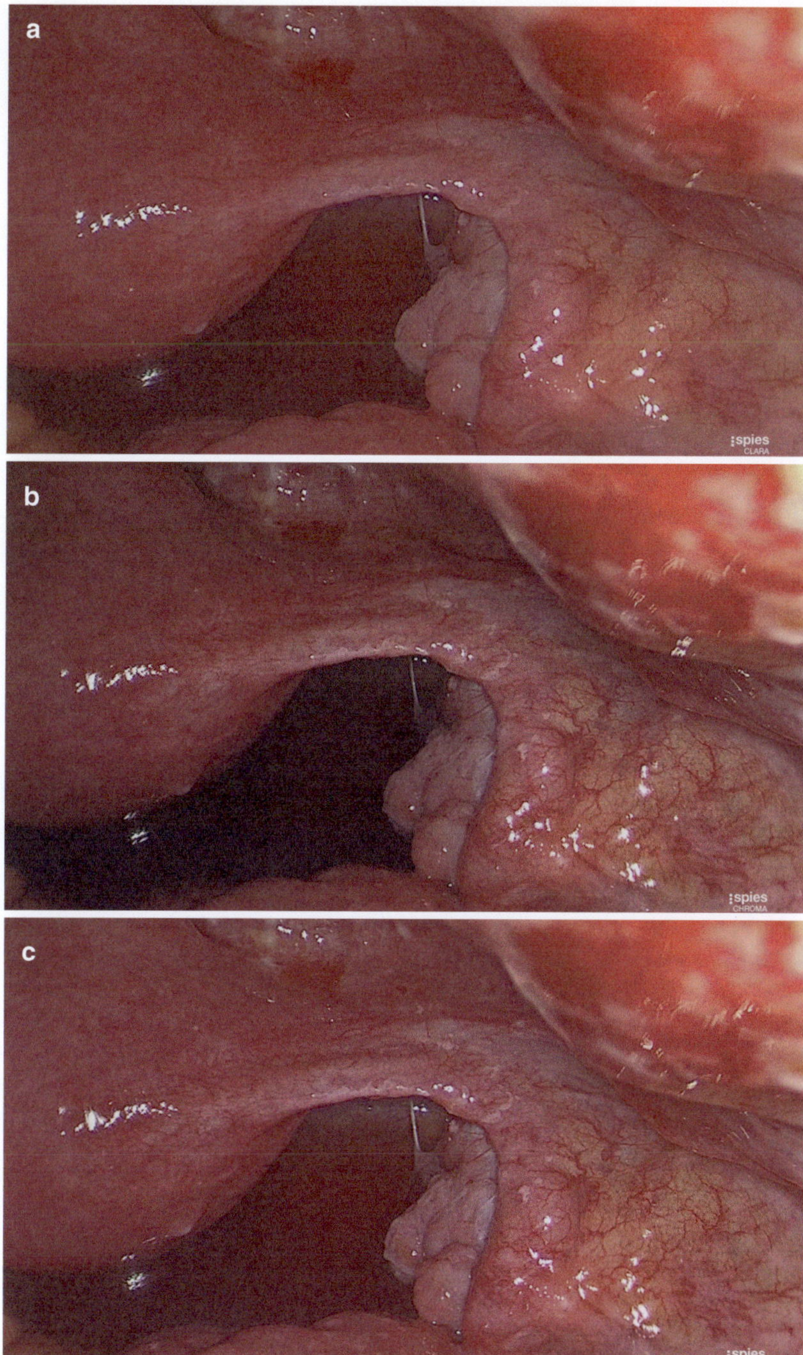

Fig. 1.23 (**a**) Gastric cancer with Krukenberg tumor (model: CLARA), (**b**) Gastric cancer with Krukenberg tumor (model: CHROMA), (**c**) Gastric cancer with Krukenberg tumor (model: CLARA+CHROMA), (**d**) Gastric cancer with Krukenberg tumor (model: SPECTA), (**e**) Gastric cancer with Krukenberg tumor (model: SPECTB)

Fig. 1.23 (continued)

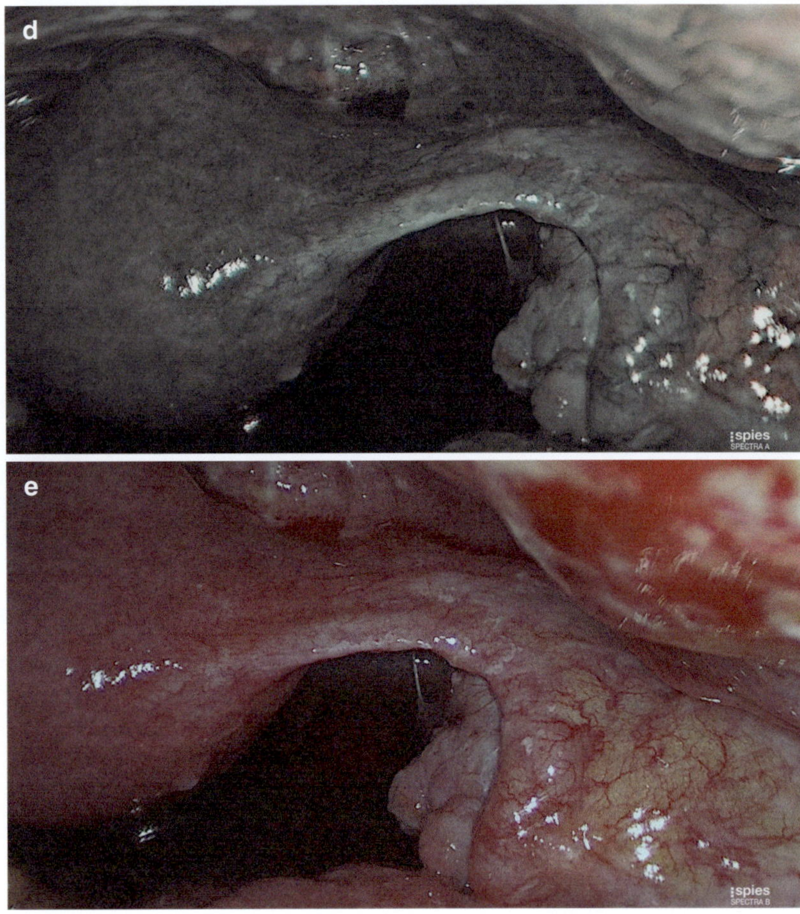

Our center also conducted a prospective, randomized, controlled study on the clinical efficacy of indocyanine green (ICG) tracer in laparoscopic gastric cancer LN dissection (NCT03050879) which will be presented in relevant chapters (Figs. 1.24 and 1.25). Written informed consent was obtained from all patients prior to their operations. This study was approved by the institutional review board of Fujian Medical University Union Hospital.

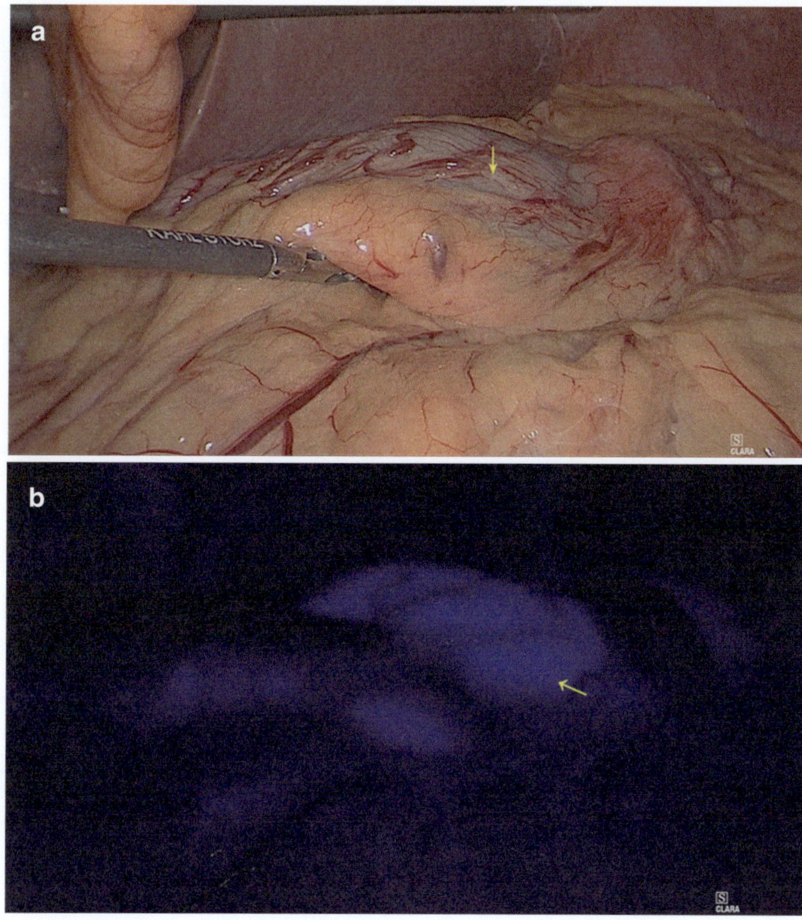

Fig. 1.24 (**a**) Preoperative injection of ICG around the tumor, (**b**) Intraoperative ICG imaging around the tumor

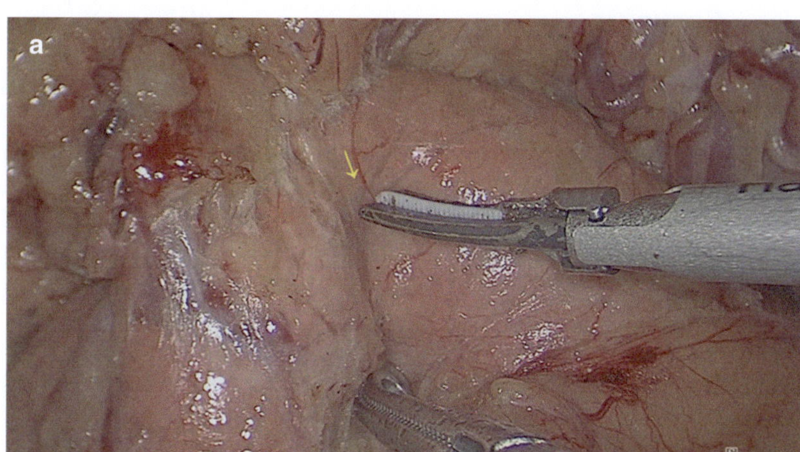

Fig. 1.25 (**a**) View with the naked eye, (**b**) ICG imaging showing gastric peripheral LNs and lymphangion (model: CLARA), (**c**) ICG imaging showing gastric peripheral LNs and lymphangion (model: SPECTA)

Fig. 1.25 (continued)

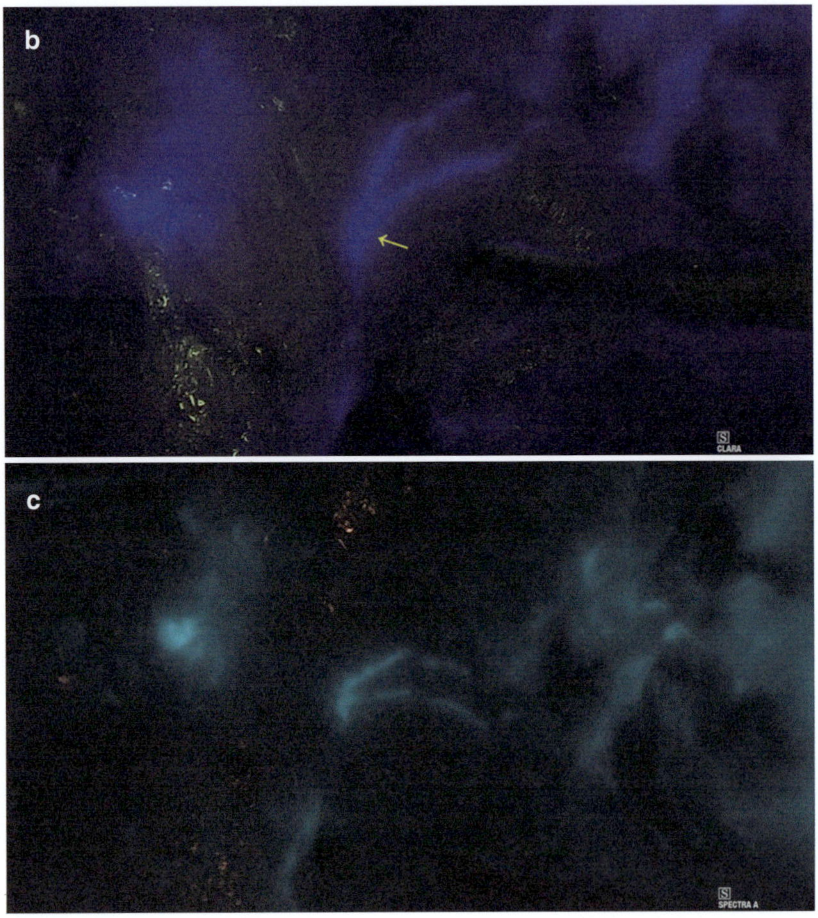

1.7 Sequence of a Lymphadenectomy

In principle, the sequence of a lymphadenectomy is from top to bottom, right to left, and a greater to lesser curvature, with the duodenum and esophagus resected in the end. The specific steps for a distal gastrectomy are as follows: No. 6 → No. 7, 9, 11p → No. 3, 1 → No. 8a, 12a, 5 → No. 4sb (Fig. 1.26).

The specific steps for a total gastrectomy are as follows: No. 6 → No. 7, 9, 11p → No. 8a, 12a, 5 → No. 1 → No. 4sb → No. 10, 11d → No. 2 (Fig. 1.27).

This lymphadenectomy sequence has a number of advantages, including: (1) the lack of need to frequently change the surgical position; (2) reducing the frequency of clamping and shifting the gastric wall; (3) an improved exposure of the surgical field; and (4) the ability to dissect whole LNs and surrounding tissue and to maximally follow the principle of 'en bloc tumor excision'.

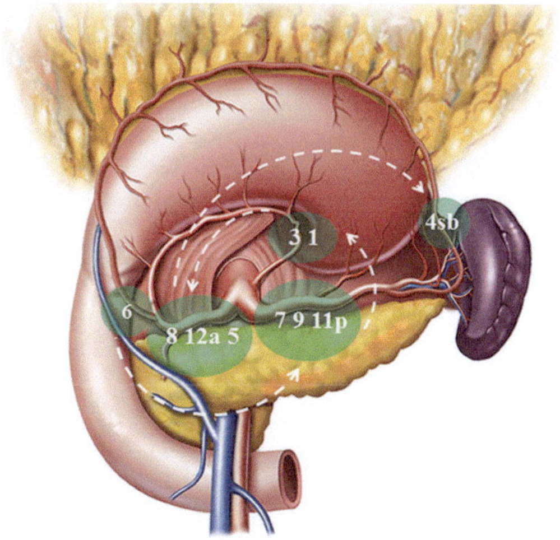

Fig. 1.26 Sequence of lymphadenectomy for laparoscopic distal gastrectomy (Reproduced with permission from [1])

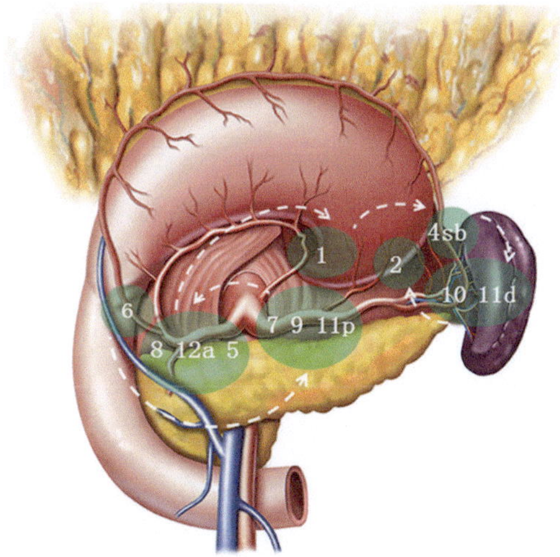

Fig. 1.27 Sequence of lymphadenectomy for laparoscopic total gastrectomy (Reproduced with permission from [1])

Clarification

All images of the chapter come from FuJian Medical University gastric surgery database and video database.

Reference

1. Huang C-M, Zheng C-H, editors. Laparoscopic gastrectomy for gastric cancer: Springer; 2015.

2 Laparoscopic Subpyloric LN Dissection for Gastric Cancer

Lymph node dissection in the subpyloric region is an important part of laparoscopic radical gastrectomy, which mainly includes the No. 6 LNs dissection, also known as the subpyloric LNs. Some cases may also require the dissection of the No.14v LNs [LNs located at the root of the superior mesenteric vein (SMV)] (Fig. 2.1).

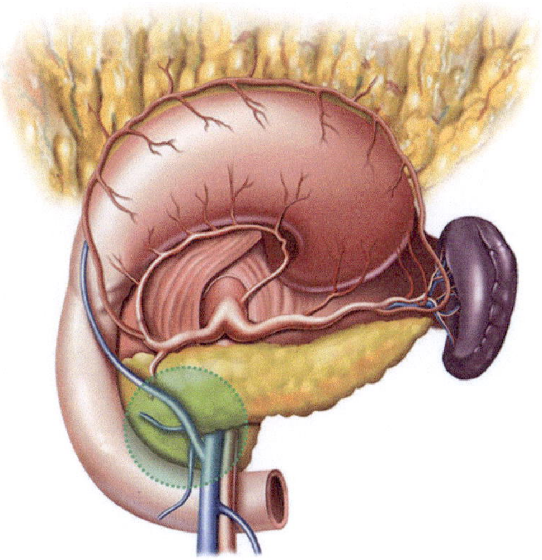

Fig. 2.1 Subpyloric Region (Reproduced with permission from [1])

C.-M. Huang et al., *Atlas of Laparoscopic Gastrectomy for Gastric Cancer*,
https://doi.org/10.1007/978-981-13-2862-6_2

2.1 Operative Steps for LN Dissection in the Subpyloric Region (Reproduced with permission from [1]

2.1.1 Resection of the Omentum Majus and Exfoliation of the Anterior Lobe of the Transverse Mesocolon (ATM)

2.1.1.1 Resection of the Omentum Majus

Surgical Approach

The approach of resection of the omentum majus is from the superior margin of the transverse colon near its central part (Fig. 2.2). This is a nonvascular zone and is where the omentum majus is thinnest.

Exposure Ways

The assistant lifts up the omentum majus and opens it on both sides by using two noninvasive grasping forceps positioned 3–5 cm away from the superior border of the transverse colon. Subsequently, the transverse colon was pressed down (counteraction) to create triangle traction and place the omentum majus under tension by the surgeon (Fig. 2.3).

Operative Procedures

From the superior margin of the transverse colon near its central part, the omentum majus is divided in the nonvascular zone using the ultrasonic scalpel (Fig. 2.4). Next, the division is

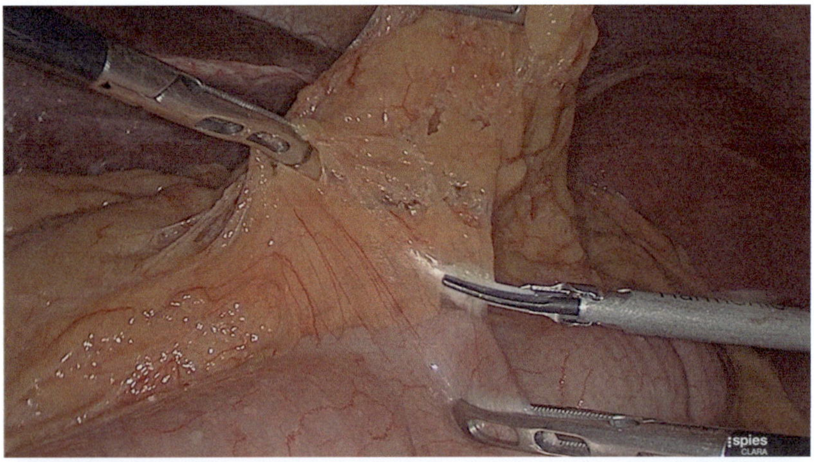

Fig. 2.2 Resection of the omentum majus is approached from the superior margin of the transverse colon near its central part

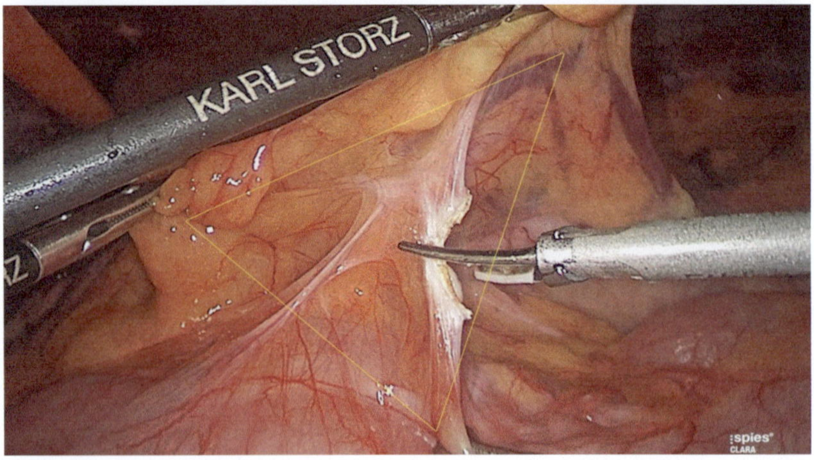

Fig. 2.3 Triangle traction tensions the omentum majus under tension

extended to the left and right. The omentum majus is disconnected to the left until the colonic splenic flexure (Fig. 2.5), then is disconnected to the right until the colonic hepatic flexure (Fig. 2.6). In this manner, the attachment of the omentum majus and transverse colon is completely free.

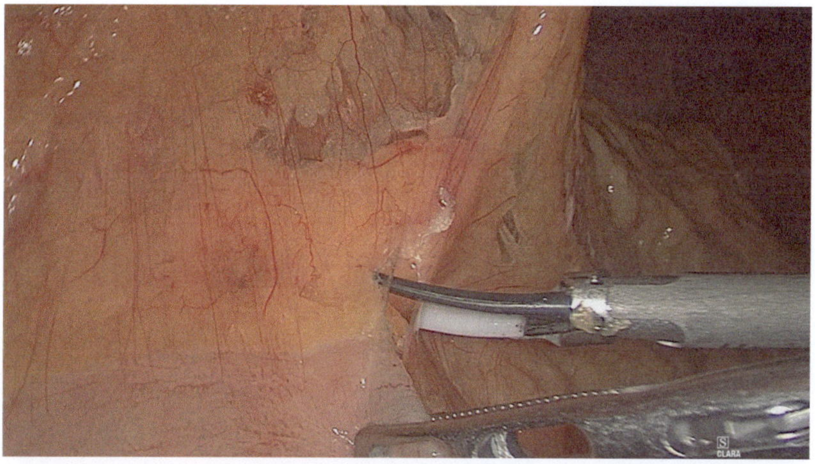

Fig. 2.4 The omentum majus is disconnected in the nonvascular zone at the superior margin of the transverse colon

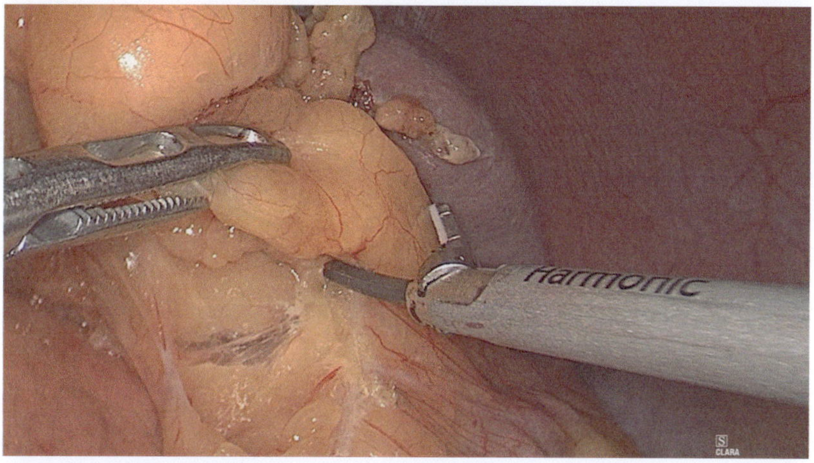

Fig. 2.5 The omentum majus is disconnected to the colonic splenic flexure

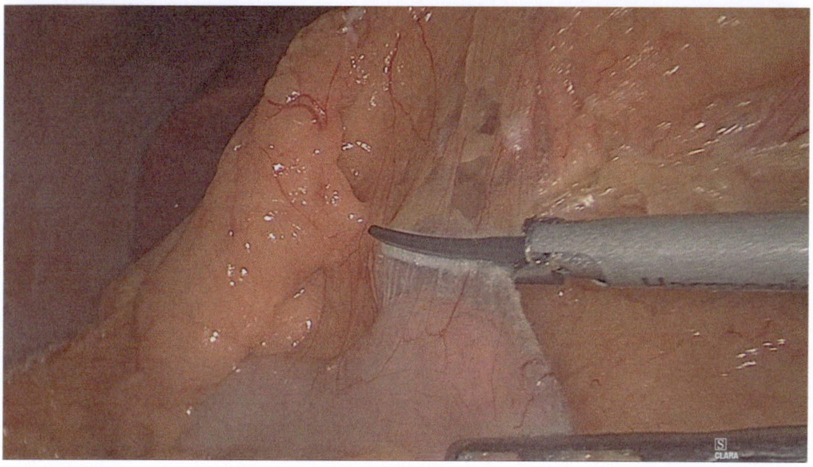

Fig. 2.6 The omentum majus is disconnected to the colonic hepatic flexure

2.1.1.2 Exfoliatling the ATM

Surgical Approach

The approach for ATM peeling is from the upper margin of the right transverse colon (Fig. 2.7). The tissues here, in the fusion gap between the ATM and posterior lobes of the transverse mesocolon (PTM), are at their most loose and have no blood vessels. Therefore, it is convenient to exfoliate the ATM from this site and not easily to cause bleeding.

Exposure Ways

RCV: Right colic vein; MCV: Middle colic vein.

The assistant pulls up the greater curvature omentum of the gastric antrum using a noninvasive left-handed grasper (Fig. 2.8) and gently lifts up the ATM (Fig. 2.9) with a right-handed grasper. Meanwhile, the TM was pressed down by the surgeon with a left-handed grasper to form a certain tension and expose the fusion space between the ATM and PTM (Fig. 2.10), which is formed by loose connective tissue. During exfoliation of the ATM, the assistant uses the atraumatic grasper to gently push the ATM up and the PTM down to help the surgeon reveal the fusion gap (Figs. 2.11 and 2.12).

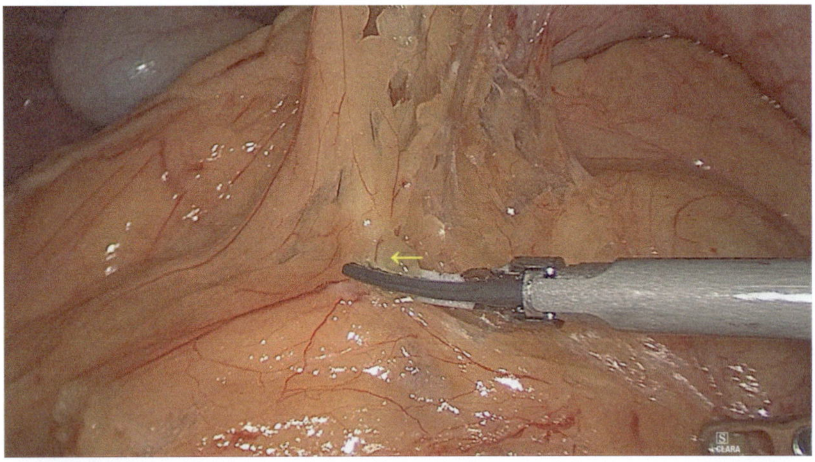

Fig. 2.7 ATM peeling is approached from the upper margin of the right transverse colon

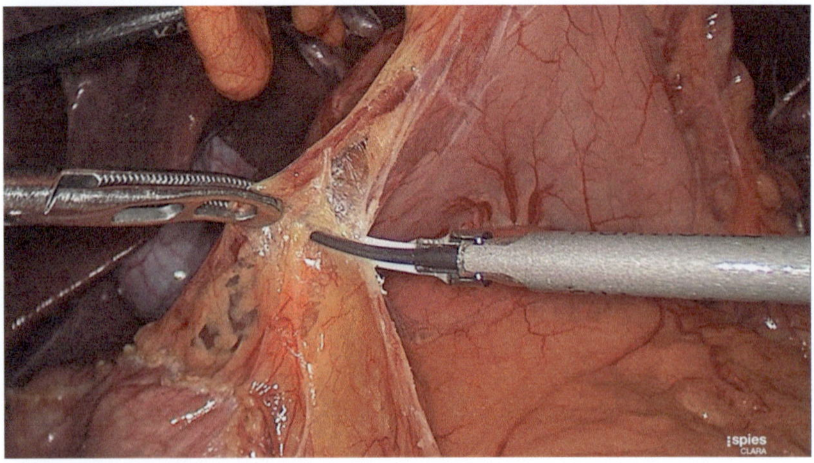

Fig. 2.8 The greater curvature omentum of the gastric antrum is lifted up by the assistant with a noninvasive left-handed grasper

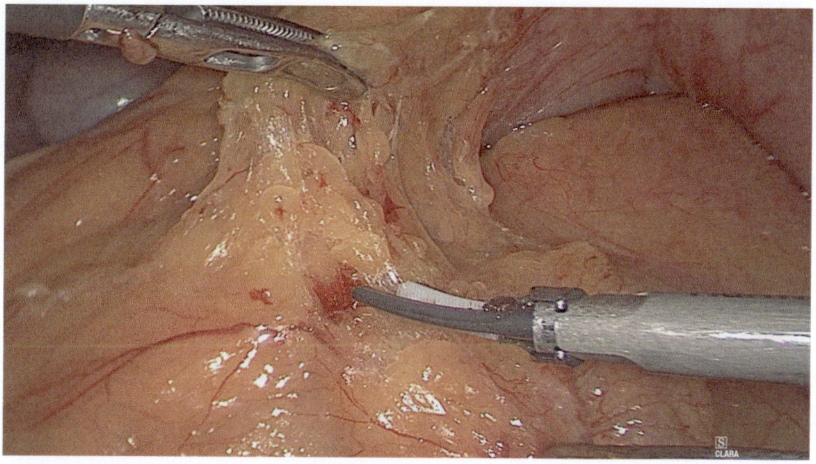

Fig. 2.9 The ATM is lifted up by the assistant with a right-landed grasper

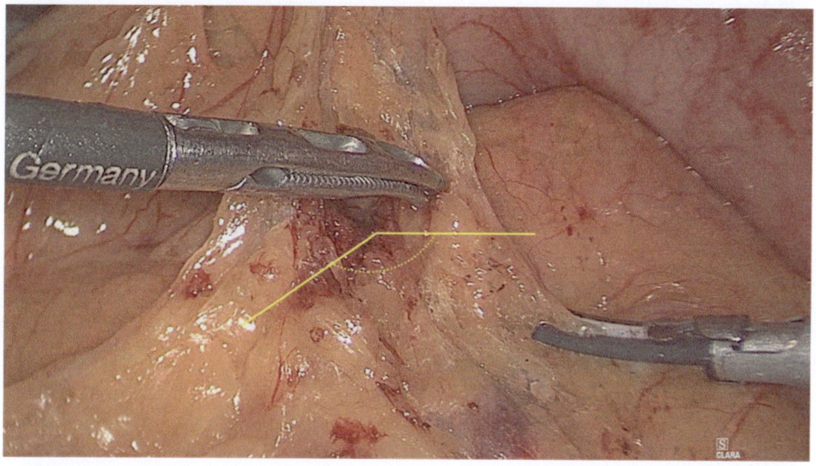

Fig. 2.10 The fusion gap between the ATM and PTM is exposed

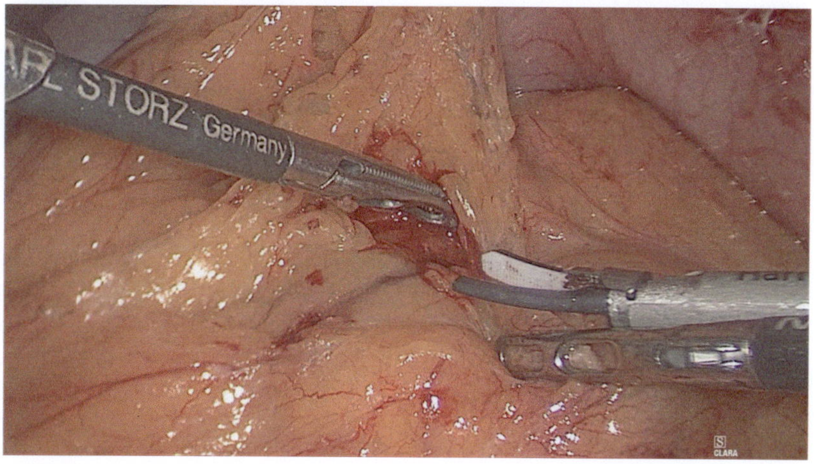

Fig. 2.11 The assistant pushes the ATM upward to assist in exposure of fusion gap

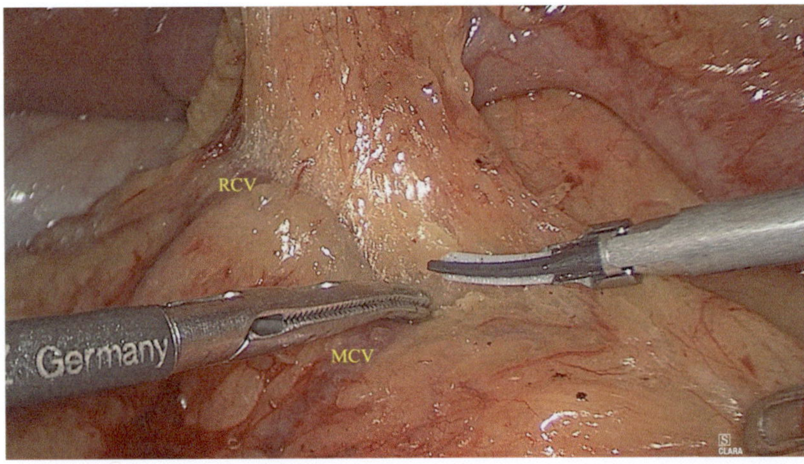

Fig. 2.12 The assistant pushes the PTM downward to assist in exposure of fusion gap

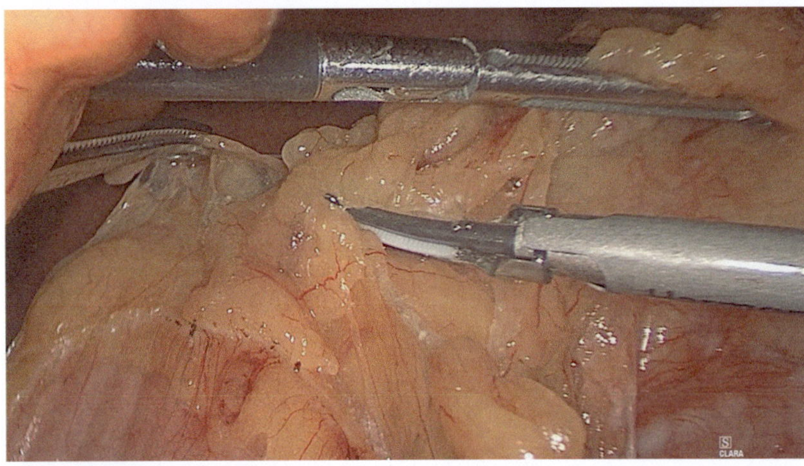

Fig. 2.13 Separation is starting from the superior margin of the right transverse colon

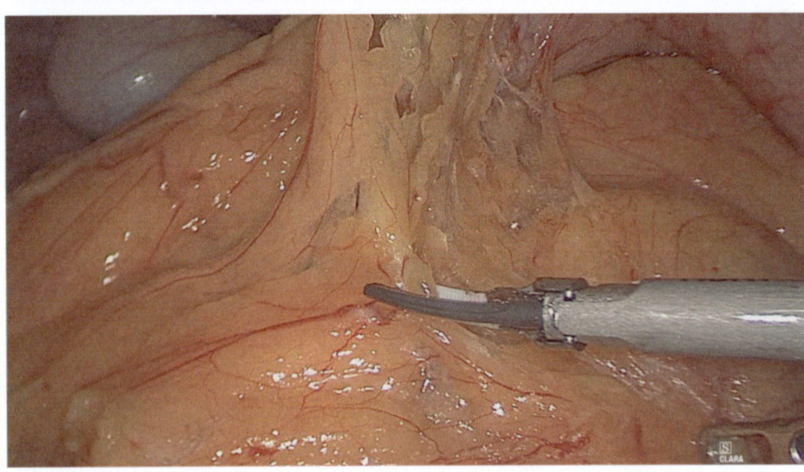

Fig. 2.14 Sharp dissection of the ATM with the ultrasonic scalpel

Operative Procedures

The separation is starting from the superior margin of the right transverse colon with the ultrasonic scalpel (Fig. 2.13). Then, alternating blunt and sharp dissection of the ATM is performed along the fusion space between the ATM and PTM (Figs. 2.14 and 2.15). Dissection is continued rightward to the medial margin of the descending duodenum (Fig. 2.16) and upwards to the inferior margin of the pancreas (Fig. 2.17).

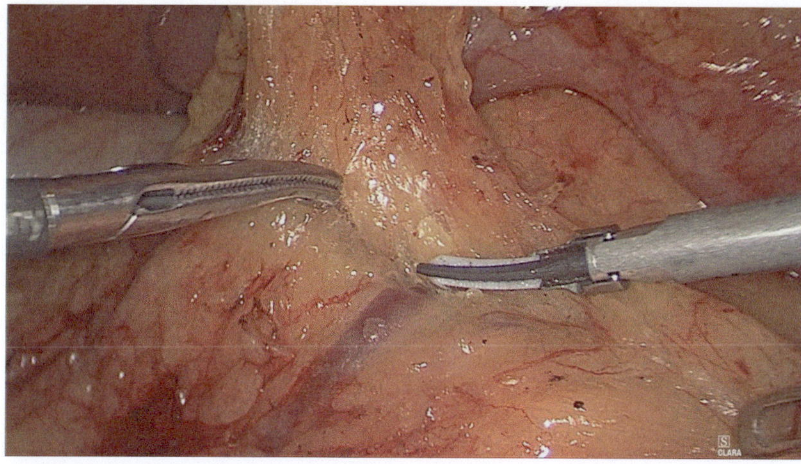

Fig. 2.15 Blunt dissection of the ATM with the ultrasonic scalpel

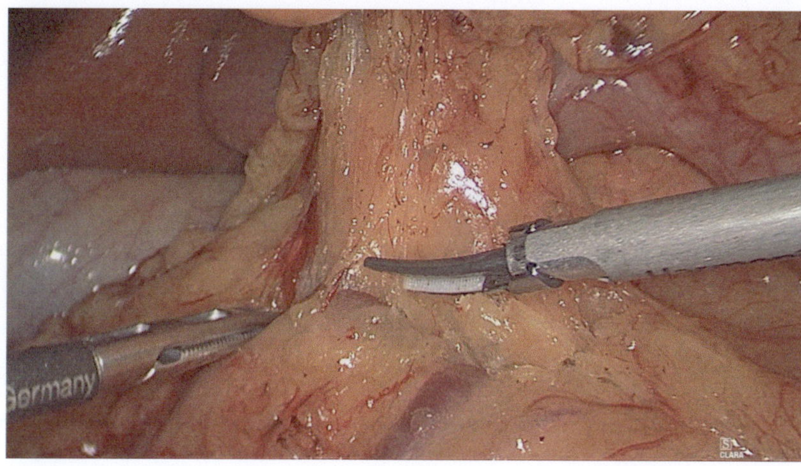

Fig. 2.16 The ATM is dissected to the medial border of the descending duodenum

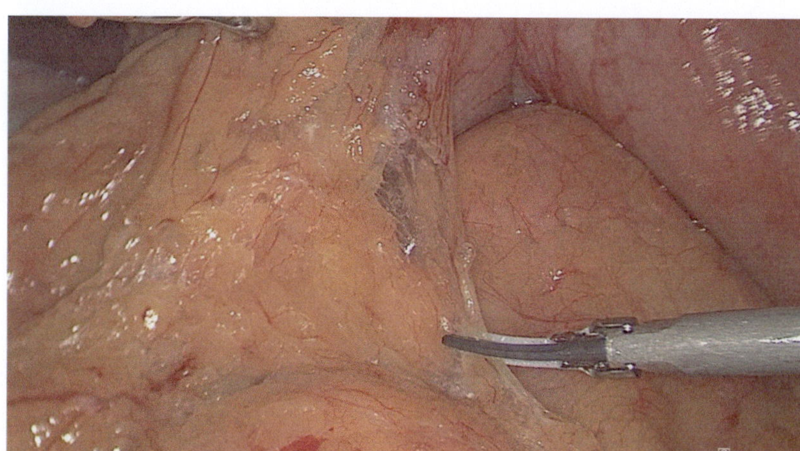

Fig. 2.17 The ATM is dissected to the inferior margin of the pancreas

2.1.2 No. 14v LNs Dissection

2.1.2.1 Surgical Approach

RCV: Right colic vein; GDV: Gastroduodenal vein; MCV: Middle colic vein.

The favored surgical approach for this dissection is from the MCV (Fig. 2.18). The MCV and the inferior margin of the pancreatic neck are the anatomical marks for the SMV during operation. The SMV can be found in the fusion gap between the ATM and PTM by following the MCV proximally up to the inferior margin of the pancreatic neck.

2.1.2.2 Exposure Ways

RCV: Right colic vein; MCV: Middle colic vein; SMV: Superior mesenteric vein.

The assistant continues to lifting up the greater curvature omentum of the gastric antrum with a noninvasive left-handed grasper, while pulling up the separated ATM with the right hand. Meanwhile, the PTM was pressed down by the surgeon to keep correct tension and reveal the MCV and the root of the SMV (Fig. 2.19).

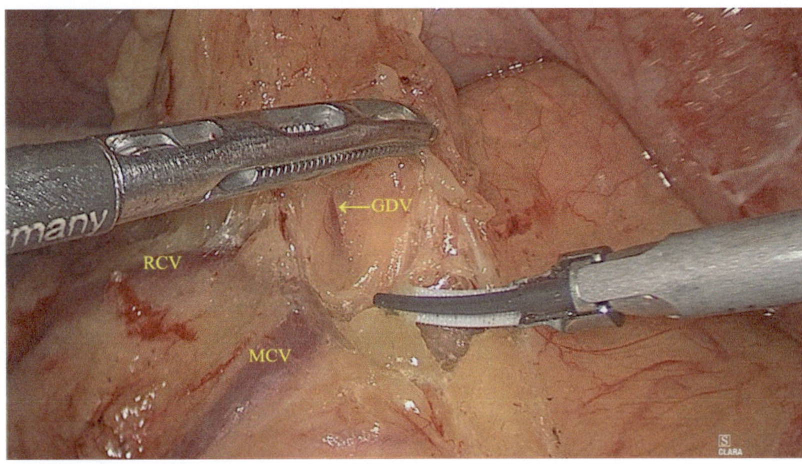

Fig. 2.18 The approach for dissection is from the MCV

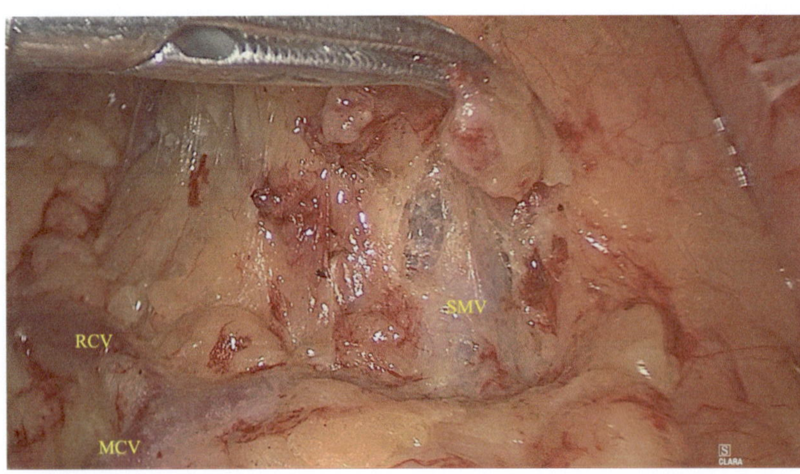

Fig. 2.19 The root of the SMV is exposed

2.1.2.3 Operative Procedures

MCV: Middle colic vein.

RCV: Right colic vein; MCV: Middle colic vein; SMV: Superior mesenteric vein.

Using the non-functional surface of the ultrasonic scalpel, the surgeon dissects the tissues along the MCV branch (Fig. 2.20) toward the inferior margin of the pancreas to reveal the confluence of the MCV and the SMV (Fig. 2.21).

GDV: Gastroduodenal vein.

The blunt and sharp dissection of tissues along the anatomic space on the surface of the SMV is continued upwards to the inferior margin of the pancreas, and then the PPDS is entered (Fig. 2.22). Then, the dissection is continued to the left up to the left border of the SMV and towards the right up to the confluence of the Henle's trunk and the SMV (Fig. 2.23).

GDV: Gastroduodenal vein; SMV: Superior mesenteric vein.

RGEV: Right gastroepiploic vessel; ASPDV: Anterior superior pancreaticoduodenal vein; SMV: Superior mesenteric vein.

SMV: Superior mesenteric vein; MCV: Middle colic vein.

Subsequently, the surgeon dissects rightward along the anatomic space on the surface of Henle's trunk to reach the confluence of the RGEV and the ARCV or RCV (Fig. 2.24), where

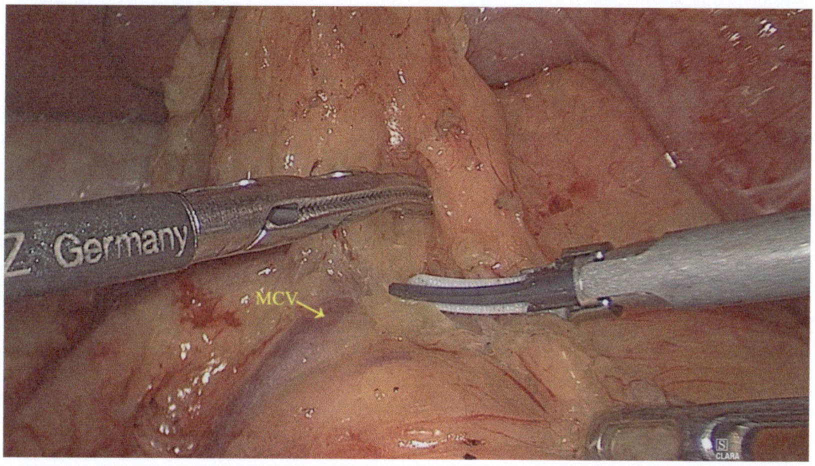

Fig. 2.20 Tissues along the MCV are dissected using the non-functional surface of the ultrasonic scalpel

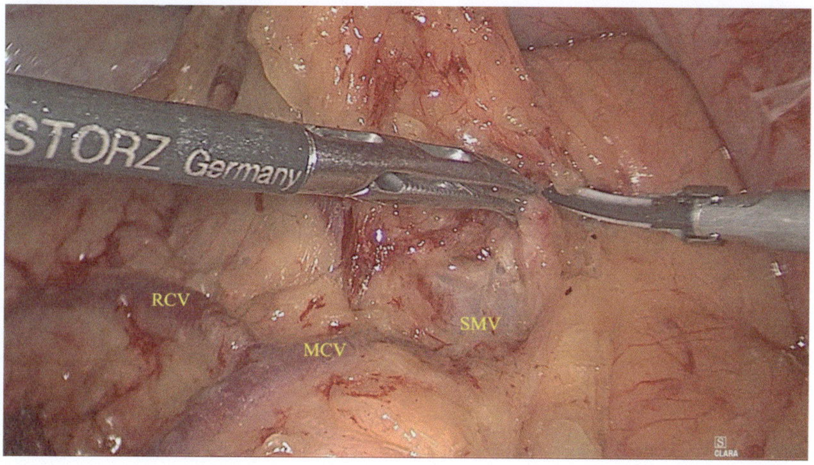

Fig. 2.21 The confluence of the MCV and the SMV is exposed

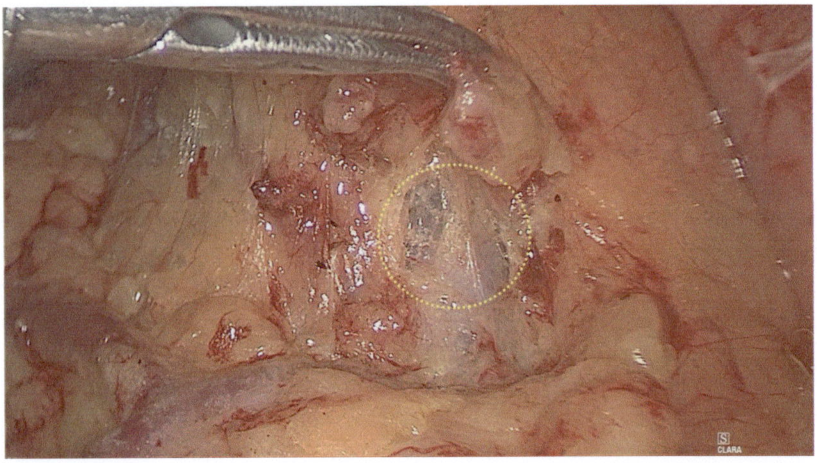

Fig. 2.22 The dissection is continued upwards to the inferior margin of the pancreas neck and enters the posterior pancreaticoduodenal space (PPDS)

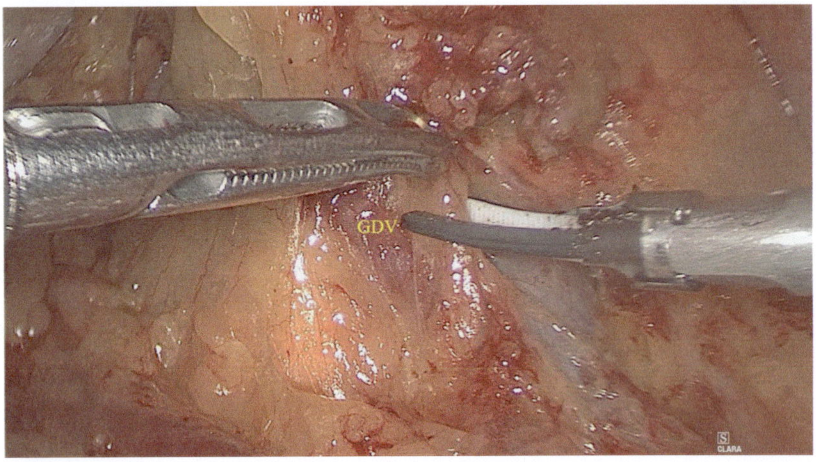

Fig. 2.23 Gastroduodenal vein or Henle's trunk is vascularized

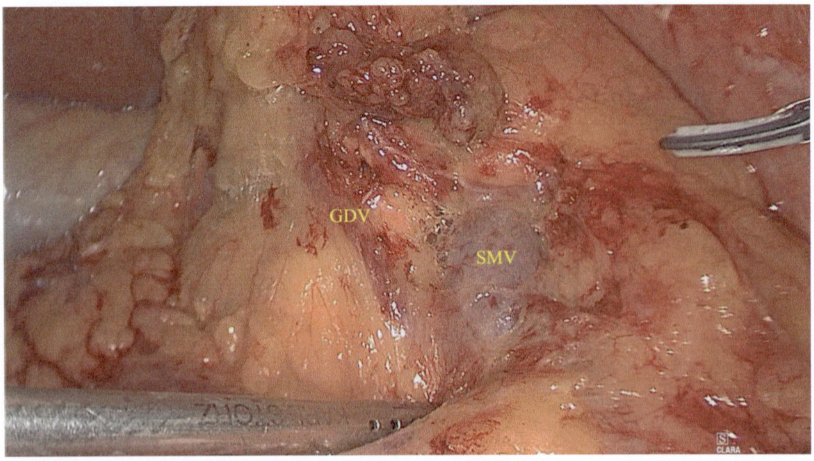

Fig. 2.24 Separation and reveal of the junction of the right gastroepiploic vessel (RGEV) and RCV or accessory right colic vein (ARCV)

the GDV can be exposed. Finally, the dissection is extended to the confluence of the RGEV and the ASPDV (Fig. 2.25). The fatty lymphatic tissue around Henle's trunk and the SMV is completely separated, which completes the dissection of No. 14v LNs (Fig. 2.26).

2.1.3 No. 6 LNs Dissection

2.1.3.1 Surgical Approach

The approach to the dissection of No. 6 LNs is from the GIS (Fig. 2.27). The junction of the RGEV and SPDV is the starting point of the dis-

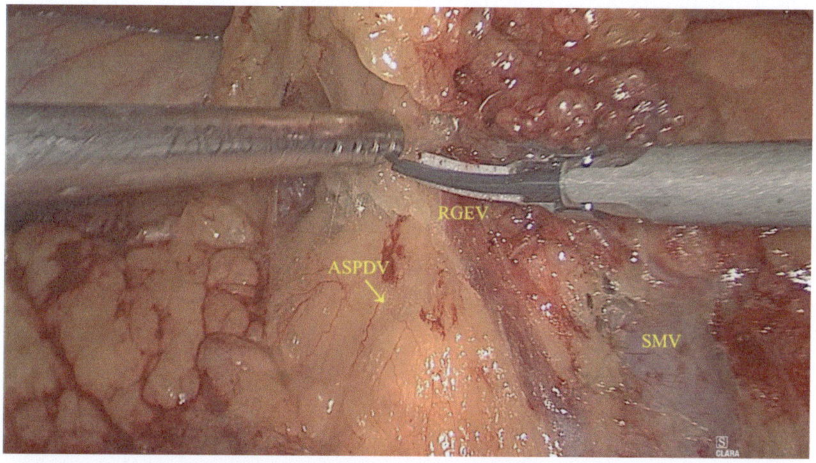

Fig. 2.25 Separation and reveal of the junction of the RGEV and ASPDV

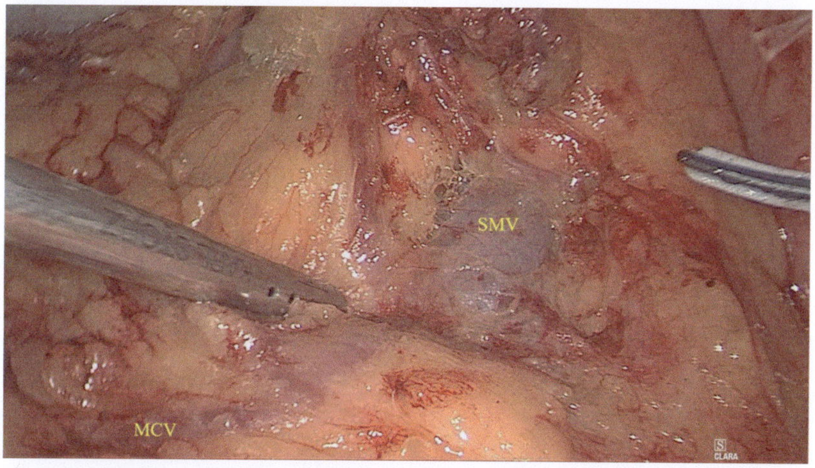

Fig. 2.26 Display of No. 14v LNs after dissection

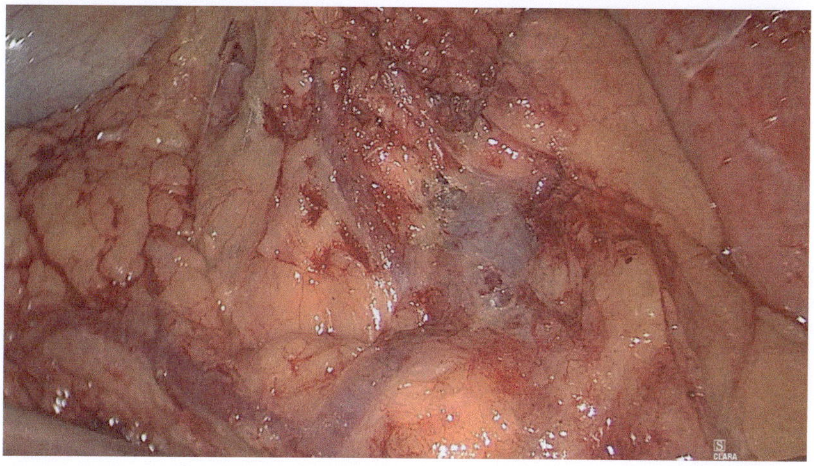

Fig. 2.27 The approach to the No. 6 LNs dissection is from the gastrocolic intrafascial space (GIS)

section. By dissecting upwards along the RGEV, the gastroduodenal artery (GDA) and the root of the right gastroepiploic artery (RGEA) can be further revealed.

2.1.3.2 Exposure Ways

The assistant lifts up the posterior wall of the gastric antrum with a left-handed grasper and gently lifts up the fatty lymphatic tissue on the surface of the vessels with the other hand. Then, the surgeon presses down the inferior margin of the pancreas (counteraction) on the root of the TM with a left-handed atraumatic grasper and a small gauze to expose the infrapyloric region. Therefore, a good vision and tension can be provided for dissecting the No. 6 LNs smoothly (Fig. 2.28).

2.1.3.3 Operative Procedures

RGEV: Right gastroepiploic vein.

The tissues on the surface of the RGEV are pulled up or retracted by the assistant with the right hand. From the confluence of the RGEV and the SPDV, the surgeon dissects these tissues along the vein distally up to the superior margin of the pancreatic head with the non-functional face of the ultrasonic scalpel (Fig. 2.29).

RGEV: Right gastroepiploic vein; SMV: Superior mesenteric vein.

After the RGEV is vascularized completely, the assistant draws the RGEV outward to separate it from the pancreas, and the surgeon disconnects it with clamps above the junction (Fig. 2.30).

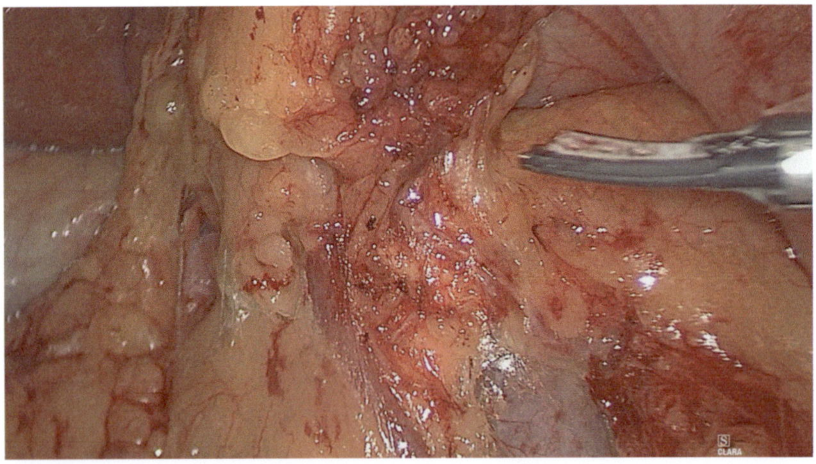

Fig. 2.28 Exposure of the infrapyloric area is convenient for the dissection of the No. 6 LNs

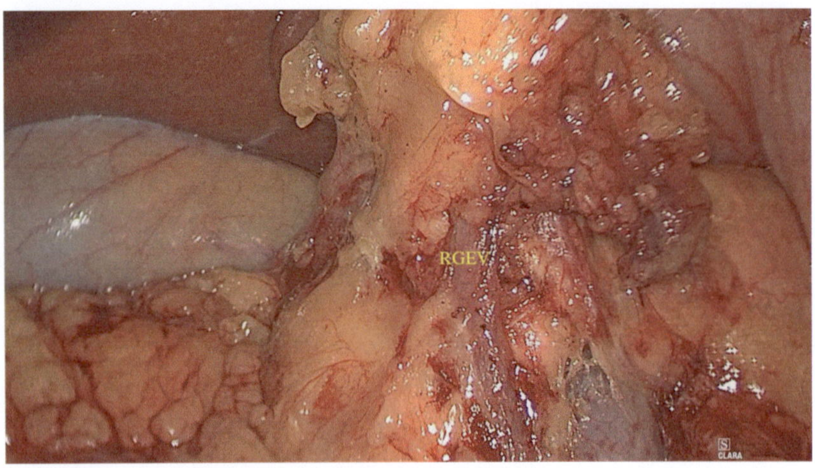

Fig. 2.29 The RGEV is dissected up to the superior margin of the pancreatic head

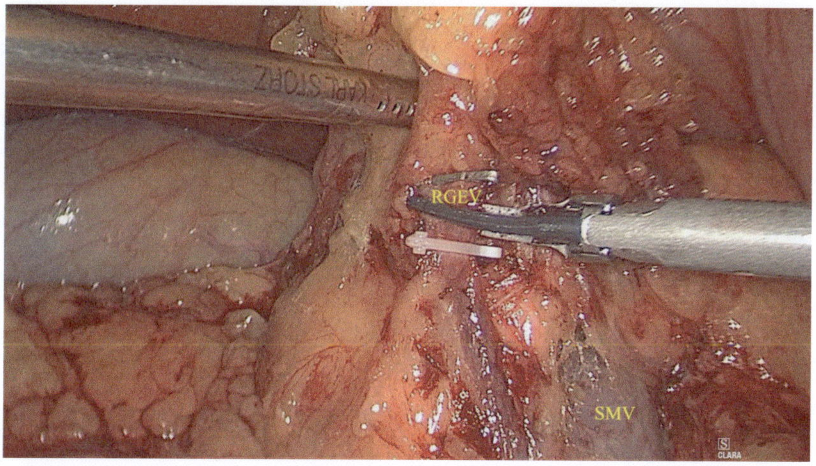

Fig. 2.30 The RGEV is disconnected above the junction of the SPDV and the RGEV

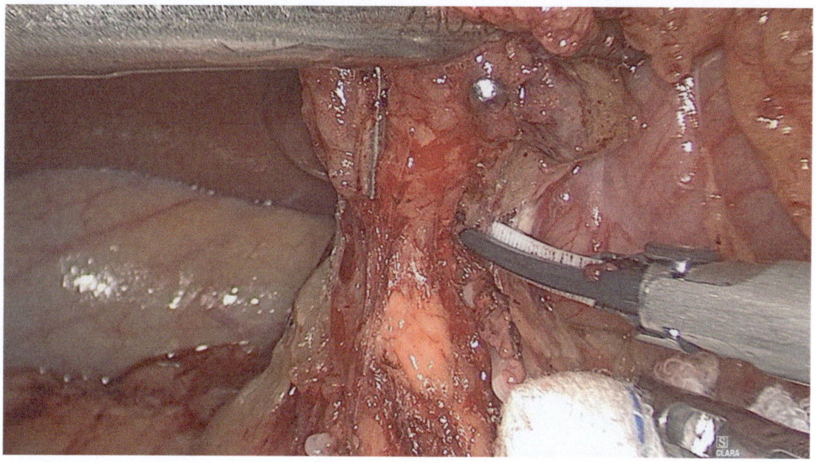

Fig. 2.31 The dissection of the fascial space between the duodenum and the pancreatic head

Then, the assistant continues to pulls the posterior wall of the antrum upwards with the left hand, while the right hand pushes the duodenal bulb outward. The surgeon gently presses the pancreas down with a small gauze on the left hand to reveal the fascial space between the duodenum and the pancreatic head (Fig. 2.31). The terminal of the GDA can then be revealed and divided (Fig. 2.32), and by dissection along it, the root of the RGEA can be exposed (Fig. 2.33).

The assistant then holds the fatty lymphatic tissue on the surface of the RGEA, and the surgeon dissects these tissues along the anatomic space on the surface of the artery toward the pylorus with the ultrasonic scalpel. Next, the root of the artery is revealed (Fig. 2.34) and disconnected with clamps (Fig. 2.35).

RGEV: Right gastroepiploic vein; RGEA: Right gastroepiploic artery.

The IPA emanates from the GDA, and should usually be severed as well. During the No. 6 LNs dissection, bleeding caused by injury of the artery should be avoided. Subsequently, from the broken end of the RGEA, the tissue along the duodenum is dissected to the pylorus using the non-functional face of the ultrasonic scalpel (Fig. 2.38). The fatty lymphatic tissue in the IPA is then divided and resected en bloc.

The No. 6 LNs dissection is then accomplished (Fig. 2.39).

RGEV: Right gastroepiploic vein; RGEA: Right gastroepiploic artery; ASPDV: Anterior superior pancreaticoduodenal vein; SMV: Superior mesenteric vein; RCV: Right colic vein).

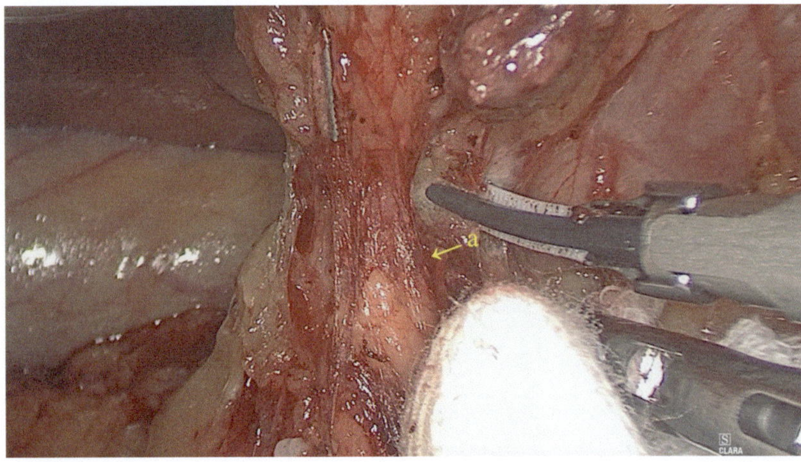

Fig. 2.32 The appearance of the terminal of the GDA (**a**)

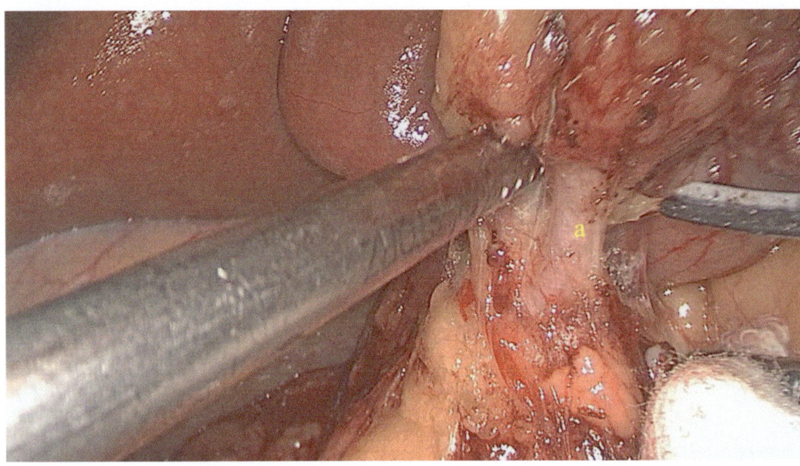

Fig. 2.33 The appearance of the root of the RGEA (**a**)

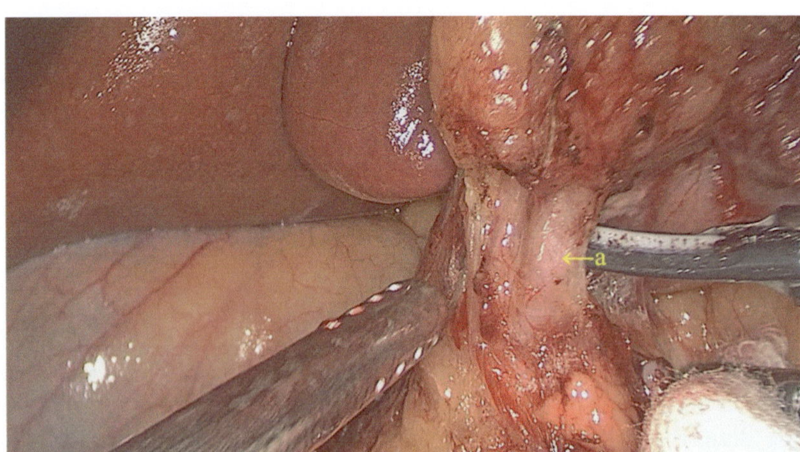

Fig. 2.34 The appearance of the RGEA (**a**)

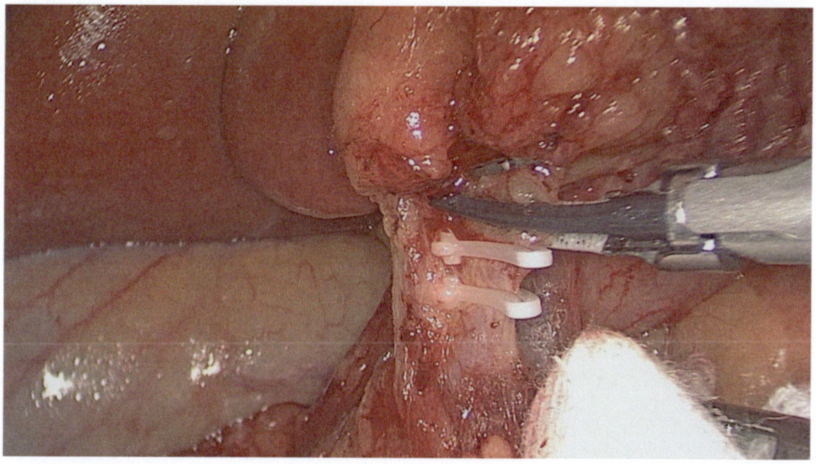

Fig. 2.35 The root of the RGEA is disconnected with clamps

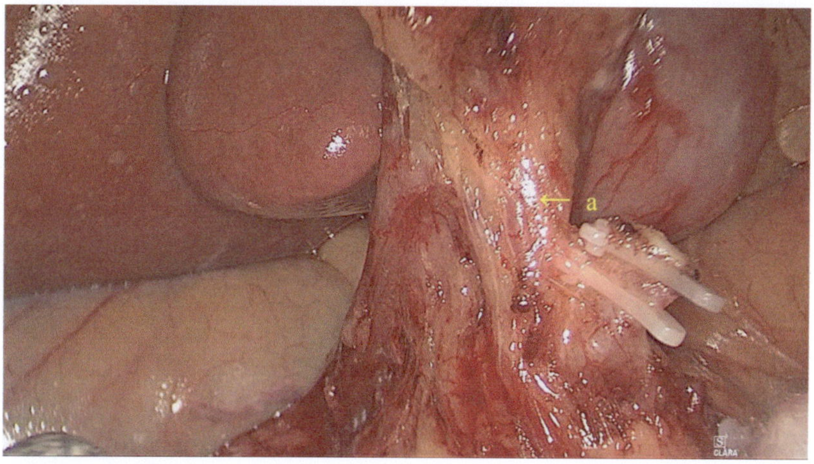

Fig. 2.36 The infrapyloric artery (IPA) (**a**) is vascularized

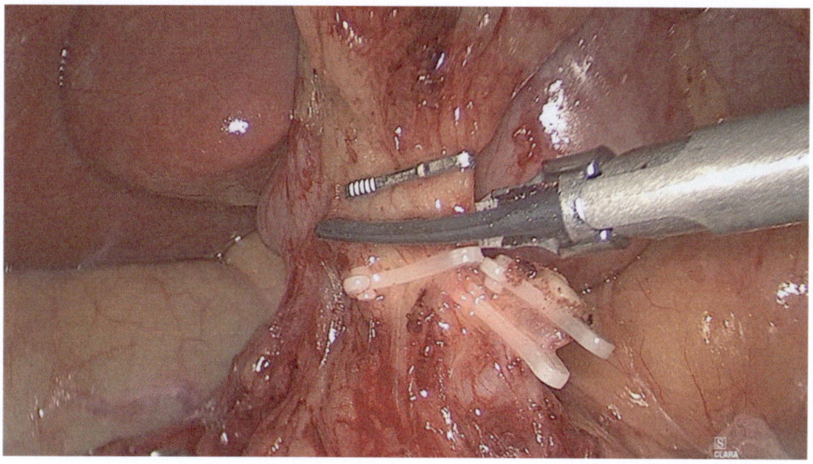

Fig. 2.37 The IPA disconnection

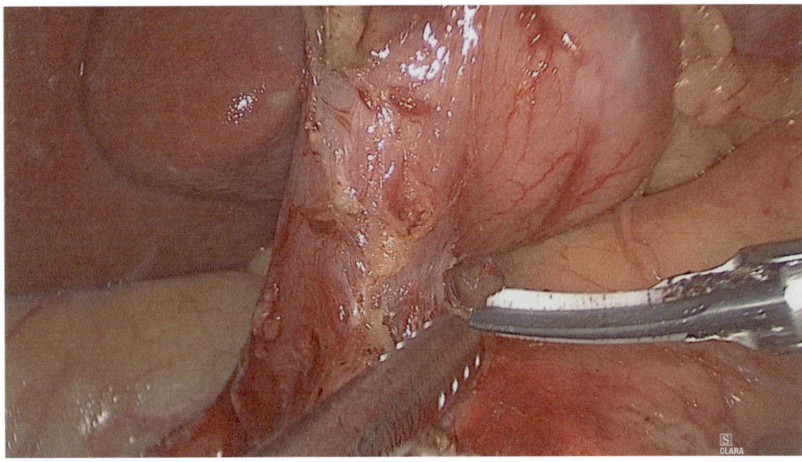

Fig. 2.38 The tissue along the duodenum is dissected to the pylorus

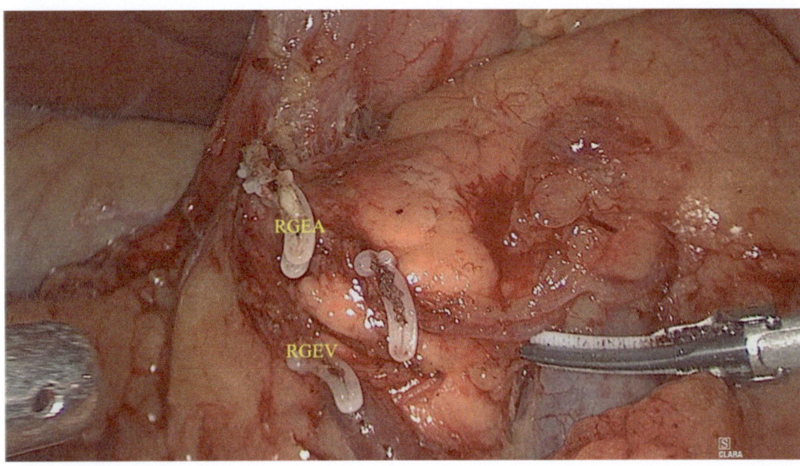

Fig. 2.39 The Display of No. 6 LNs after dissection

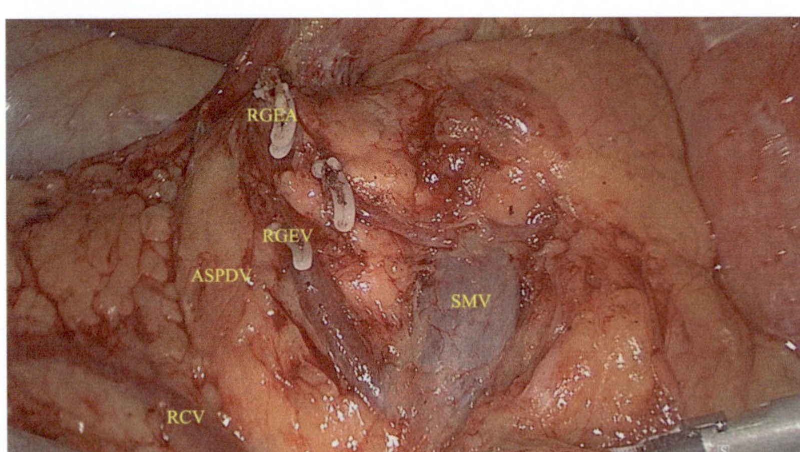

Fig. 2.40 The Display of No. 14v and No. 6 LNs after dissection

2.2 Operative Announcements of Laparoscopic Subpyloric LN Dissection for Gastric Cancer

2.2.1 Intraoperative Anatomy of the Subpyloric LN Dissection

2.2.1.1 Fascia Space in the Subpyloric Region

Omentum Majus

The omentum majus is a four-layered fold of peritoneum. It extends rightward as far as the initial segment of the duodenum, and extends leftward to the gastrosplenic ligament (GSL) (Figs. 2.41 and 2.42).

Gastrocolic Intrafascial Space (GIS)

GIS, Gastrocolic intrafascial space.

The two posterior layers of the omentum majus and the TM fuse together near the pylorus to form a potential fusion space called the GIS, which is a nonvascular zone filled with loose connective tissue and some fatty tissue. By opening this space, the right gastroepiploic and infrapyloric vessels can be exposed and then the No. 6 LNs can be dissected (Figs. 2.43 and 2.44).

TM

The two posterior layers of the omentum majus wrap the transverse colon and then attach upwards to the posterior abdominal wall to form the TM (Figs. 2.45 and 2.46).

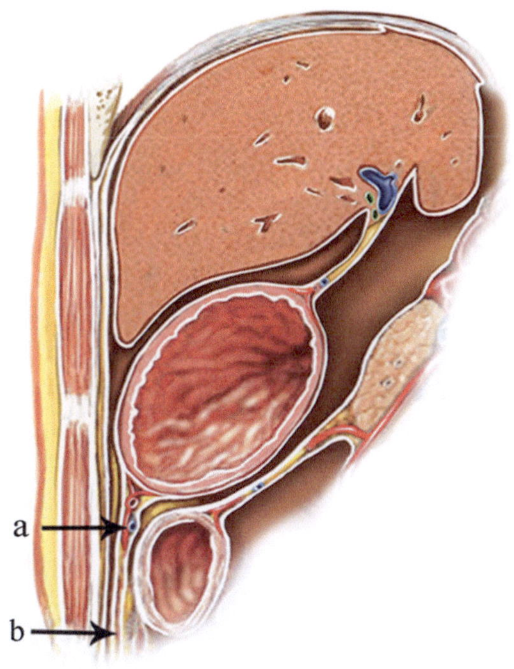

Fig. 2.41 Gastric and colonic ligaments (GCL) (**a**) and omentum majus (**b**) (Reproduced with permission from [1])

Fig. 2.42 Intraoperative view of the omentum majus

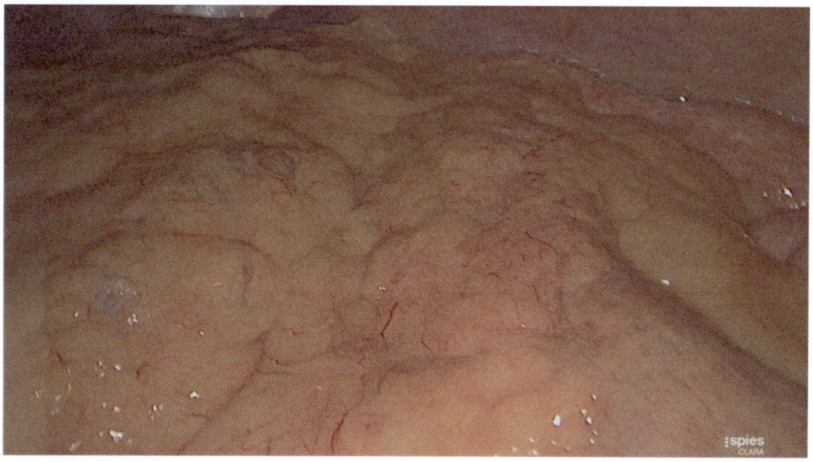

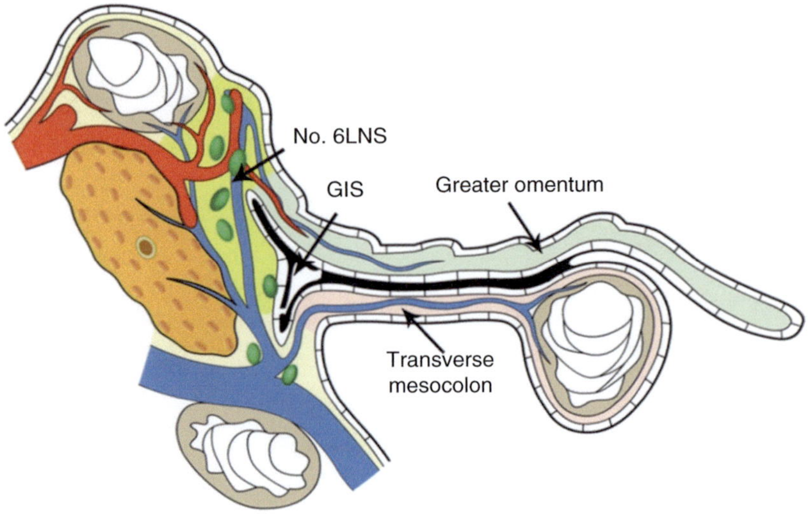

Fig. 2.43 Sketch of the GIS (Reproduced with permission from [1])

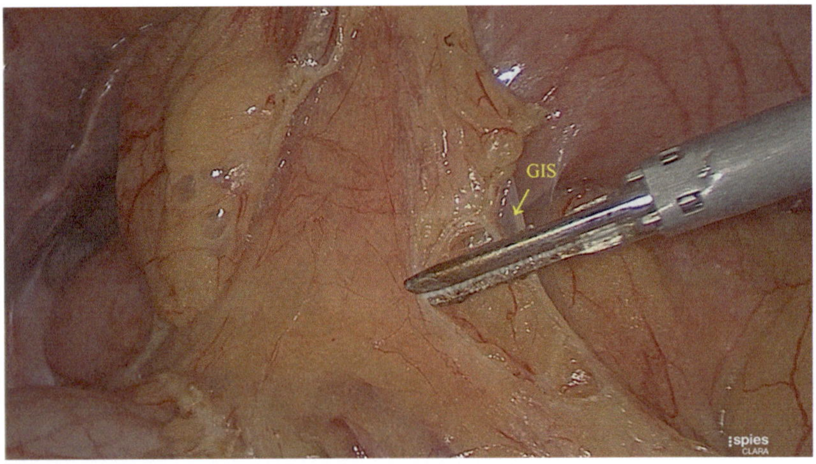

Fig. 2.44 GIS

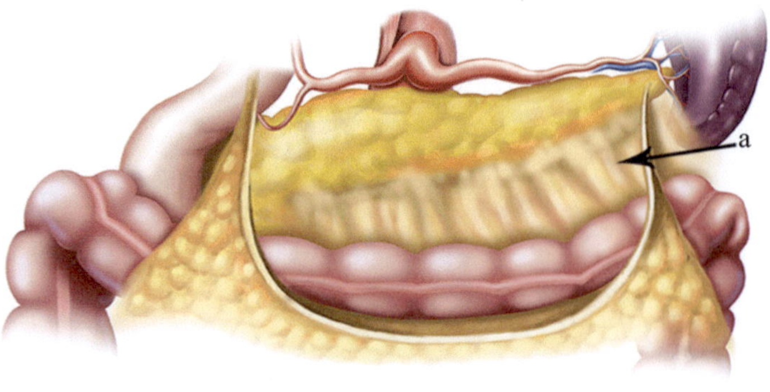

Fig. 2.45 TM (Reproduced with permission from [1])

Pancreaticoduodenal Fascia (PDF) and its Intrafascial Space

The PDF is derived from the posterior layer of the dorsal mesogastrium (DM). It wraps around the pancreatic head and the second part of the duodenum, and it mixes together with the mesocolon ascendens. The intrafascial space between the posterior PDF and the inherent pancreatic fascia is called the posterior pancreaticoduodenal space (PPDS), which contains the SMV, portal vein (PV), and No. 14v LNs (Fig. 2.47).

2.2.1.2 Arteries Associated with the Subpyloric LN Dissection

Right Gastroepiploic Artery (REGA)

The RGEA with the largest diameter is the main blood supply vessel in the gastric antrum region, and it's one of the terminal branches of the GDA in the subpyloric region. The RGEA has no notable anatomic variations. Its root can usually be confirmed by identifying the GDA and dissecting along the arterial trunk (Fig. 2.48).

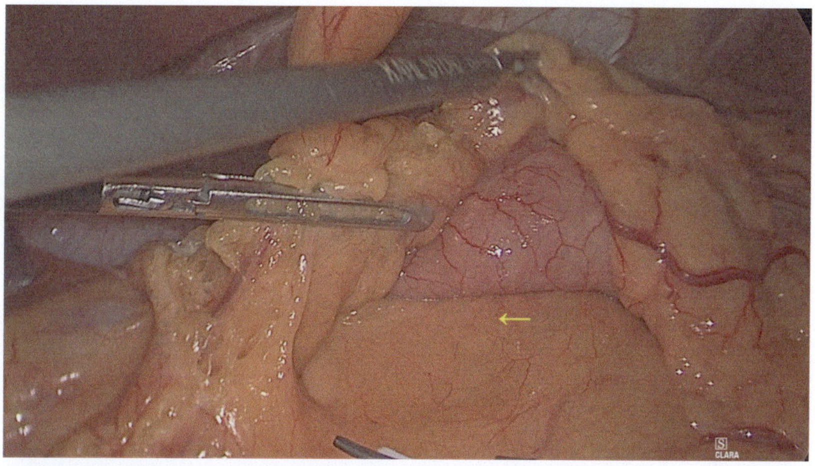

Fig. 2.46 TM

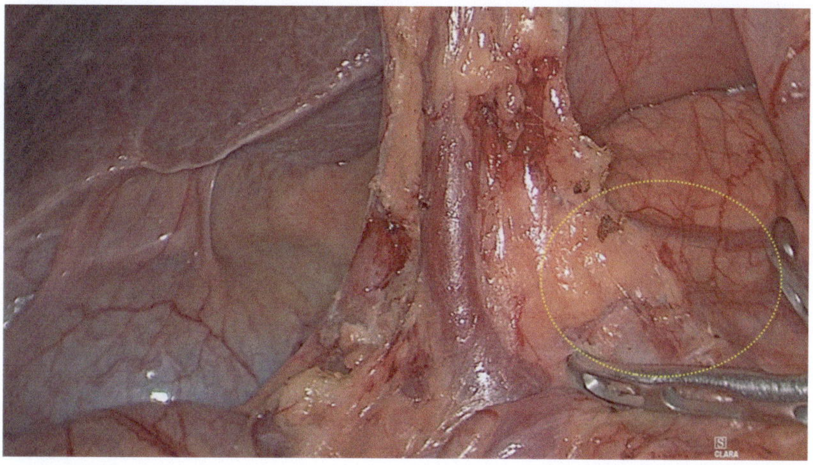

Fig. 2.47 PPDS

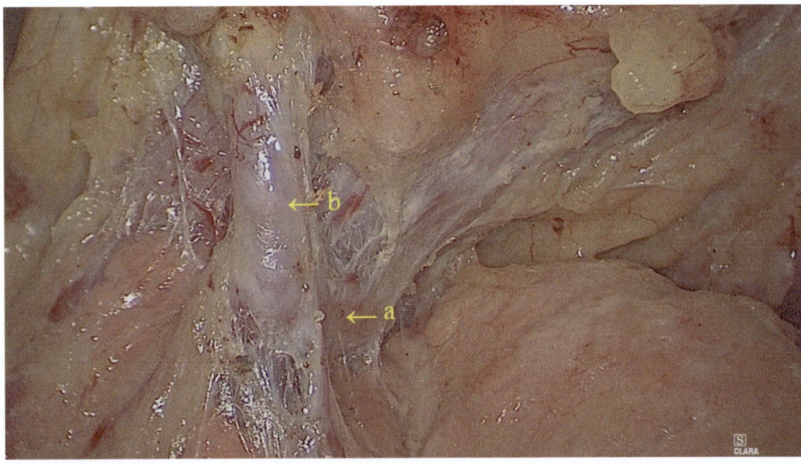

Fig. 2.48 The GDA (**a**) branches out of the RGEA (**b**)

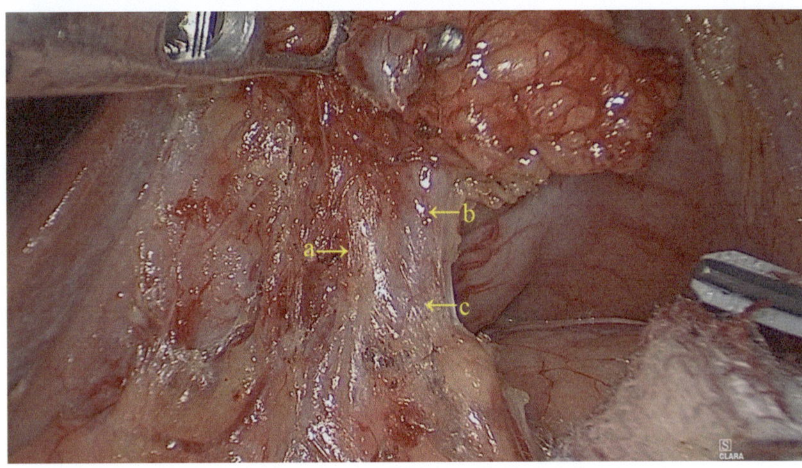

Fig. 2.49 The IPA (**a**) and the RGEA (**b**) both arise from the GDA (**c**)

IPA

About 85% of the IPA arises from the GDA (Fig. 2.49).

About 15% of the IPA arises from the RGEA (Fig. 2.50), which mainly supplies the pylorus.

Superior Pancreaticoduodenal Artery (SPDA)

The GDA gives off two terminal branches, the RGEA and the SPDA, at the inferior border of the pylorus. The latter emits the anterior and posterior branches (Fig. 2.51).

2.2.1.3 Veins Associated with the Subpyloric LN Dissection

Right Gastroepiploic Vein

RGEV: Right gastroepiploic vein; ASPDV: Anterior superior pancreaticoduodenal vein.

RGEV: Right gastroepiploic vein; ASPDV: Anterior superior pancreaticoduodenal vein; GDV: Gastroduodenal vein.

IPV: Infrapyloric vein.

The RGEV accompanies the homonymic artery, but they diverge from each other under the

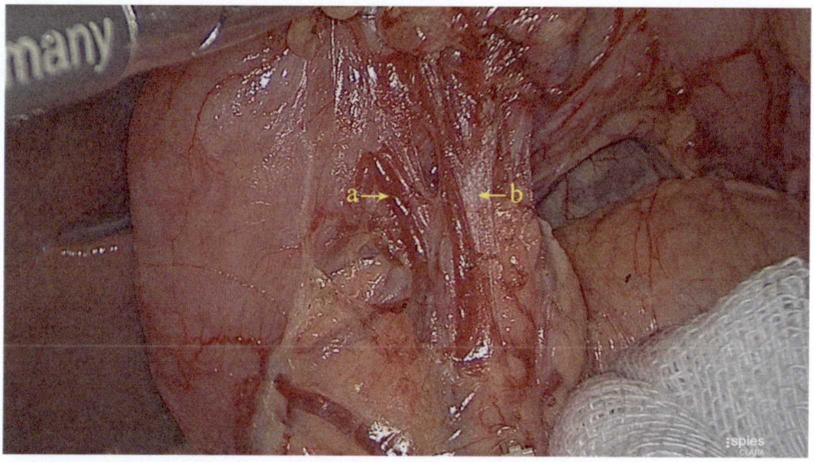

Fig. 2.50 The IPA (**a**) arises from the REGA (**b**)

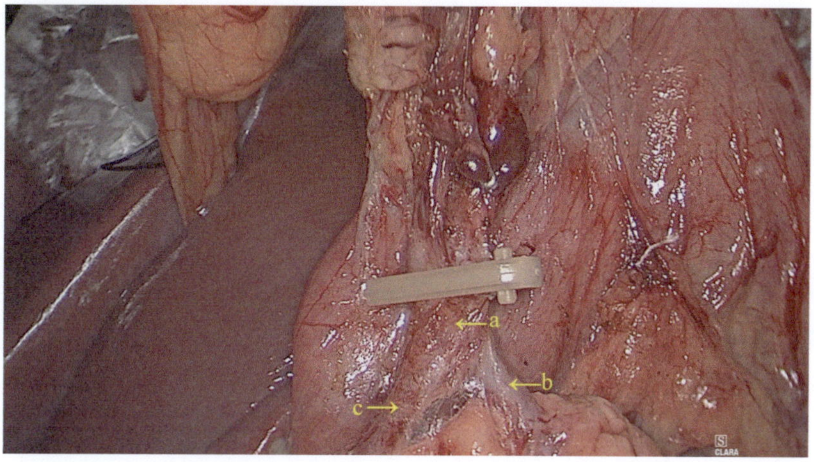

Fig. 2.51 The SPDA (**a**) branches into anterior (**b**) and posterior (**c**) branches

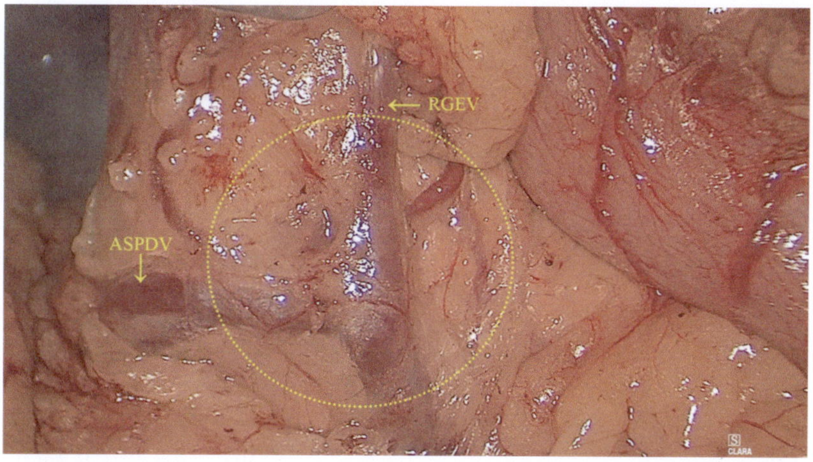

Fig. 2.52 The RGEV joins the ASPDV and combines with the RCV

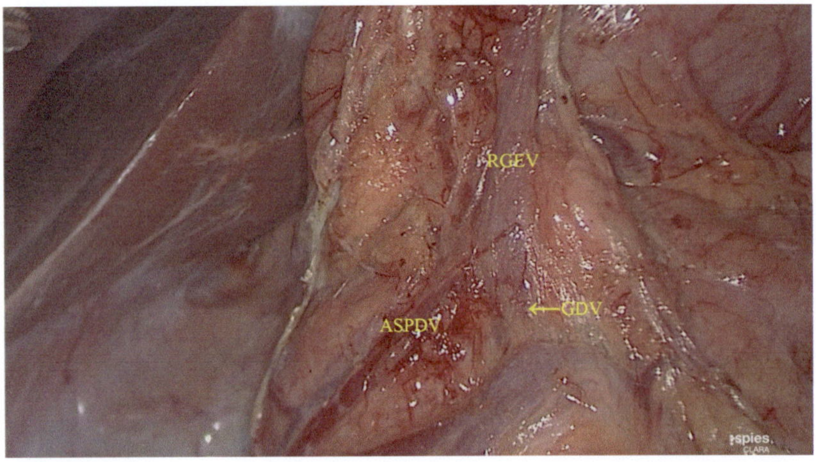

Fig. 2.53 The RGEV joins the ASPDV to form the GDV

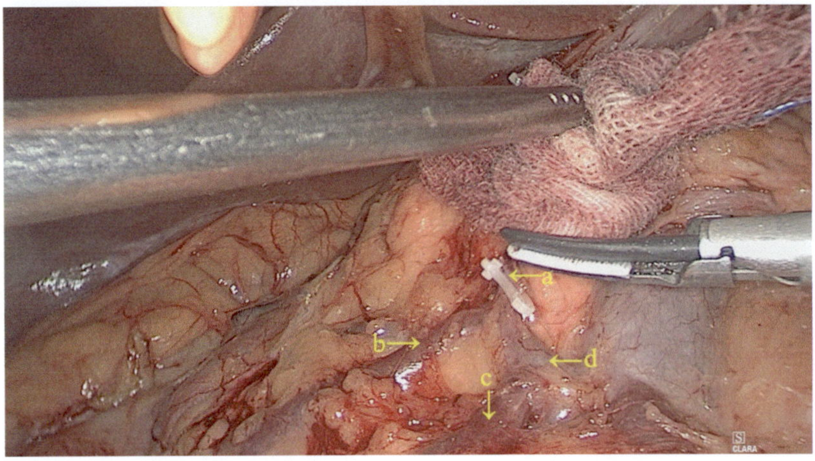

Fig. 2.54 The RGEV (**a**) joins the ASPDV (**b**) to form Henle's trunk (**d**) together with the RCV (**c**)

pylorus. At the front of the pancreatic head, the vein turns downwards to join the ASPDV and form the GDV. The GDV forms Henle's trunk together with the RCV or ARCV, flows into the SMV, and finally drains into the portal system (Fig. 2.55).

SMV

RGEV: Right gastroepiploic vein; RGEA: Right gastroepiploic artery.

The SMV is located in the mesentery and lies to the right of the corresponding artery. It is located behind the neck of the pancreas and joins the splenic vein (SpV) to form the PV (Fig. 2.56).

MCV

The MCV usually runs alongside its homonymic artery. It is an important anatomic mark for finding the SMV during the operation.

2.2.1.4 Anatomy of Lymph Nodes in the Infrapyloric Area

No. 6 Group Lymph Nodes (Infrapyloric Lymph Nodes)

Definition of No. 6 group lymph nodes.

No. 6 group lymph nodes are located between the anterior and posterior layer of gastric mesentery in the greater curvature under the pylorus. This group includes the infrapyloric and

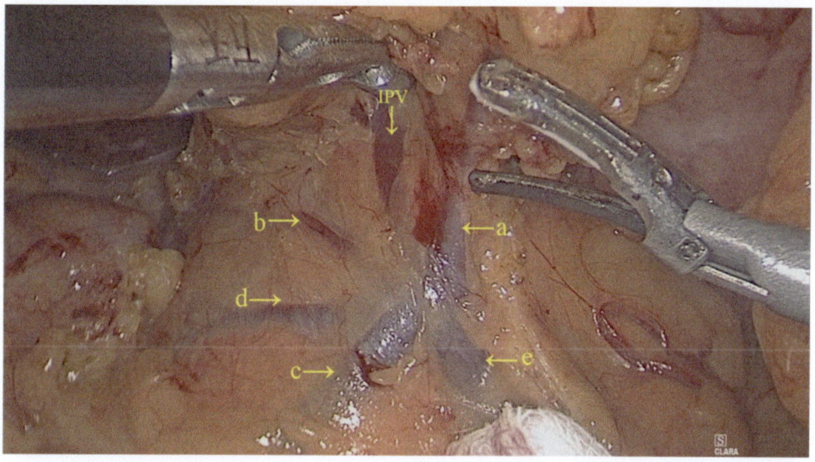

Fig. 2.55 The RGEV (**a**) joins the ASPDV (**b**), the RCV (**c**), and the ARCV (**e**) to form Henle's trunk (**d**)

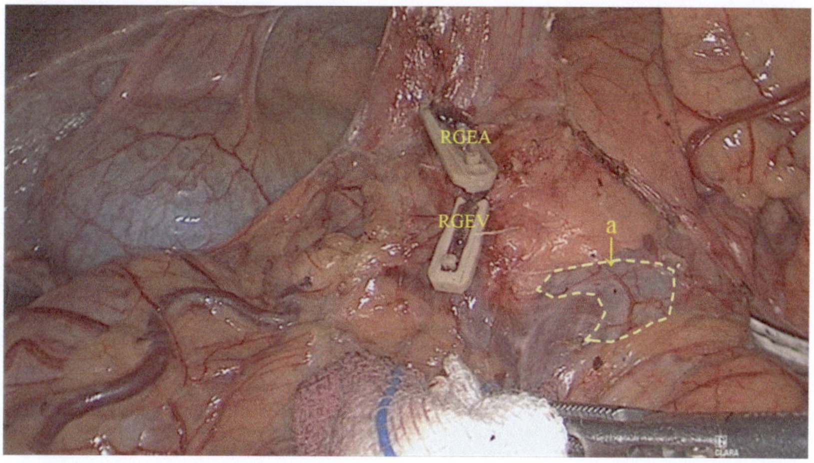

Fig. 2.56 Root of the SMA (**a**)

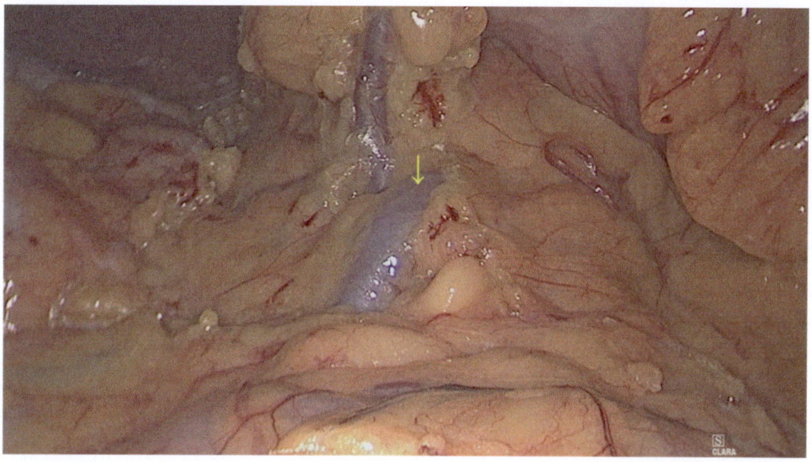

Fig. 2.57 The MCV

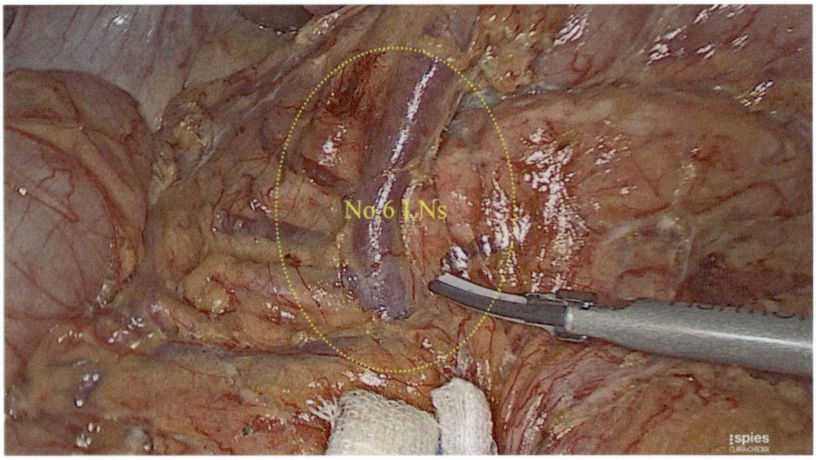

Fig. 2.58 The region of the No. 6 group lymph nodes

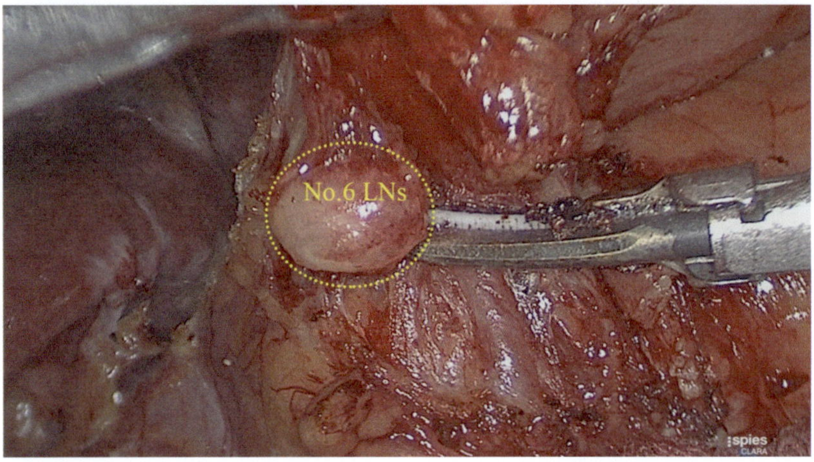

Fig. 2.59 No. 6 group lymph nodes

retropyloric lymph nodes along the surface of infrapyloric vessels, and the lymph nodes distributed in the convergent site of ASPDV and RGEV (Figs. 2.58 and 2.59).

No. 6 group lymph node metastasis cases are shown in Figs. 2.60, 2.61, and 2.62.

IPA: Infrapyloric artery; RGEA: Right gastroepiploic artery; RGEV: Right gastroepiploic vein.

Imaging of No. 6 group lymph nodes was developed using ICG fluorescence (Figs. 2.63, 2.64, 2.65, 2.66, 2.67, and 2.68).

HST: Henle's trunk; RCV: Right colic vein; RGEV: Right gastroepiploic vein.

ASPDA: Anterior superior pancreaticoduodenal artery; RGEA: Right gastroepiploic artery.

No. 14v Group Lymph Nodes at the SMV Root

Definition of No. 14v group lymph nodes.

RGEV: Right gastroepiploic vein; RGEA: Right gastroepiploic artery.

SMV: Superior mesenteric vein.

No. 14v group lymph nodes are part of the superior mesenteric lymph nodes. This group contains lymphatic drainage along with SMVs and the branch vessels. The lymph nodes distributed in front of the root of the SMV are known as No.14v lymph nodes; the upper boundary is the lower pancreatic margin, the right boundary is near the left of the RGEV and ASPDV convergent site, the left boundary is near the left of the

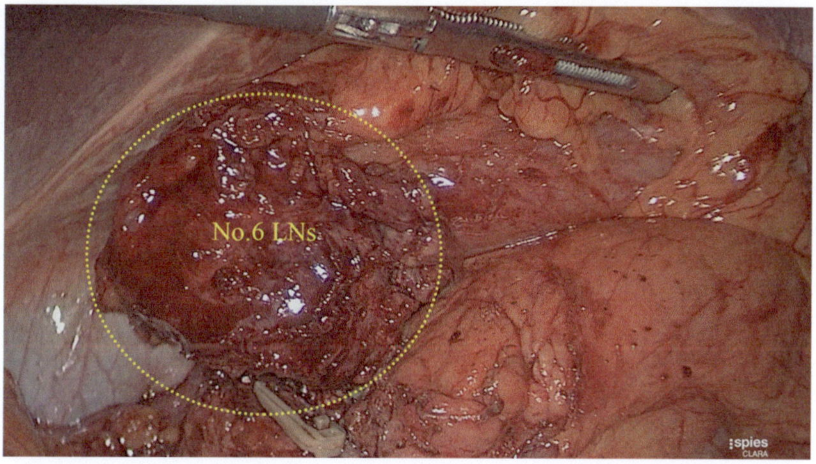

Fig. 2.60 Intraoperative appearance of No. 6 group lymph node metastasis

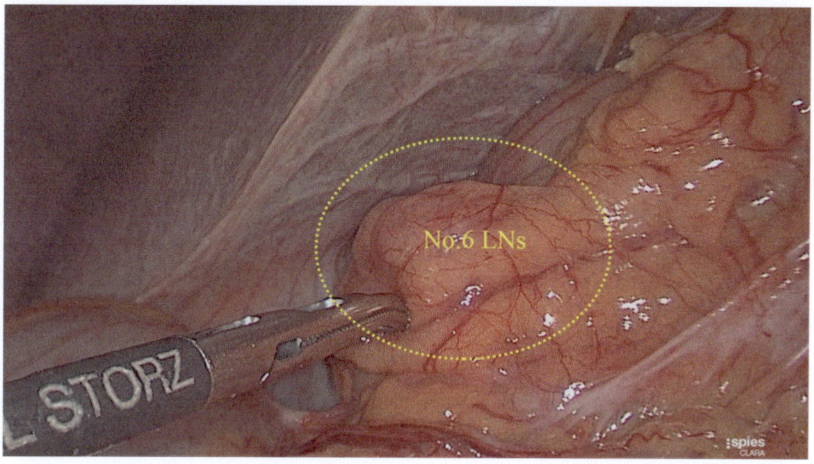

Fig. 2.61 Intraoperative appearance of swollen No. 6 group lymph nodes

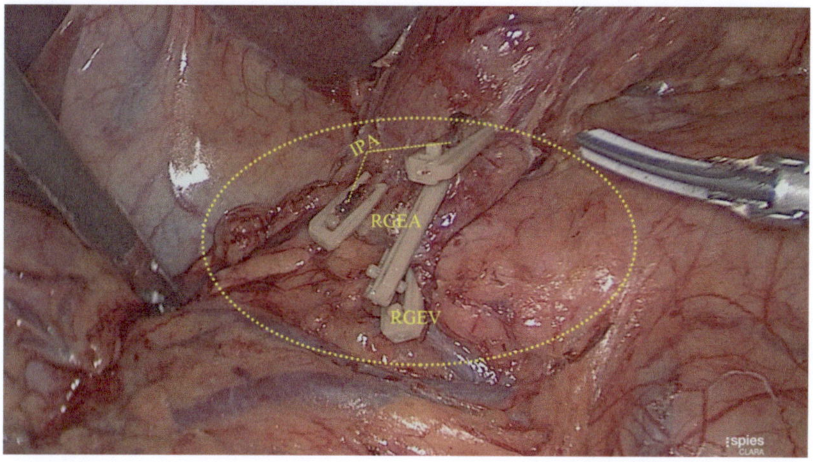

Fig. 2.62 Display of No. 6 group lymph nodes after dissection

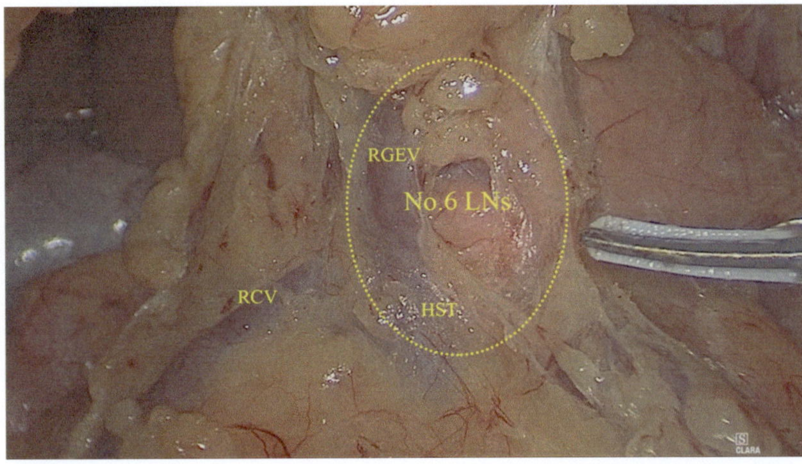

Fig. 2.63 Intraoperative appearance of No. 6 group lymph nodes by the naked eye

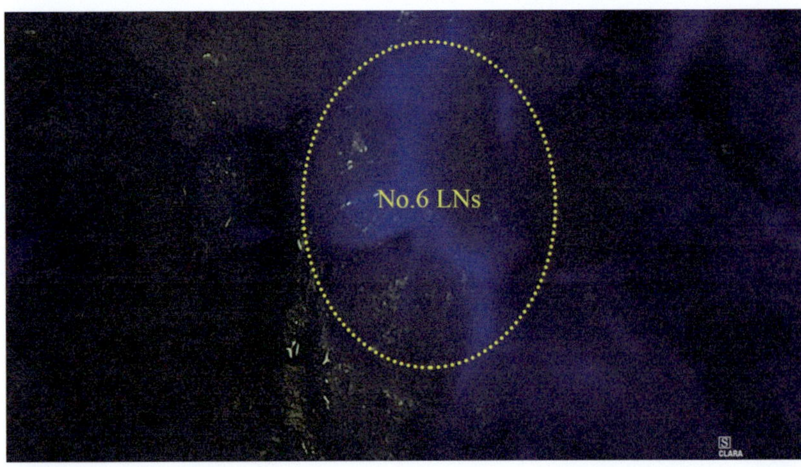

Fig. 2.64 Intraoperative developing of No. 6 group lymph nodes using ICG fluorescence imaging

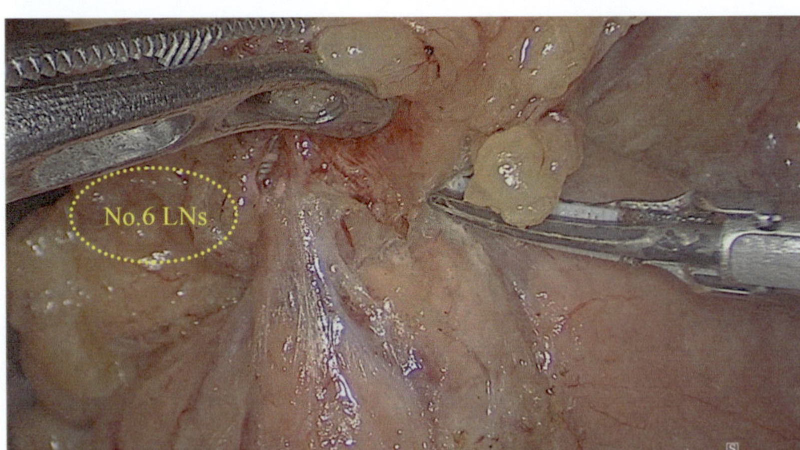

Fig. 2.65 Intraoperative appearance of No. 6 group lymph nodes by the naked eye

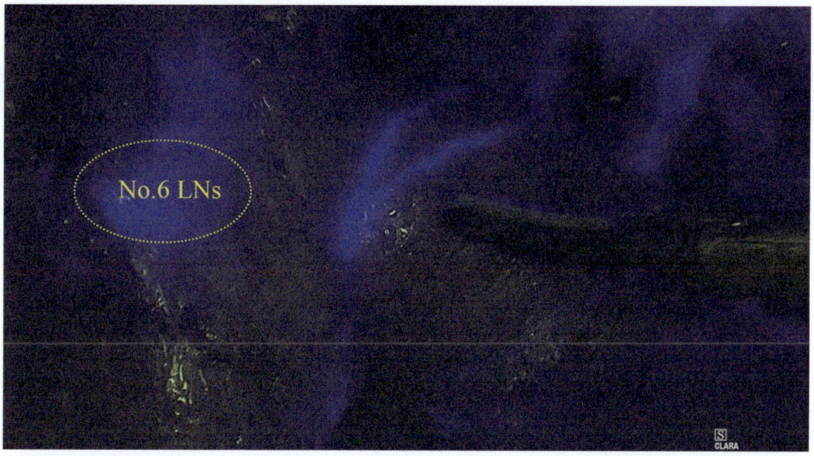

Fig. 2.66 Intraoperative developing of No. 6 group lymph nodes using ICG fluorescence imaging

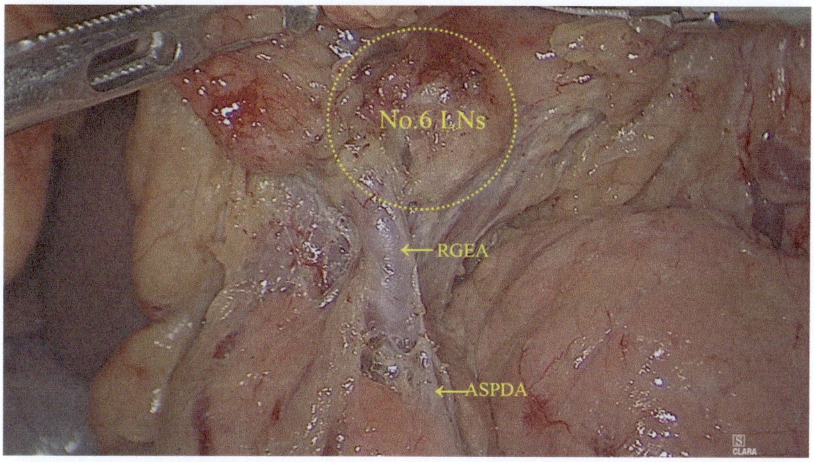

Fig. 2.67 Intraoperative appearance of No. 6 group lymph nodes

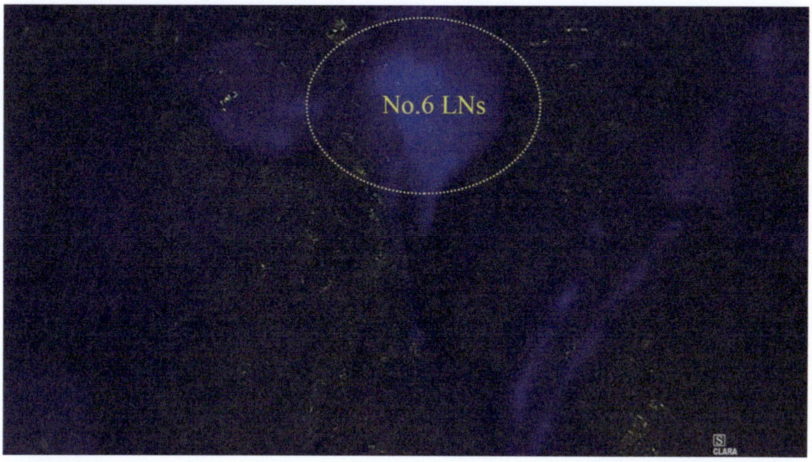

Fig. 2.68 Intraoperative developing of No. 6 group lymph nodes using ICG fluorescence imaging

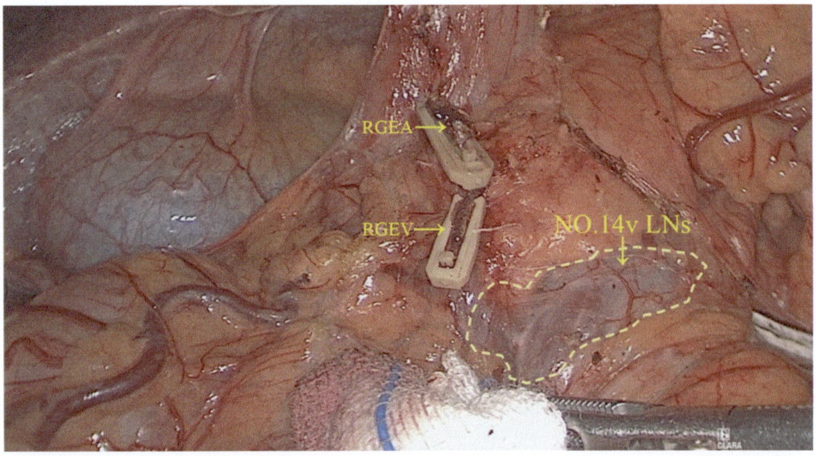

Fig. 2.69 The region of No. 14v group lymph nodes

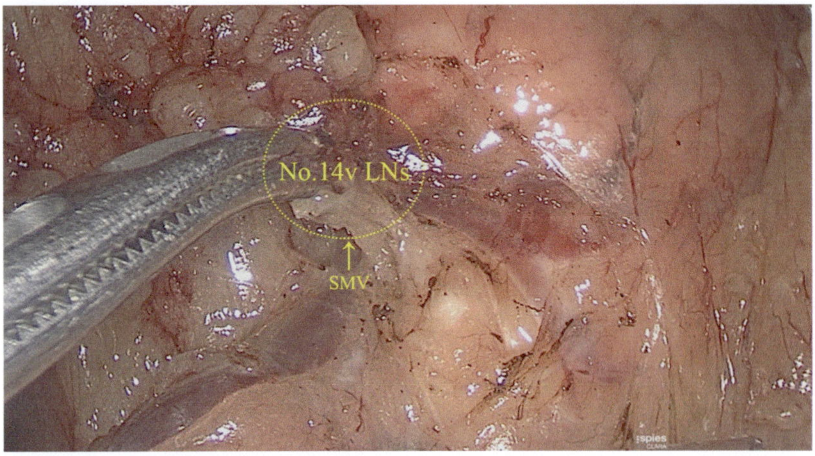

Fig. 2.70 No. 14v group lymph nodes

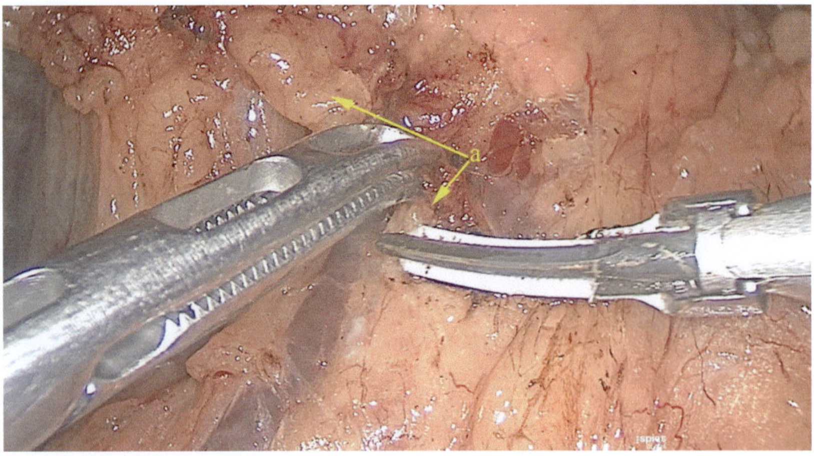

Fig. 2.71 Intraoperative appearance of No. 14v group lymph node metastasis (**a**)

SMV, the lower boundary is the bifurcation of the MCV (Figs. 2.69 and 2.70).

No. 14v group lymph node metastasis cases are shown in Figs. 2.71, 2.72, and 2.73.

SMV: Superior mesenteric vein.

MCV: Middle colic vein.

Imaging of No. 14v group lymph nodes was developed using ICG fluorescence imaging (Figs. 2.74 and 2.75).

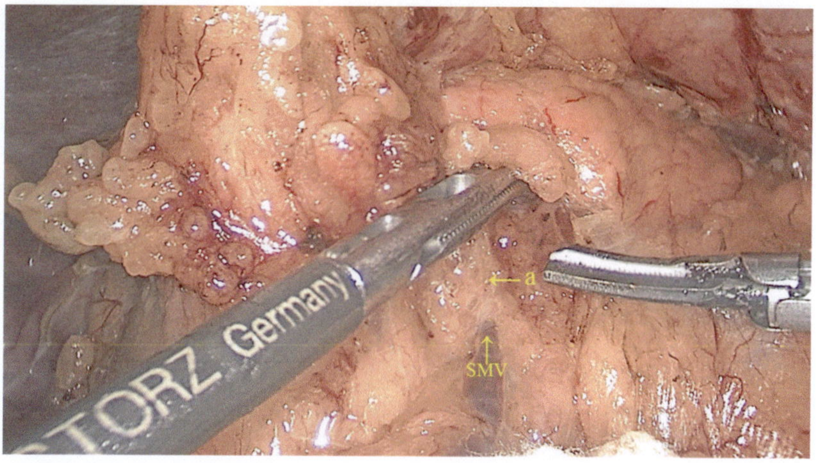

Fig. 2.72 Intraoperative appearance of No. 14v group lymph nodes (**a**)

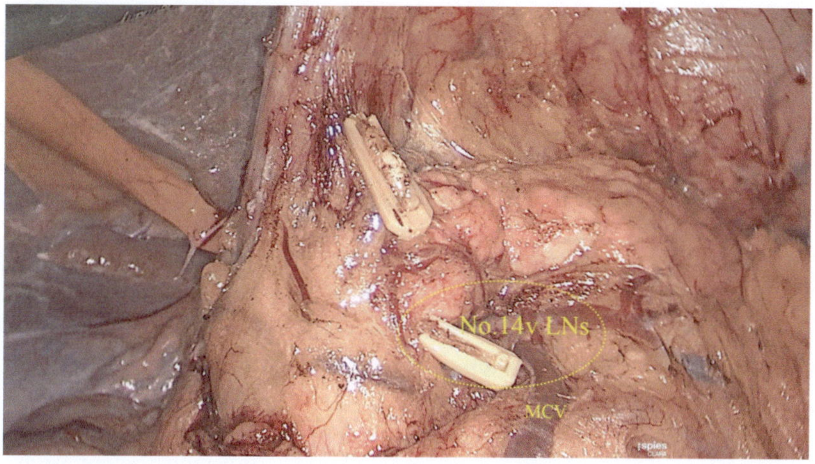

Fig. 2.73 Appearance after No. 14v group LN dissection

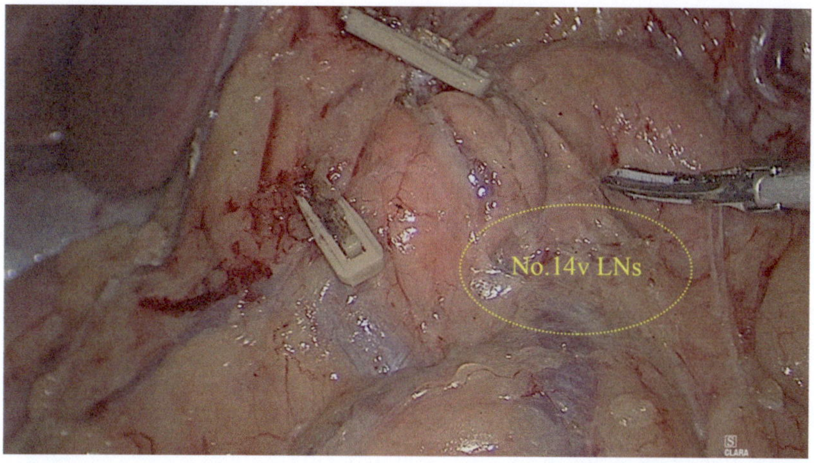

Fig. 2.74 Appearance of No. 14v group lymph nodes as seen by the naked eye

Fig. 2.75 Intraoperative developing of No. 14v group lymph nodes using ICG fluorescence imaging

2.2.2 Operative Announcements of Laparoscopic Gastric Cancer Lymph Node Dissection in Infrapyloric Area

2.2.2.1 Matters Needing Attention when Resecting the Greater Omentum and Dividing the Anterior TM

Matters Needing Attention when Resecting the Greater Omentum

Before the omentum is separated, the condition of the abdominal cavity should be explored. Abdominal adhesions are often present in patients with a history of abdominal surgery. However, adhesions may also be present in patients with no surgical history (Figs. 2.76 and 2.77).

Obese patients have a thicker omentum, and are prone to adhesions. Additionally, the transverse colon is often covered by a large omentum, so it is not easy to expose. When detaching the omentum, blunt and sharp separation should be used alternately to prevent damage to the colon (Fig. 2.78).

The separation of the gastrocolic membrane should be close to the stomach wall (Fig. 2.79).

Because of the good mobility of colon, separating omentum along transverse colon readily identifies the hepatic flexure; pulling the hepatic flexure outward then better exposes the duodenum inside (Fig. 2.80).

Matters Needing Attention when Dividing the Anterior TM

When separating the anterior TM to the lower pancreatic margin, the assistant should lift the antrum upwards and the surgeon should pull the TM downwards. This can form an obtuse angle between the anterior and the posterior TM planes. The loose connective tissue between the two planes is the surgical separated plane (Fig. 2.81).

If the space is not obvious, the right-hand grasping forceps of assistant can be used gently to bluntly separate the TM to the inferiority of pancreatic head to help exposing the space (Fig. 2.82).

Since the fascial space between the anterior and the posterior TM contains no blood vessels, it is easy to separate and less prone to bleeding. If repetitive small blood vessel bleeding occurs during the separation process, this suggests that the plane of separation is either too deep or not deep enough. In such cases, re-finding the operation plane is necessary (Fig. 2.83).

The interior edge of the duodenum is close to the right boundary of the anterior TM. Therefore, the boundary needs to be separated when the anterior TM is fully divided. The adhesions of the duodenal bulb and the

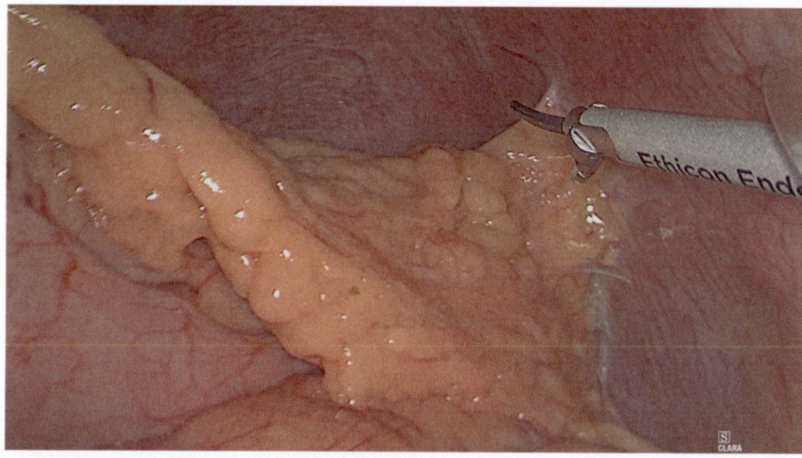

Fig. 2.76 Before excising the greater omentum, the adhesion should be divided first

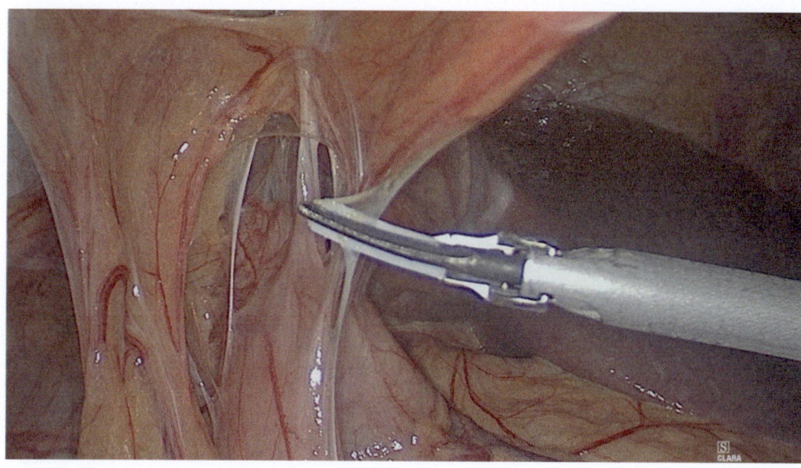

Fig. 2.77 Adhesions may exist even in patients with no previous abdominal surgical history

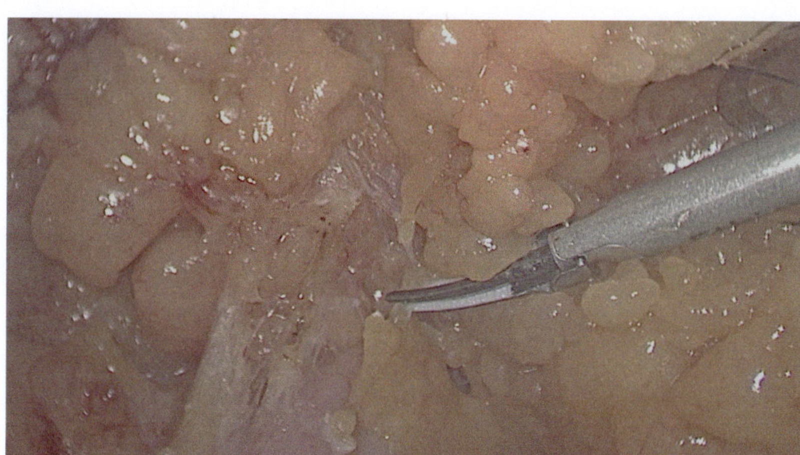

Fig. 2.78 Care should be taken during surgery of obese patients because the transverse colon will be covered by a large omentum

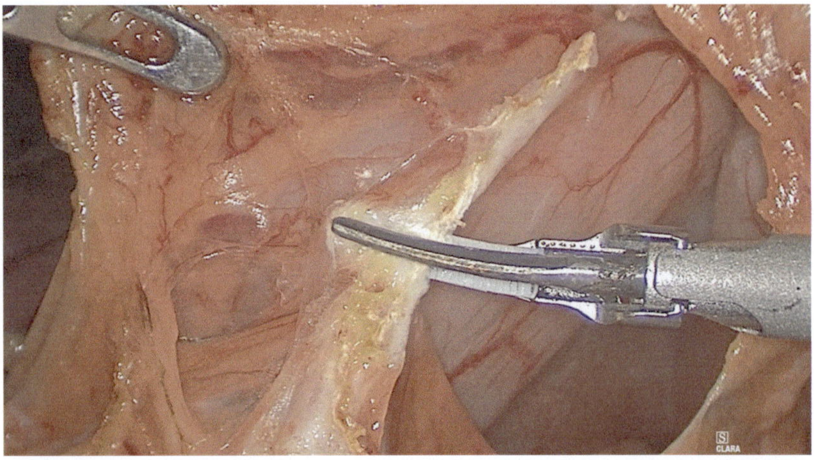

Fig. 2.79 Separation of the gastrocolic membrane should be close to the stomach wall

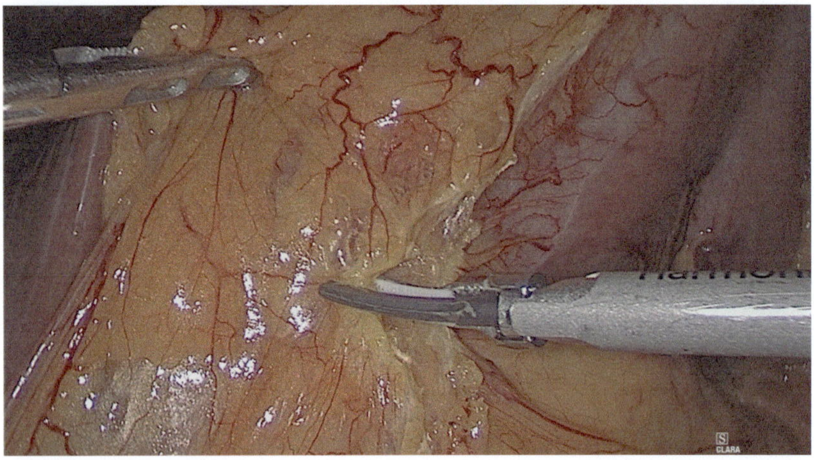

Fig. 2.80 When dragging the hepatic flexure out, the duodenum will be easily exposed

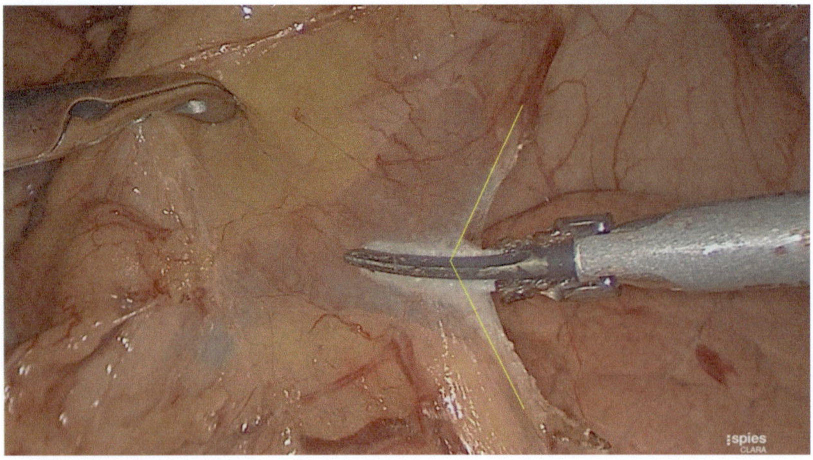

Fig. 2.81 The obtuse angle between the anterior and the posterior TM planes

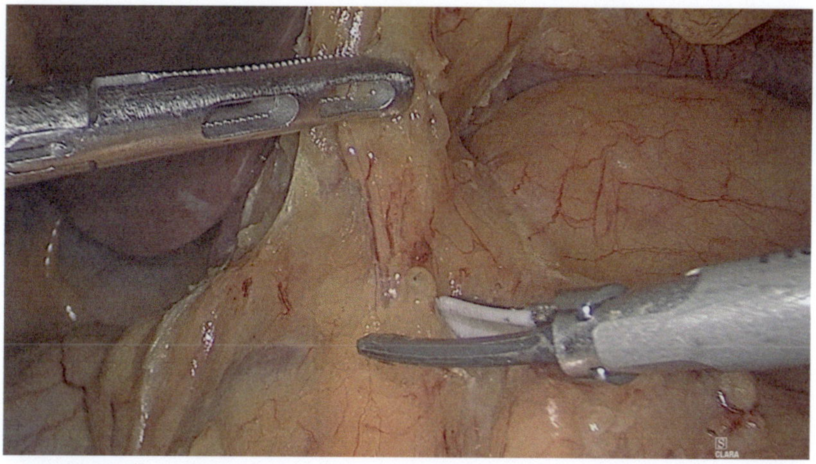

Fig. 2.82 Use of grasping forceps by the assistant gently and bluntly separates the TM inferior to the pancreatic head to assist in exposing the space

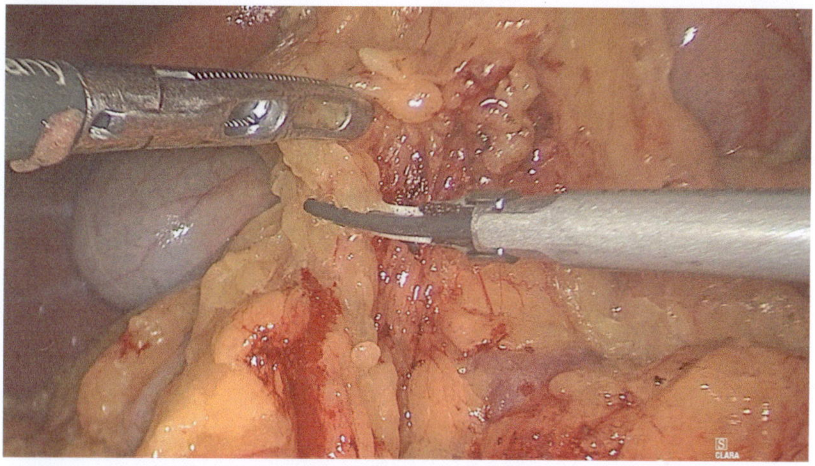

Fig. 2.83 Bleeding indicates the plane of separation is either too deep or not deep enough. In such cases, re-finding the operation plane is necessary

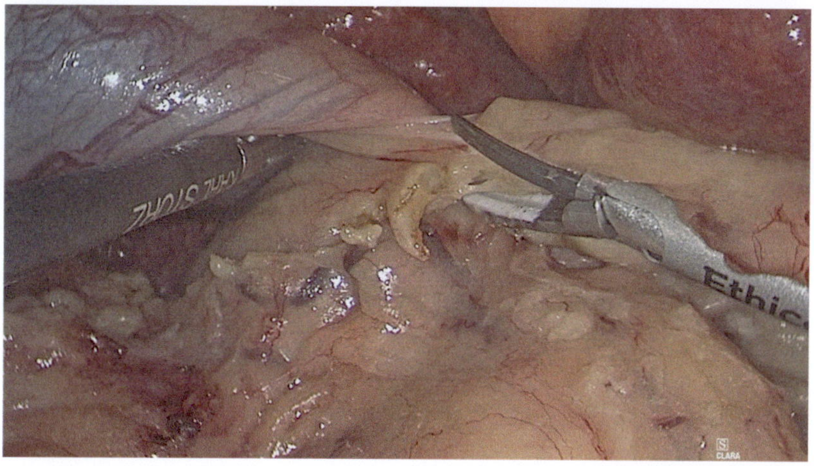

Fig. 2.84 The adhesions of the duodenal bulb and the descending duodenum to the colonic hepatic flexure must be completely separated firstly

descending duodenum to the colonic hepatic flexure must be completely separated firstly. so that the assistant can pull the antrum upwards making dissection of the infrapyloric region easier (Fig. 2.84).

When the anterior TM is separated, the mesentery may be broken because it has been entered too deeply (Fig. 2.85).

When the TM is lifted, it should be separated adjacent to the gastric wall, and the plane of

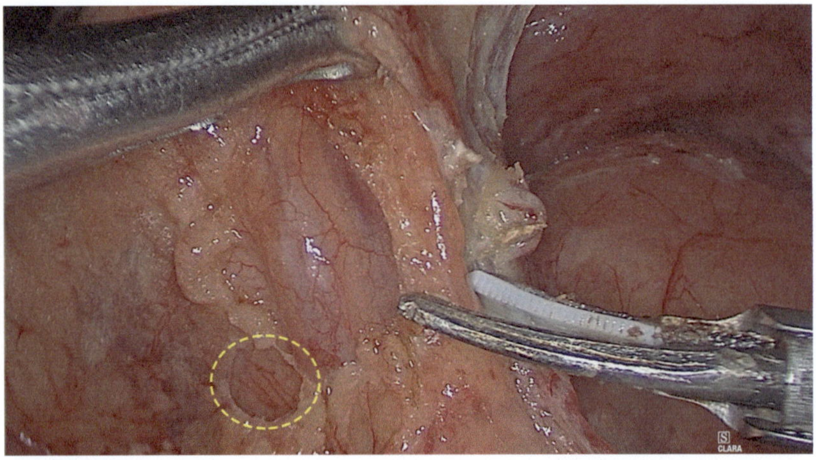

Fig. 2.85 Breakage of the TM

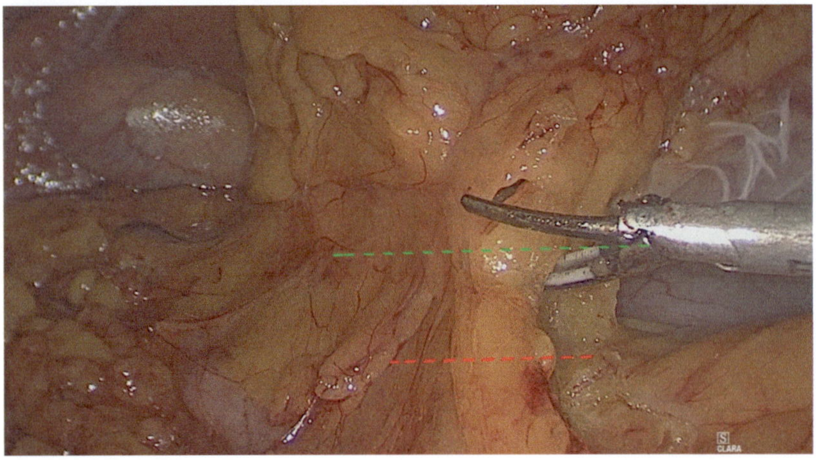

Fig. 2.86 Because the TM is lifted, it should be separated adjacent to the gastric wall (line with green color)

separation must be correctly confirmed to prevent damage to either the TM or its blood vessels (Fig. 2.86).

2.2.2.2 Matters Needing Attention when Dissecting No. 14v Group Lymph Nodes

When seeking and making the anatomical space obvious, one of the assistant's grasping forceps should be used to drag the posterior antral wall upwards, and another grasping forceps should pull against the operator's grasper to slightly tighten the tissue to be separated. This makes the anatomical space easier to expose and facilitates operation of the ultrasonic scalpels (Fig. 2.87).

RCA: Right colic artery.

For obese patients or patients with deep SMV that are difficult to expose, the RGEV can be found at the inferior edge of the pancreas. Along the RGEV and the MCV, the site of entry of both veins into the SMV can be visualized. After entering into the post-pancreatic space at this site; the SMV can be revealed (Fig. 2.88).

For overweight patients, fat and lymph nodes are often not easily distinguished from pancreatic tissue. Therefore, it is important to carefully discriminate between fat, lymph nodes, and pancreatic tissue when dissecting lymph nodes near the SMV root at the lower pancreatic edge. It is best way to dissect the lymph nodes on the pancreatic surface to help prevent the occurrence of postoperative pancreatic fistulae (Fig. 2.89).

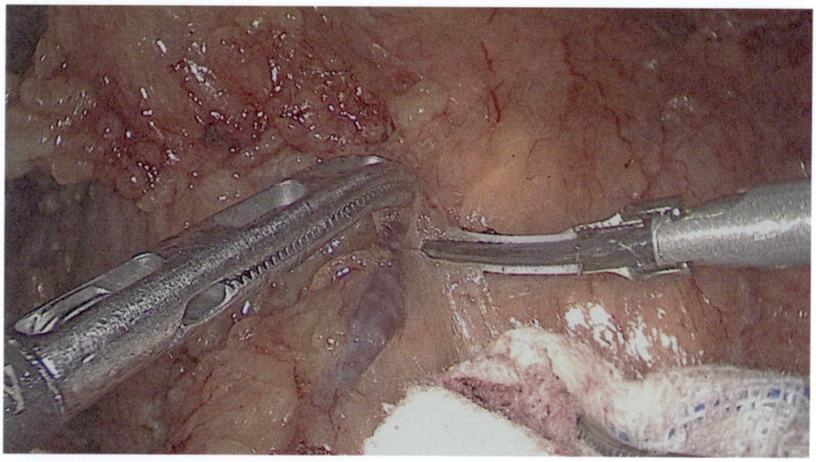

Fig. 2.87 Cooperation between the surgeon and the assistant makes exposing the anatomical space easier, enabling greater operation accuracy

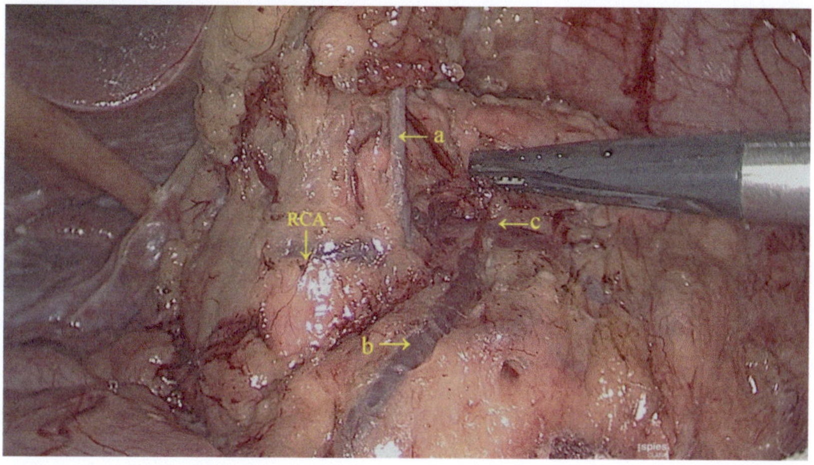

Fig. 2.88 Along the RGEV (**a**) and the MCV (**b**), the site of entry of both veins into the SMV (**c**) can be exposed

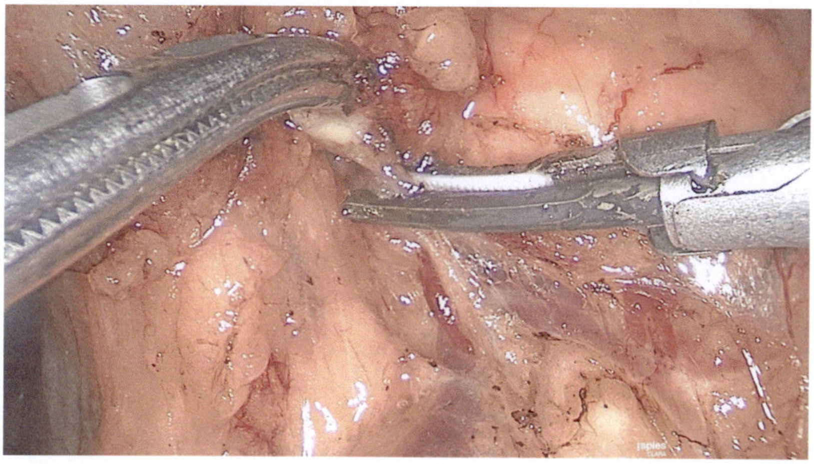

Fig. 2.89 It is best to dissect the lymph nodes on the pancreatic surface to help prevent the occurrence of postoperative pancreatic fistulae

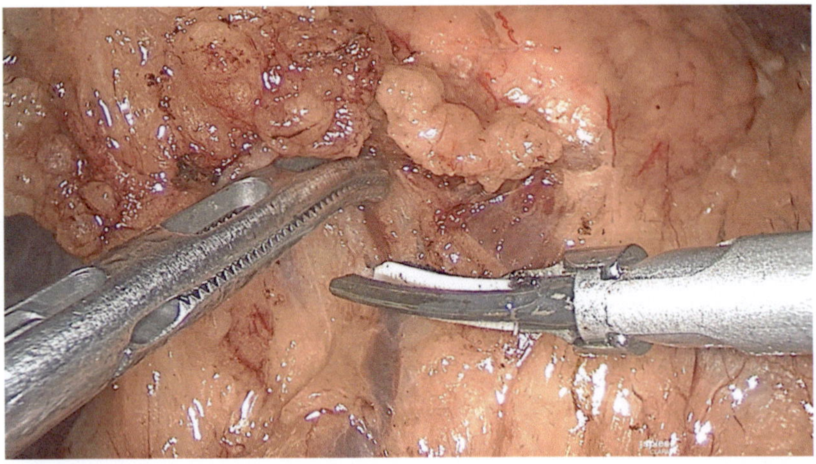

Fig. 2.90 As the anterior TM is separated, the SMV can be easily revealed

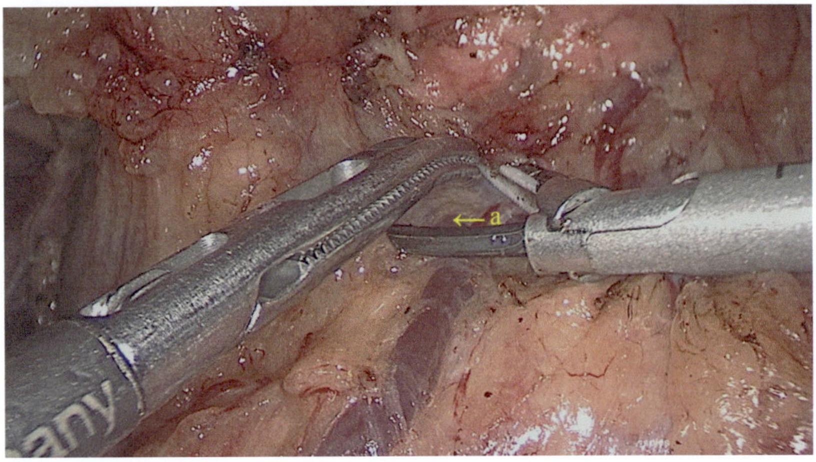

Fig. 2.91 Using an ultrasonic scalpel to open the tissue ahead the SMV (**a**)

It is necessary to expand the anatomic plane surrounding the MCV fully. As the anterior TM is separated, the SMV will be naturally exposed (Fig. 2.90).

The surgeon should pull the MCV and the transverse mesocolon downwards to make the space exposed between the fat, lymphoid tissue, and blood vessels, facilitating convenient dissection (Fig. 2.91).

Because the walls of the veins are relatively thin, dissection of lymph nodes along the SMV must be gentle. The best way is to dissect using ultrasonic scalpels directly, with the non-functional face put near the wall of veins; blunt dissection should be used as little as possible to prevent vascular injury (Fig. 2.92).

At the lower pancreatic edge, the SMV often contains some venules (Fig. 2.93). Because the pressure of the SMV is relatively high and the wall of the vein is thin, it is improper to transect these venules when dissecting No. 14v group lymph nodes to prevent bleeding.

RGEA: Right gastroepiploic artery; IPA: Infrapyloric artery.

In a small proportion of patients, the branches of the SPDA are superficial and exposed on the surface of the pancreas. Care should be taken when separating the pancreatic membrane and dissecting No. 14v group lymph nodes to prevent injury to these arterioles (Fig. 2.94).

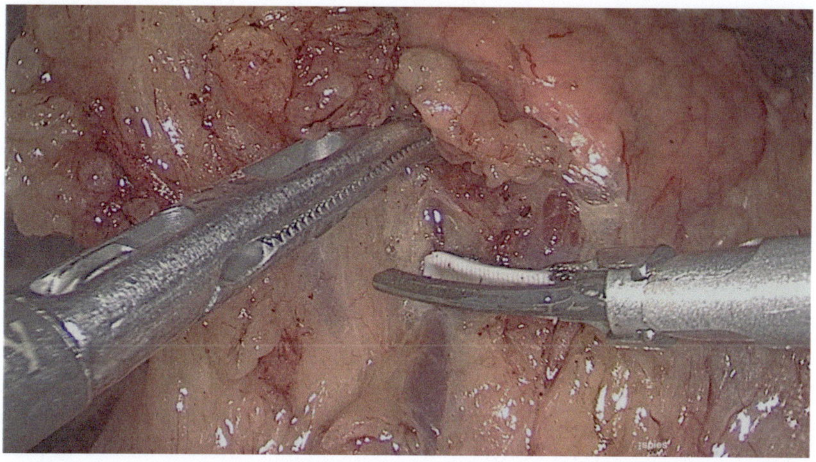

Fig. 2.92 The best way is to dissect using ultrasonic scalpels directly, with the non-functional face put near the wall of veins

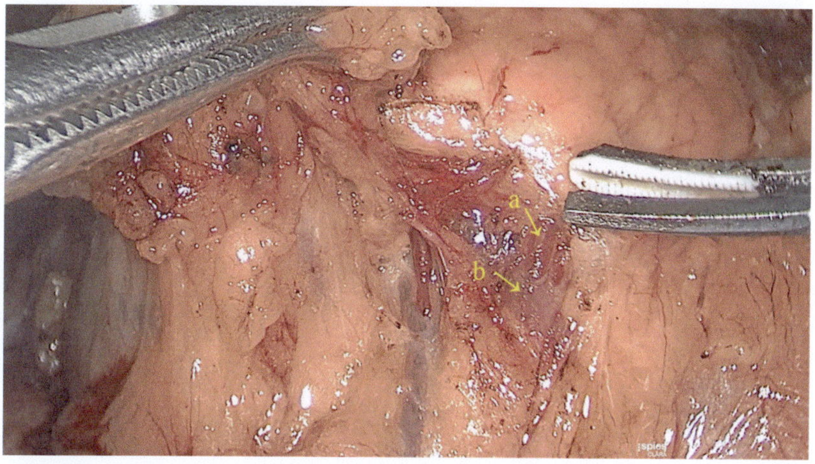

Fig. 2.93 At the lower pancreatic edge, the SMV (**b**) often contains some venules (**a**)

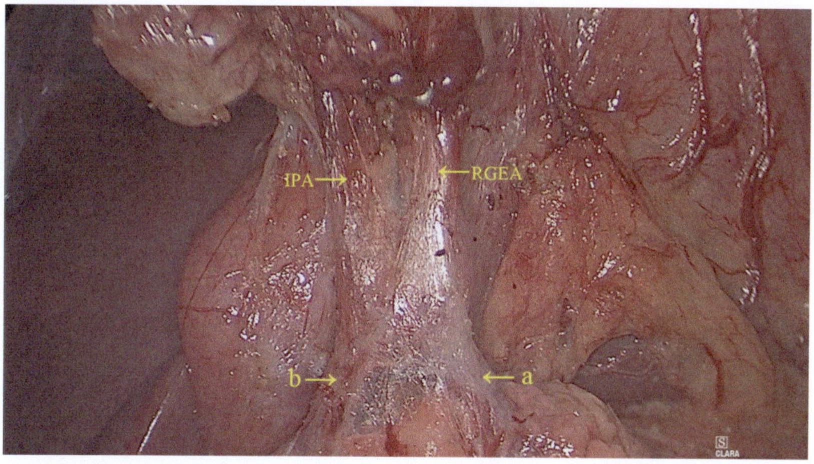

Fig. 2.94 The upper anterior SPDA (**a**) and the upper posterior SPDA (**b**) are two branches of the SPDA

2.2.2.3 Common Intraoperative Situations and Matters Needing Attention When Dissecting No. 6 Group Lymph Nodes

When the tumor in the antrum is much large, the wall of the gastric antrum may not be easily grasped by the assistant. At this point, atraumatic grasping forceps can be used to hold the posterior antral wall or to hold more omentum. This enables exposure of the anatomical space (Fig. 2.95).

When large amounts of adipose and lymphoid tissue are present in the infrapyloric region, small gauze can make free fat between the duodenum and the liver fixed to better expose the infrapyloric region (Figs. 2.96 and 2.97).

RGEV: Right gastroepiploic vein; SMV: Superior mesenteric vein.

For overweight patients or whose No. 6 group lymph nodes are swollen, it is not easy to determine the confluent site of the ASPDV and the RGEV which is known as an optimal surgical approach. In such cases, the SMV and Henle's trunk should be exposed first. Then, tissues should be separated on the pancreatic head from an upwards to downwards position to show the initial position of the RGEV (Fig. 2.98).

In the process of mobilizing the duodenum, attention must be paid to the boundaries between different tissues to prevent accidental injuries of other organ tissues (e.g. the gallbladder, colon, or pancreas). When the assistant aids the surgeon in

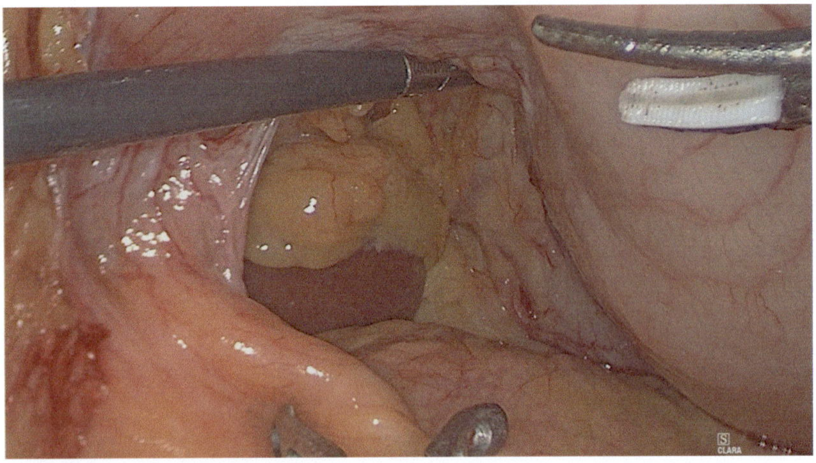

Fig. 2.95 When the tumor in the antrum is much large, atraumatic grasping forceps can be used to hold the posterior wall of the antrum

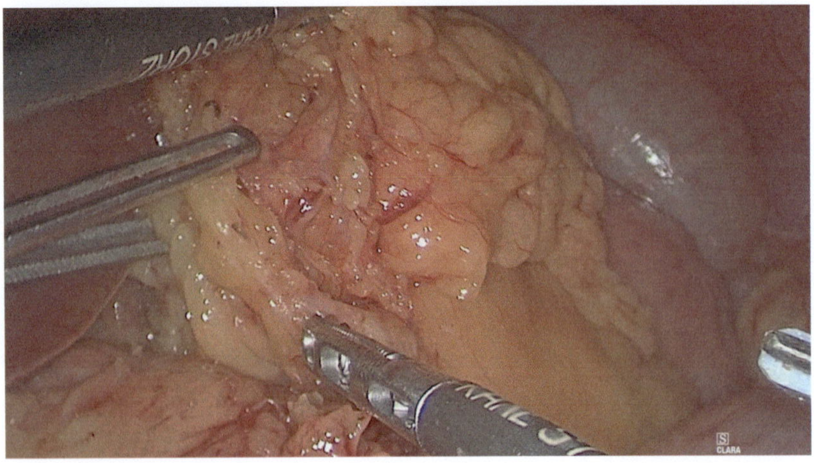

Fig. 2.96 In the infrapyloric region, exposing the operating scope before rotating the body of the stomach is difficult because of the free adipose tissue

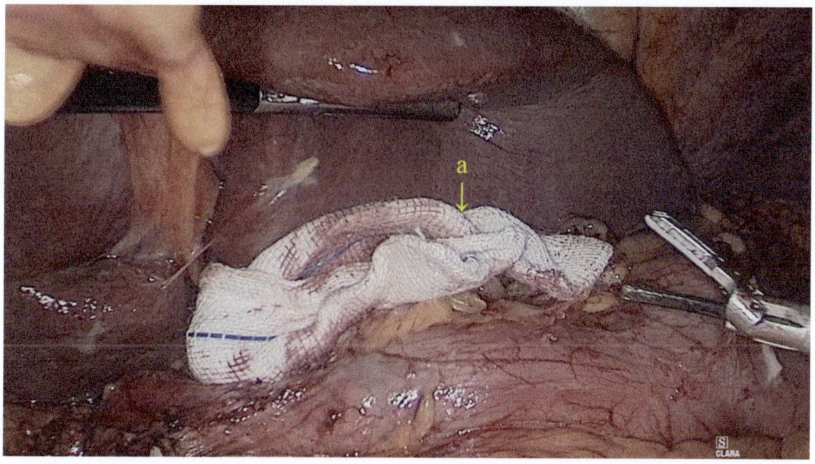

Fig. 2.97 Adipose tissues can be fixed between the liver and duodenum by a piece of gauze (**a**)

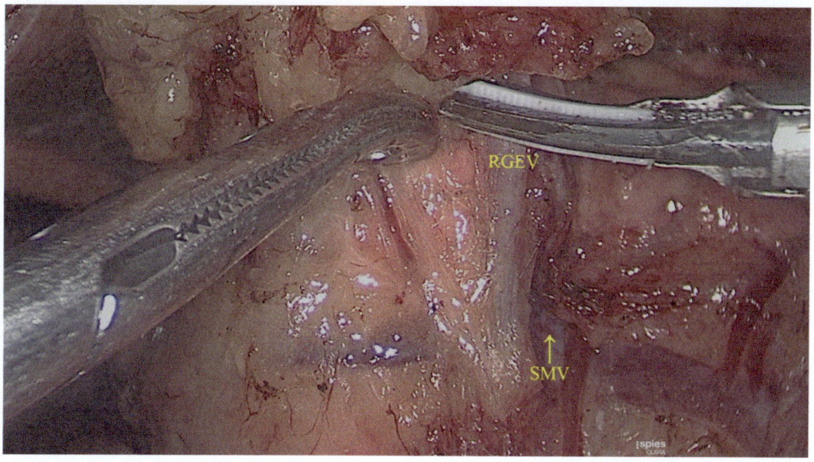

Fig. 2.98 The first vein to be exposed is SMV, and then followed by the RGEV

the process of exposure, retraction of the omentum should involve appropriate tension to avoid tearing the omentum, causing bleeding (Fig. 2.99).

Separation should be performed alternately along the horizontal and vertical axes of the RGEV to completely dissociate the backface of the RGEV (Figs. 2.100 and 2.101).

RGEV: Right gastroepiploic vein; RGEA: Right gastroepiploic artery; IPV: Infrapyloric vein.

RGEV: Right gastroepiploic vessel.

Aberrant or heterogenic pancreatic lobes are often present in the infrapyloric area in some patients, and need to be differentiated from enlarged lymph nodes and fat in this area. The former can be removed, while the latter should be preserved to avoid bleeding or postoperative pancreatic fistulae (Figs. 2.102, 2.103, and 2.104).

RGEA: Right gastroepiploic artery; RGEV: Right gastroepiploic vein.

The area between the RGEV and RGEA is drained by No. 6 group lymph nodes. Since the planes of dividing the RGEA and the RGEV are distinguishing (the former above the pancreatic head surface, while the latter below it), the two vessels should be divided at different sites. And the RGEV should be ligated first so as to avoid bleeding caused by tearing during separation (Figs. 2.105 and 2.106).

The severing plane of the RGEV lies above the convergent site with the ASPDV. Hence,

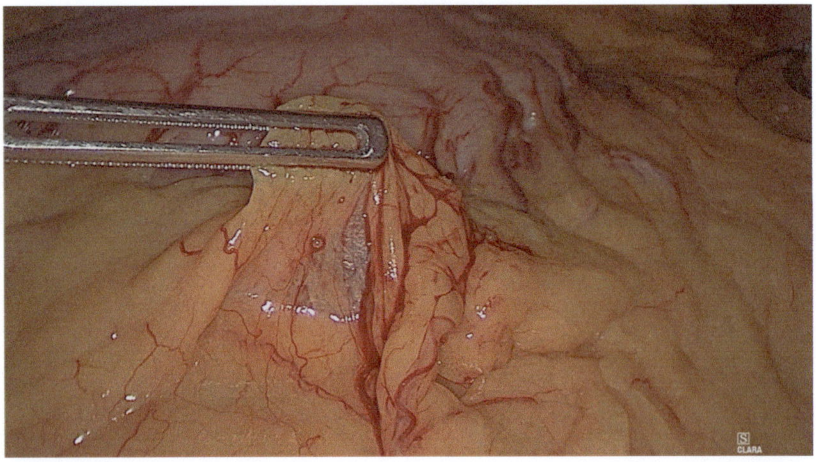

Fig. 2.99 Retracting the omentum without proper tension may cause bleeding of the omental tissues

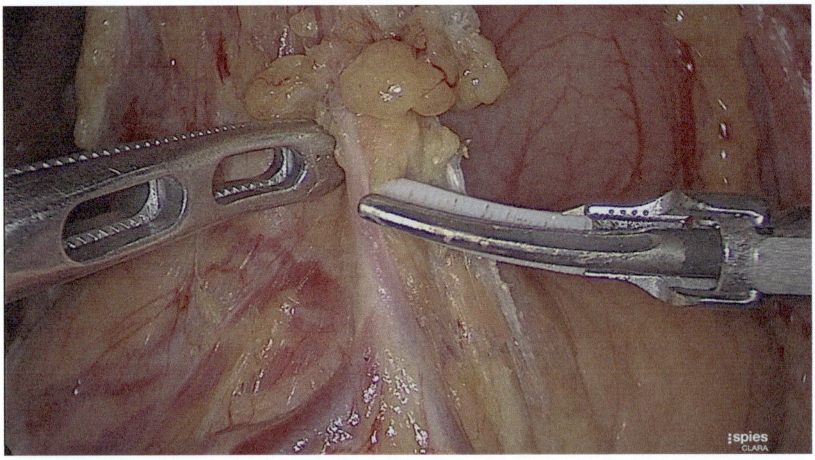

Fig. 2.100 An ultrasonic scalpel is used along the vertical axis of the blood vessel to dissect the tissues

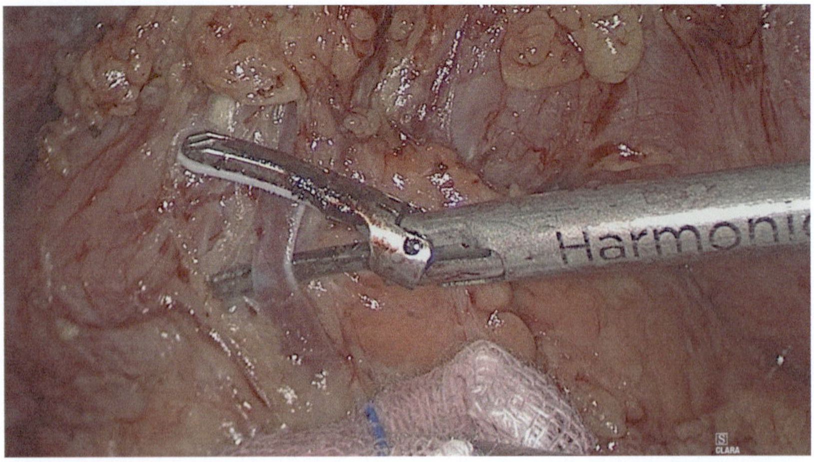

Fig. 2.101 The vessel is completely denuded with an ultrasonic scalpel

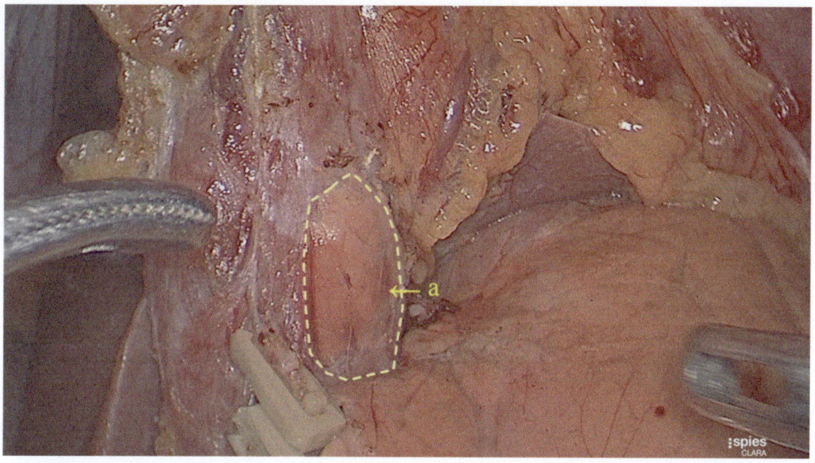

Fig. 2.102 The heterogenic pancreatic tissue (**a**)

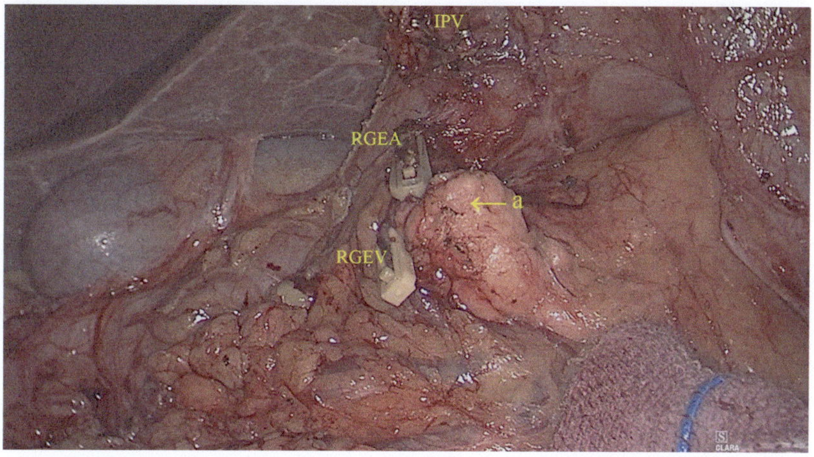

Fig. 2.103 The heterogenic pancreatic tissue (**a**) should be preserved during surgery

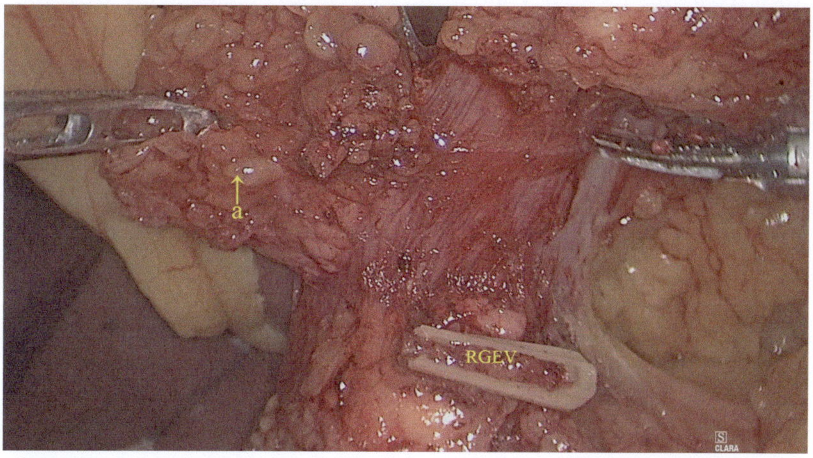

Fig. 2.104 Aberrant pancreatic tissue (**a**) on the antral wall

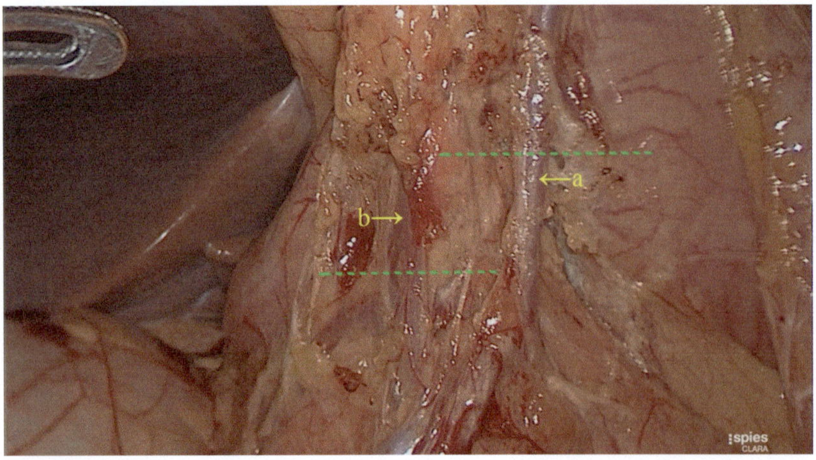

Fig. 2.105 Planes of sever the RGEV (**b**) and the RGEA (**a**) are different

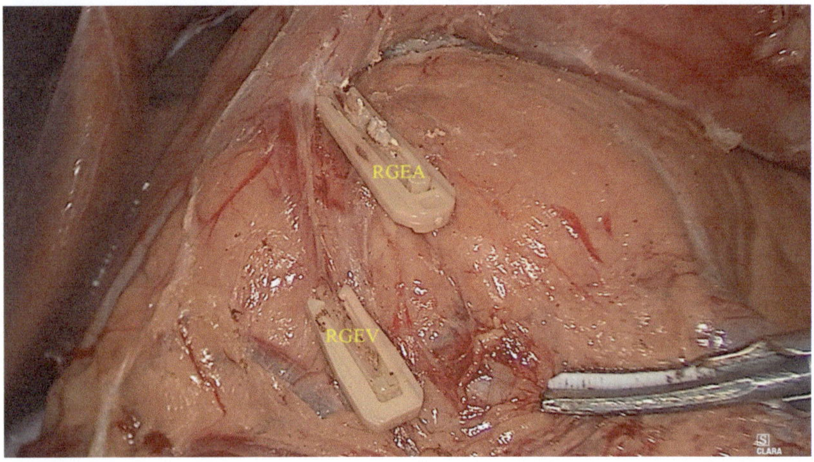

Fig. 2.106 After severing appearances of the RGEV and the RGEA

when separating the RGEV along the pancreatic head surface, attention must be paid to the ASPDV which may come from the right, at the back of the pancreatic head (Fig. 2.107).

When the RGEV directly joins to the SMV, it can be ligated at the lower pancreatic edge. When the RGEV root did not be exposed well, if the ASPDV, the RCV, and the RGEV form the Henle's trunk near the right site of SMV, attention must be paid not to ligate or severe the ASPDV and the Henle's trunk (Figs. 2.108 and 2.109).

After the RGEV has been divided, the assistant should pull the RGEA upwards. The SPDA and the GDA may also move up together at this time. Ligation of the root of the RGEA should be performed after the gastroduodenal arteria branches off to the SPDA. And the ligation plane should not be too low to prevent ischemia caused by mistaken ligation of the SPDA (Figs. 2.110 and 2.111).

Behind the RGEA, the GDA often give out the IPA. Therefore, it is necessary to pay attention to the existence of the artery after dividing the RGEA. The IPA is relatively thin and branched, making its exposure difficult. It should be ligated first and then divided using the ultrasonic scalpel's minimum gear (Fig. 2.112).

Clarification

All images of the chapter come from FuJian Medical University gastric surgery database and video database.

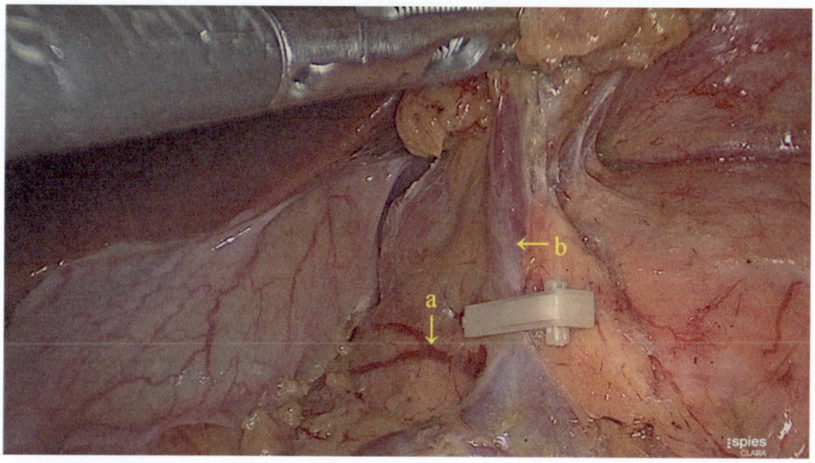

Fig. 2.107 Above the convergent site with the ASPDV (**a**) is the severing plane for the RGEV (**b**)

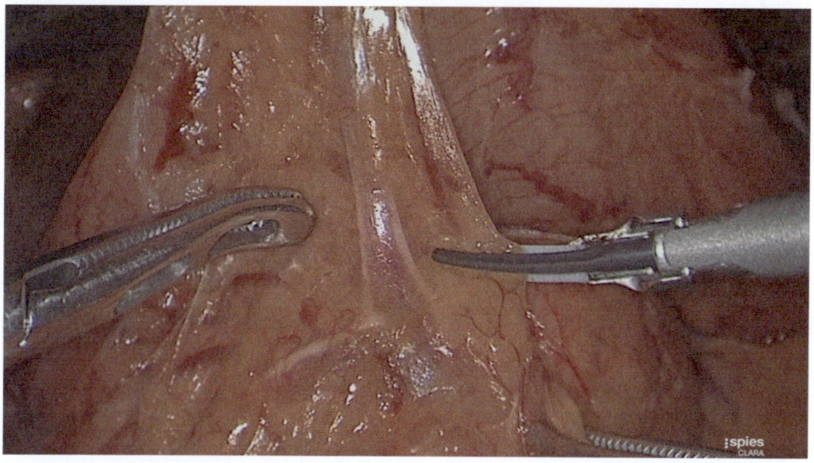

Fig. 2.108 Insufficient exposure of the RGEV

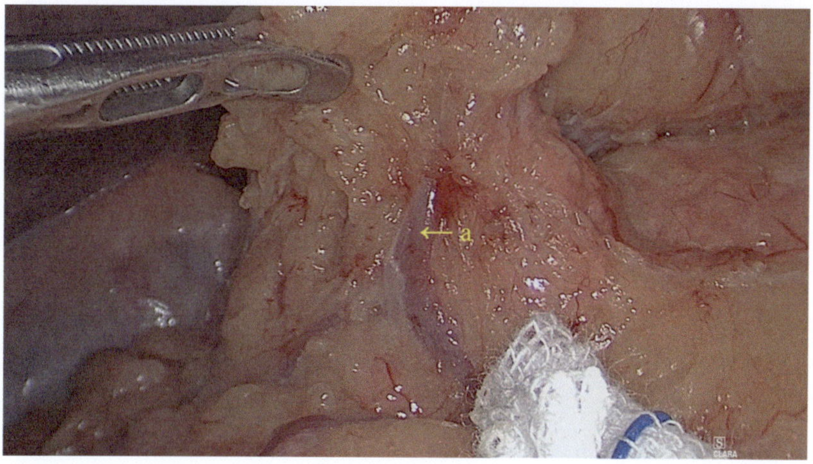

Fig. 2.109 Sufficient exposure of the RGEV (**a**)

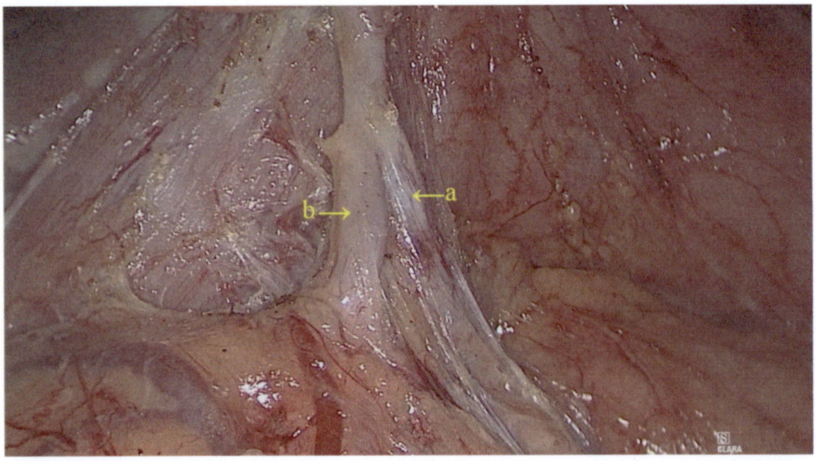

Fig. 2.110 The GDA (**a**) and the SPDA (**b**) may be mistakenly severed because of improper traction

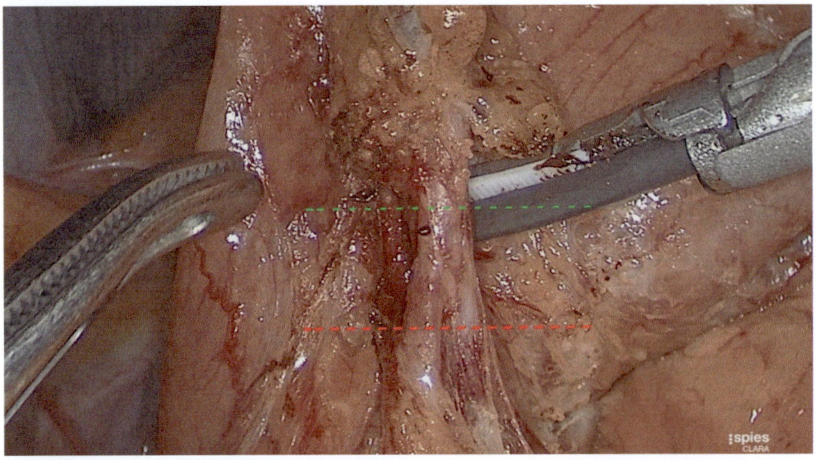

Fig. 2.111 The green line indicates the RGEA's severing plane

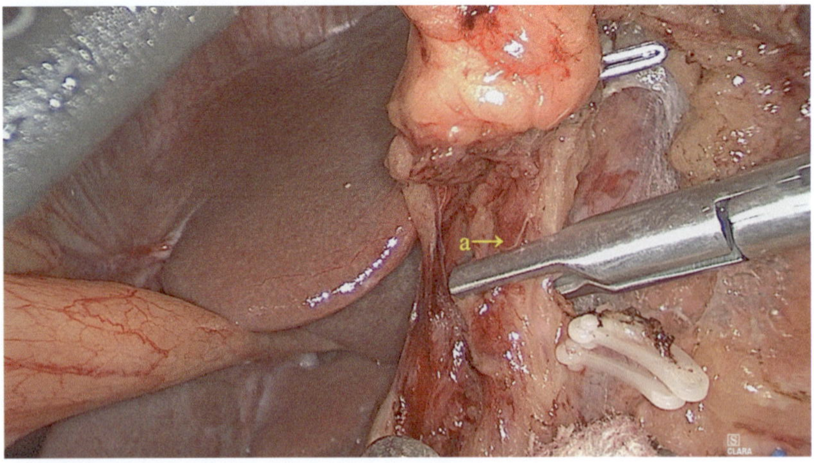

Fig. 2.112 Ligation of the IPA (**a**)

Reference

1. Huang C-M, Zheng C-H, editors. Laparoscopic gastrectomy for gastric cancer: Springer; 2015.

3 Laparoscopic Suprapancreatic Area LN Dissection for Gastric Cancer

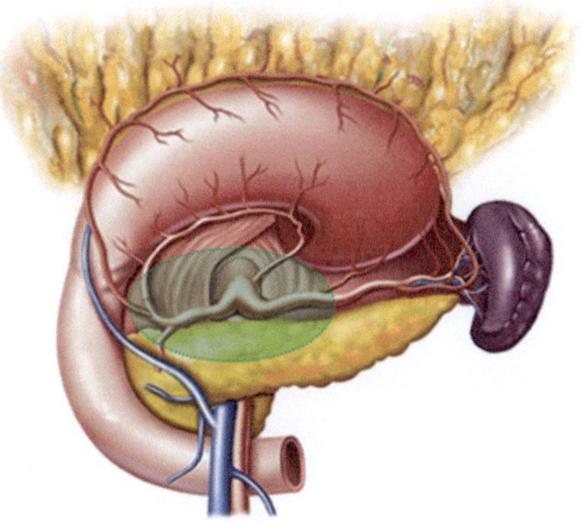

Fig. 3.1 Suprapancreatic area (Reproduced with permission from [1])

3.1 Operative Steps for LN Dissection in the Suprapancreatic Area

SpA: Splenic artery.

LNs requiring dissection in the suprapancreatic area include group No. 5, 7, 8a, 9, 11p, and 12a. When LN dissection is performed in this area, we do not first transect the duodenum. Instead, we use the HGL to keep back the left lateral liver, and dissect the vessels and fatty lymphatic tissue from behind the stomach. This enables the LNs to be completely removed (Fig. 3.2). Simulataneously, we dissect the LNs from the left to the right side: No. 11p → No. 9 → No. 7 → No. 8a → No. 5 → No. 12a. The first LN dissection also facilitates the next one.

3.1.1 Dissection of No. 7, 8a, 9, and 11p LNs

3.1.1.1 Operative Procedures

SpA: Splenic artery.

CHA: Common hepatic artery; GDA: Gastroduodenal artery; LGA: Left gastric artery; SpA: Splenic artery.

RGA: Right gastric artery; CHA: Common hepatic artery; LGA: Left gastric artery; CV: Coronary vein; SpA: Splenic artery.

Dissection is approached from the left side mainly because the initial segment of the SpA (Fig. 3.3) has low anatomic variation (Fig. 3.4) and is the closest artery to the suprapancreatic area. It is also easy to expose after peeling away the pancreatic capsule (Fig. 3.5).

C.-M. Huang et al., *Atlas of Laparoscopic Gastrectomy for Gastric Cancer*,
https://doi.org/10.1007/978-981-13-2862-6_3

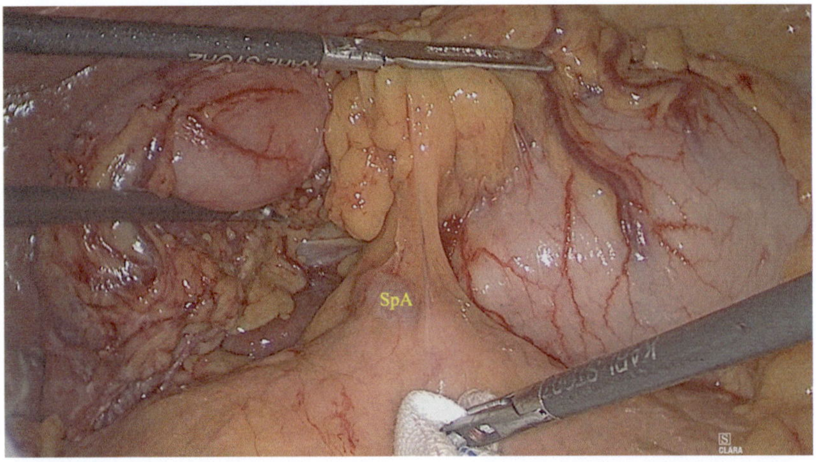

Fig. 3.2 Dissecting LNs from behind the stomach using the hepatogastric ligament (HGL) to keep back the left lateral liver

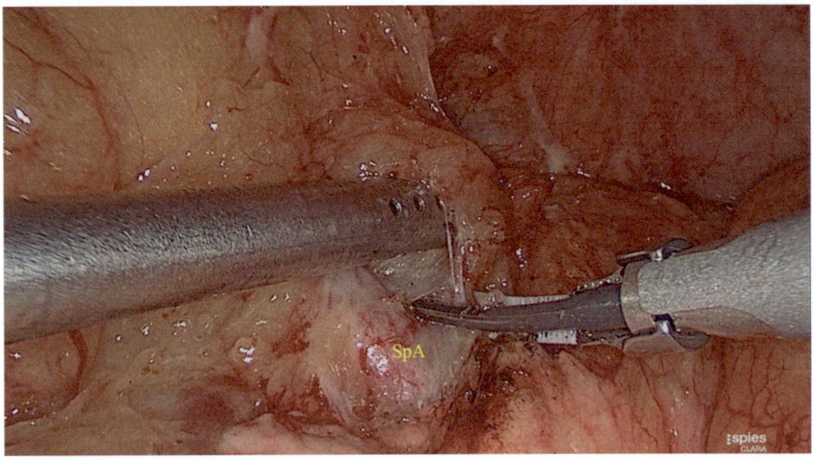

Fig. 3.3 The starting point of the left approach to dissection

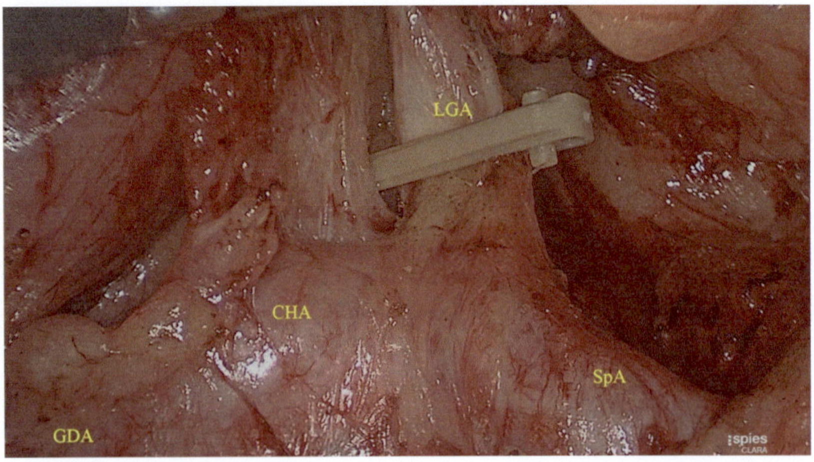

Fig. 3.4 The location of the initial SpA segment is constant with low anatomic variation

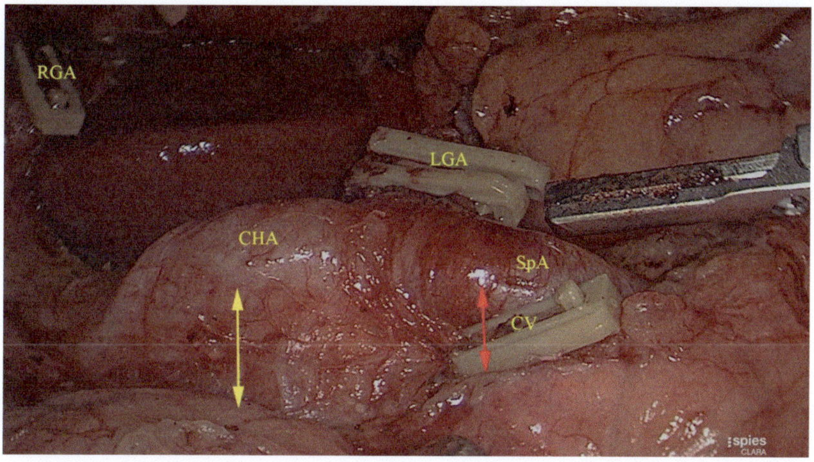

Fig. 3.5 The initial SpA segment is the closest artery to the suprapancreatic area and is easy to expose

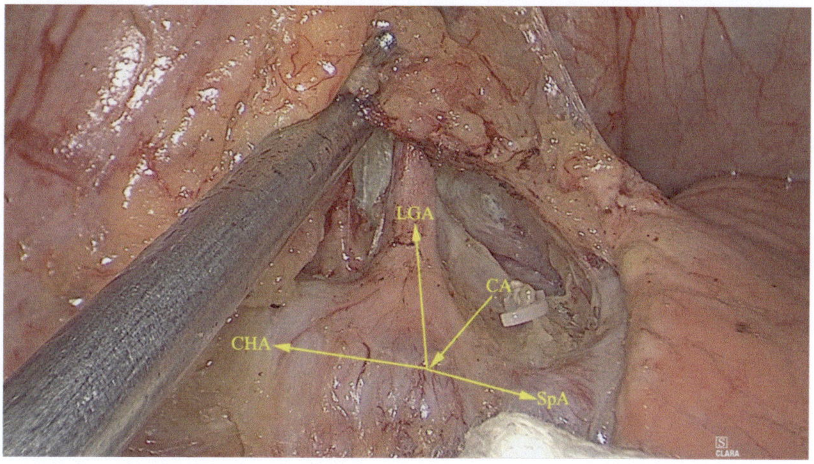

Fig. 3.6 Further exposing the CA, LGA, and CHA on the right side of the SpA

CHA: Common hepatic artery; LGA: Left gastric artery; SpA: Splenic artery; CA: Celiac artery.

LGA: Left gastric artery; CV: Coronary vein; SpA: Splenic artery.

We use the initial segment of the SpA as an anatomic marker to further expose the CA, the LGA, and the CHA to the right (Fig. 3.6). This approach provides a large space for surgery, and because the area is almost avascular it is associated with a low risk of bleeding (Fig. 3.7).

3.1.1.2 Exposure Methods

The assistant places the amputated omentum on the left upper abdomen between the anterior wall of the stomach and the lower margin of the left liver, and flips the great curvature of the gastric body to the cephalic side. The assistant's left hand then lifts up the GPF by clamping the junction of its upper and middle segments (Fig. 3.8). The right hand pulls out the posterior wall of the duodenal bulb. The surgeon then gently presses down the body of the pancreas on the uppermost point with a small gauze.

3.1.1.3 Operative Procedures

SpA: Splenic artery.

Close to the surface of the pancreas, the ultrasonic scalpel carefully peels the pancreatic capsule up to the superior border of the pancreas, and the GPF is opened to enter the RPS. The HPF is opened to the right (Fig. 3.9). The assistant then lifts the separated pancreatic capsule on the left side of the GPF with the aid of the right hand,

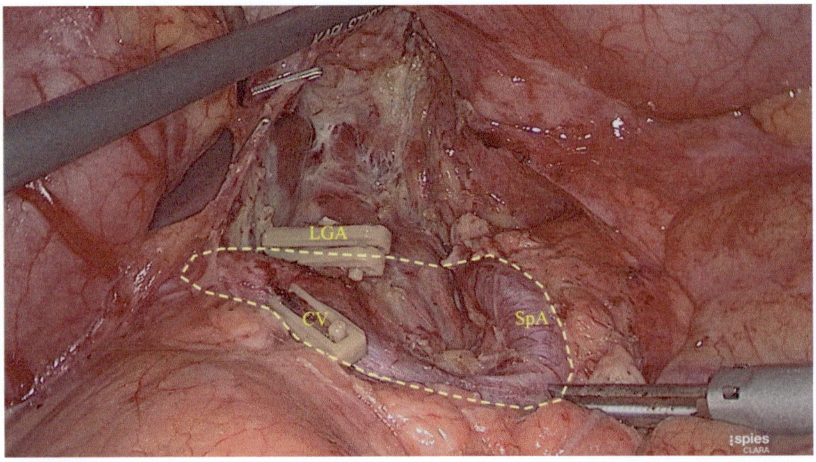

Fig. 3.7 This area is almost avascular, resulting in a low risk of bleeding

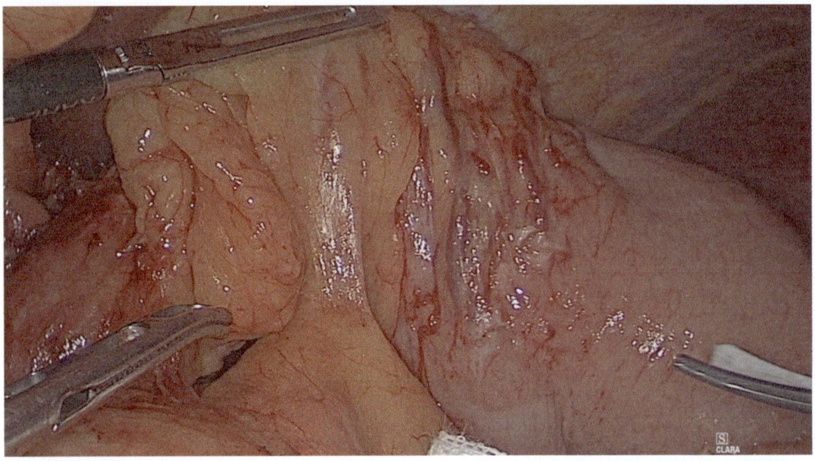

Fig. 3.8 The assistant's left hand lifts up the gastropancreatic fold (GPF) by clamping the junction of its upper and middle segment

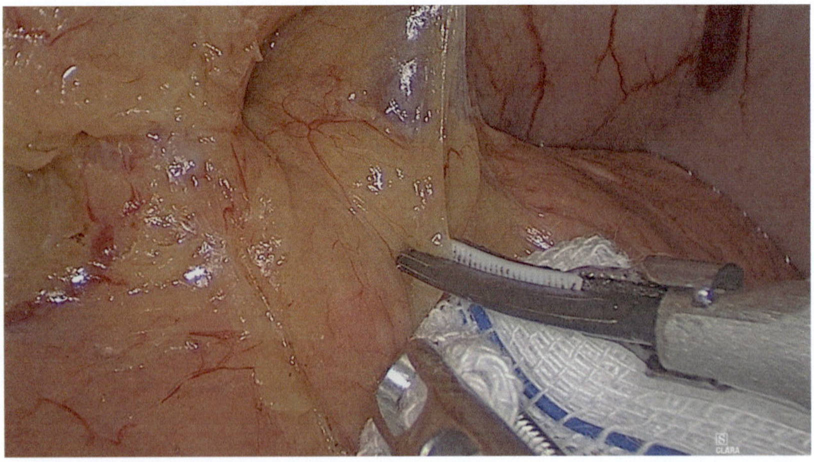

Fig. 3.9 Separation from the left side of the GPF into the retropancreatic space (RPS)

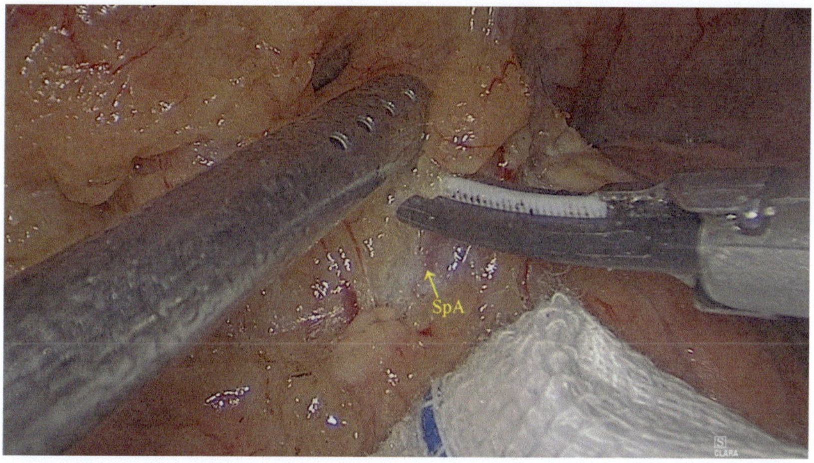

Fig. 3.10 Separating and exposing the initial segment of the SpA from the left side of the GPF

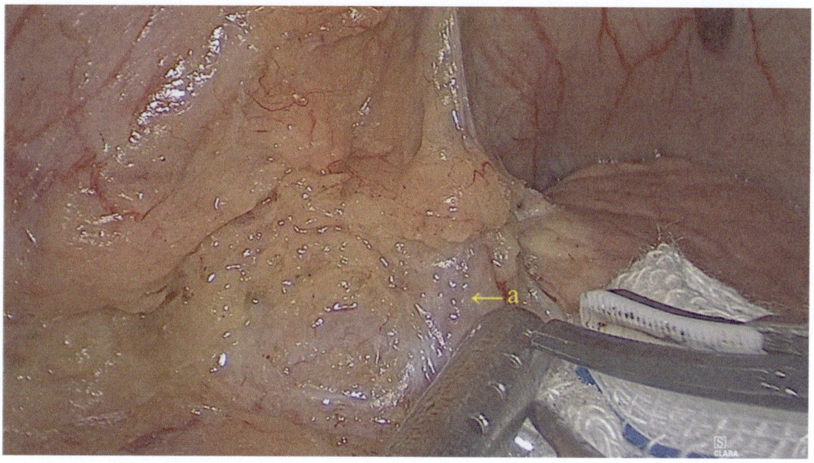

Fig. 3.11 Exposing the initial segment of the SpA (**a**)

and the ultrasound scalpel further separates the initial segment of the SpA (Figs. 3.10 and 3.11).

The assistant then lifts the isolated fatty lymphatic tissue away from the surface of the SpA. The surgeon uses the non-functional surface of the ultrasound scalpel to dissect this lymphatic tissue along the anatomical space of the SpA, exposing the origin of the CHA (Fig. 3.12).

CV: Coronary vein.

CV: Coronary vein.

CHA: Common hepatic artery.

The ultrasound scalpel dissects the CV from the origin of the CHA along the surface of the right margin of the CA (Fig. 3.13). The fatty lymphoid tissue around the CHA is dissected at the upper margin of the CHA, and the CV is vascularized and separated at its root between the clips (Figs. 3.14 and 3.15).

CHA: Common hepatic artery; CV: Coronary vein.

After determining the course of the SpA along the superior border of the pancreatic body, the assistant's right hand continues to pull up the fatty lymphatic tissue on the surface of the SpA. The surgeon uses the ultrasonic scalpel to meticulously dissect the lymphatic tissue along the SpA until the origin of the posterior gastric artery (PGA) is reached (Fig. 3.16). Then the fatty

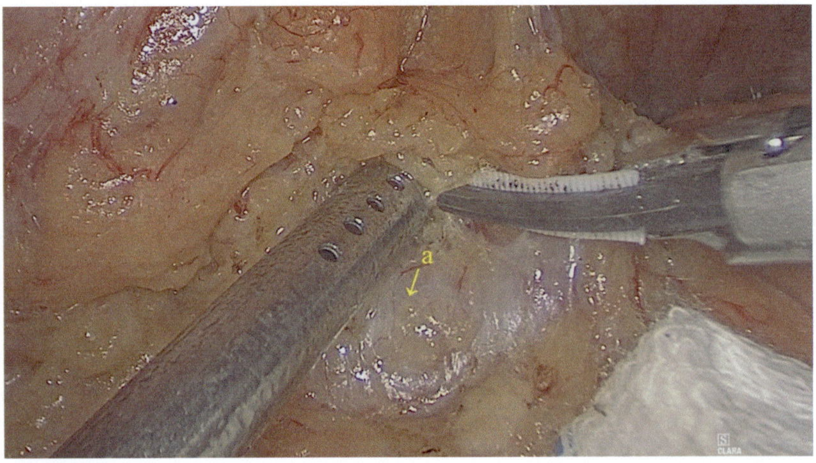

Fig. 3.12 Separating and exposing the origin of the CHA from the initial segment of the SpA (**a**)

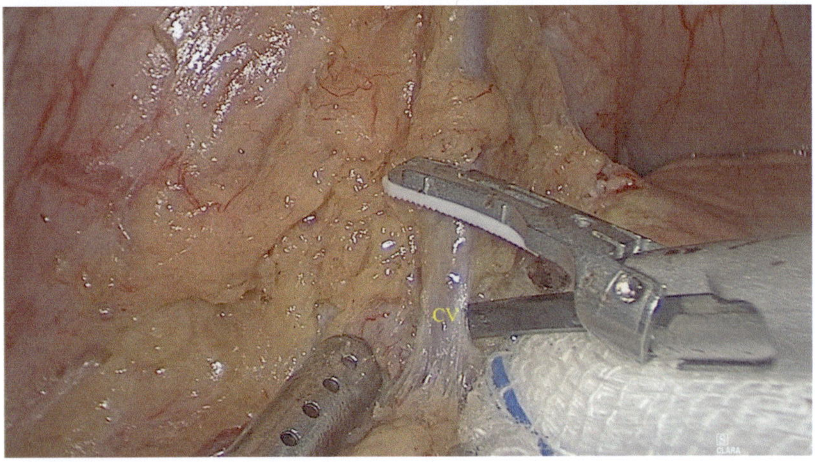

Fig. 3.13 Exposure of the CV

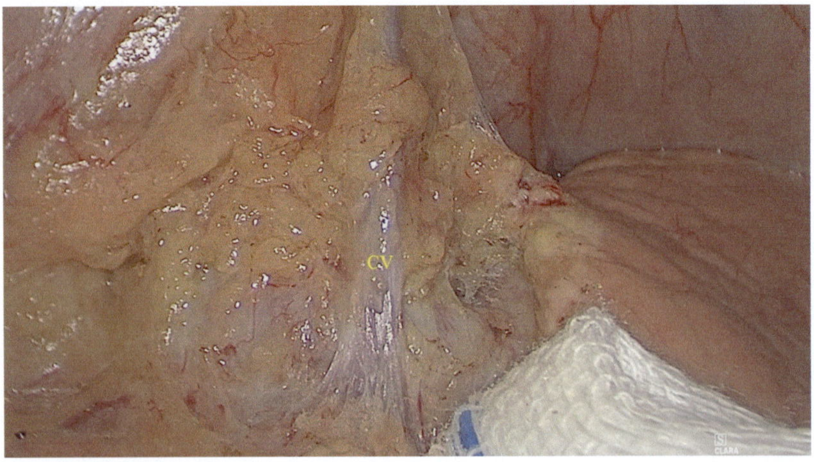

Fig. 3.14 CV

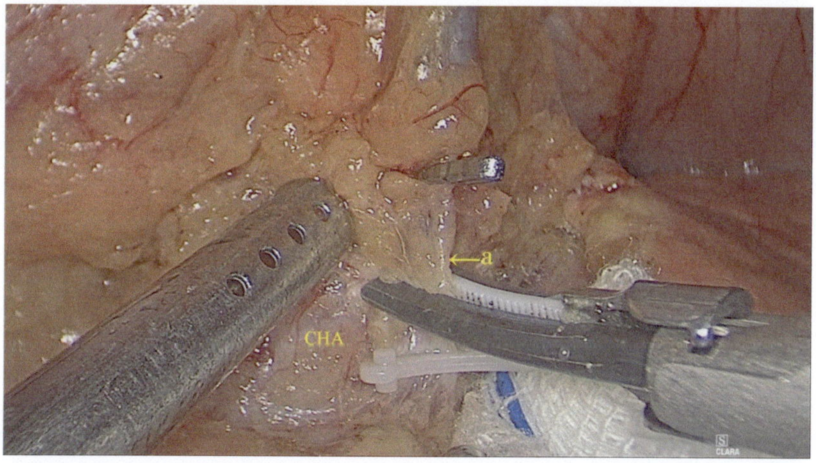

Fig. 3.15 Mutilation of the CA on the upper border of the CHA (**a**)

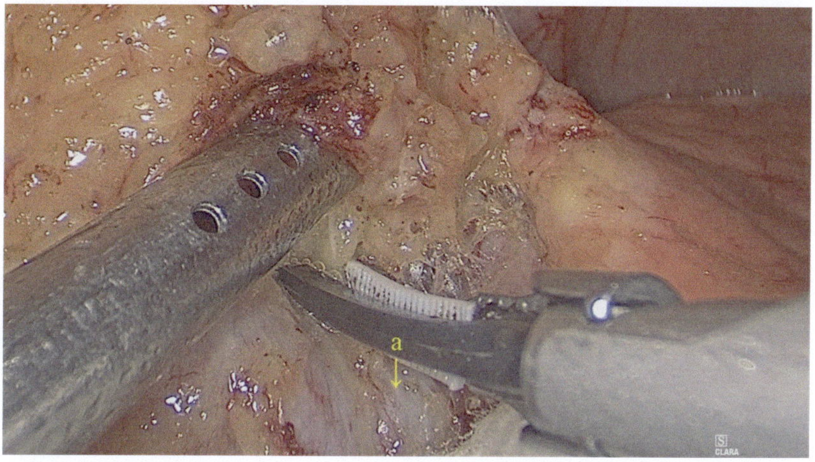

Fig. 3.16 No. 11p LN dissection is along the superior border of the pancreas on the surface of the SpA (**a**)

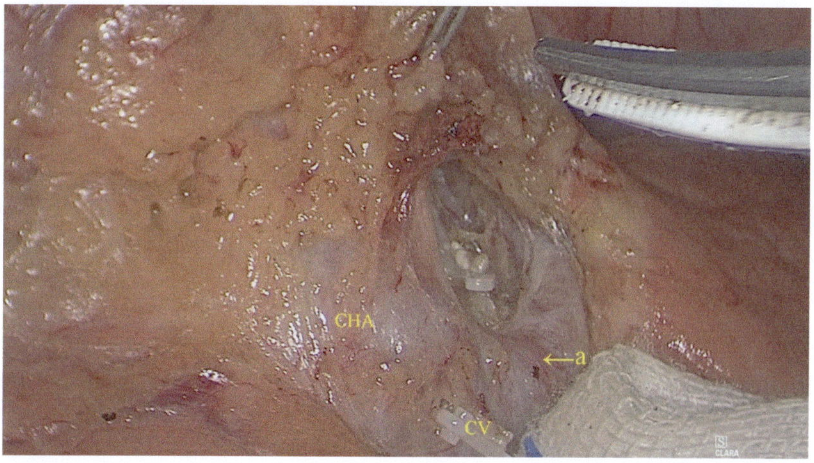

Fig. 3.17 No. 11p LN dissection and exposing the proximal end of the SpA (**a**)

lymphatic tissue around the proximal end of the SpA is removed and the No. 11p LN is dissected (Fig. 3.17).

LGA: Left gastric artery.

The dissection of No. 9 LNs starts from the origin of the SpA. The assistant lifts the isolated fatty lymphatic tissue on the left side of the GPF with their right hand. The ultrasound scalpel

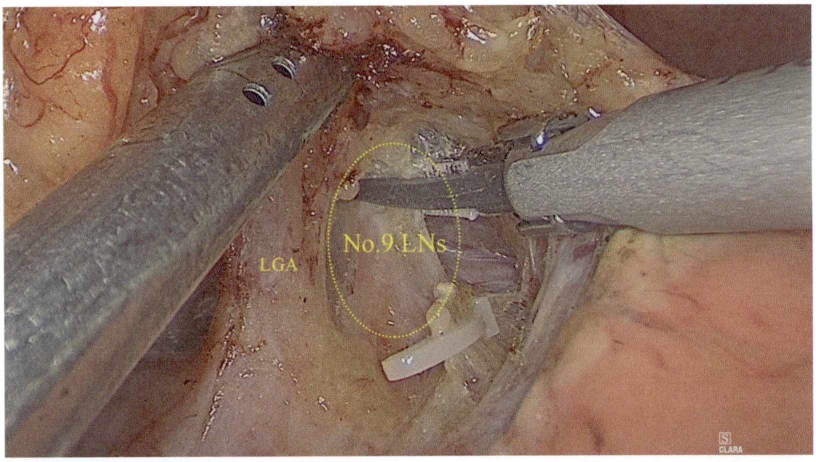

Fig. 3.18 Dissection of the No. 9 LNs is along the left margin of the CA

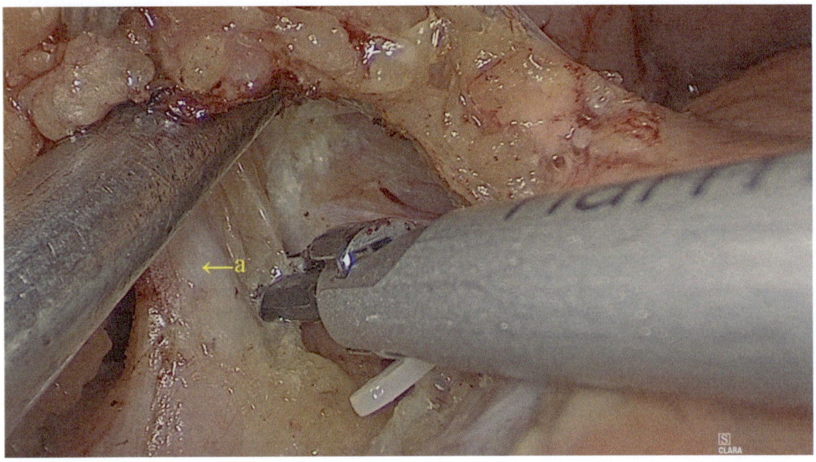

Fig. 3.19 Exposing left margin of the root of the LGA (**a**)

follows the anatomic space on the surface of the left margin of the CA (Fig. 3.18), dissecting the fatty lymphatic tissue on its surface in the direction of the diaphragm. The left margin of the root of the left gastric artery is then exposed (Fig. 3.19) until the gastrophrenic ligament is opened (Fig. 3.20).

CHA: Common hepatic artery.

CHA: Common hepatic artery.

CHA: Common hepatic artery; LGA: Left gastric artery; SpA: Splenic artery.

CHA: Common hepatic Artery; LGA: Left gastric artery.

The surgeon uses the ultrasonic scalpel to separate and expose the left gastic vein (LGV) by dissecting along the anatomic space on the surface of the right margin of the CA starting from the origin of the CHA (Fig. 3.21). The soft tissues around the LGV are dissected on the superior margin of the CHA. The LGV (Fig. 3.22) is vascularized and divided at its root between the clips (Fig. 3.23) to achieve dissection of No. 7 and No. 9 LNs. Next, the assistant's right hand pulls out the posterior wall of the duodenum and the surgeon's left hand gently presses down on the pancreas with gauze to expose the general course of the CHA on the superior border of the pancreas (Fig. 3.24).

LGA: Left gastric artery.

CHA: Common hepatic artery.

The assistant's right hand pulls up the isolated fatty lymphatic tissue on the surface of the

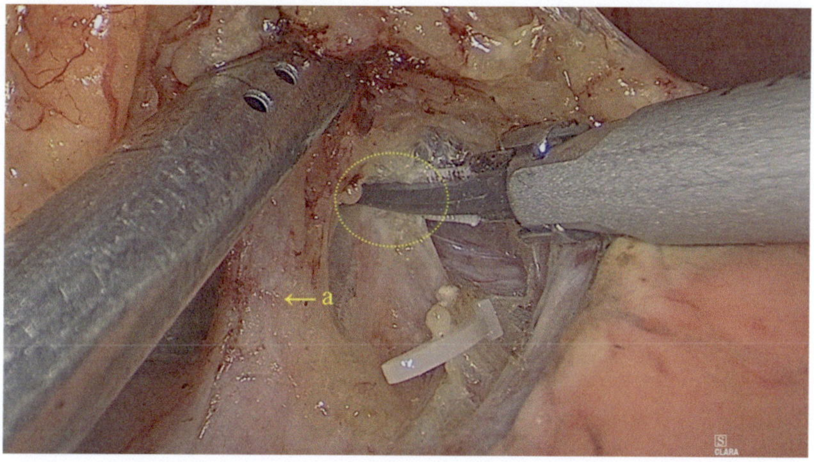

Fig. 3.20 The gastrophrenic ligament (GPL) is opened at the left margin of the LGA (**a**)

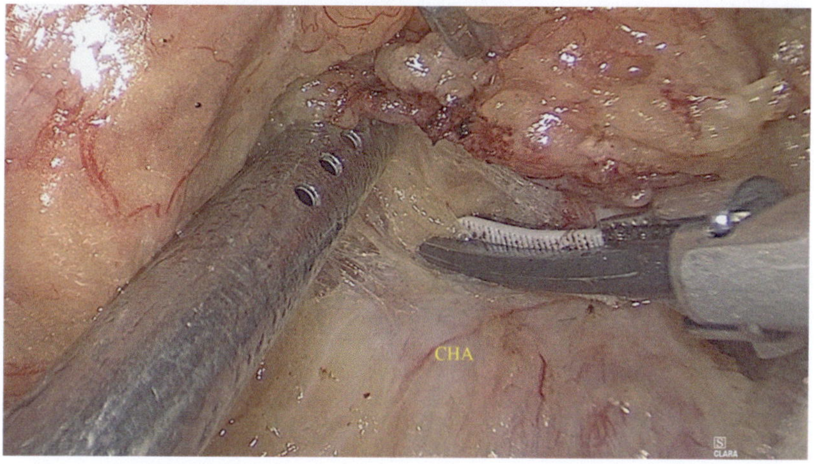

Fig. 3.21 Dissect the lymphatic fatty tissue along the right margin of the CA surface

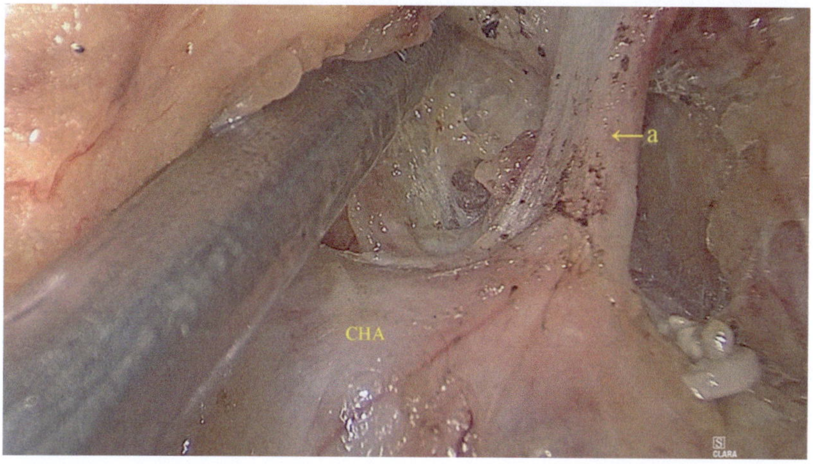

Fig. 3.22 The right margin of the LGA (**a**) is denuded

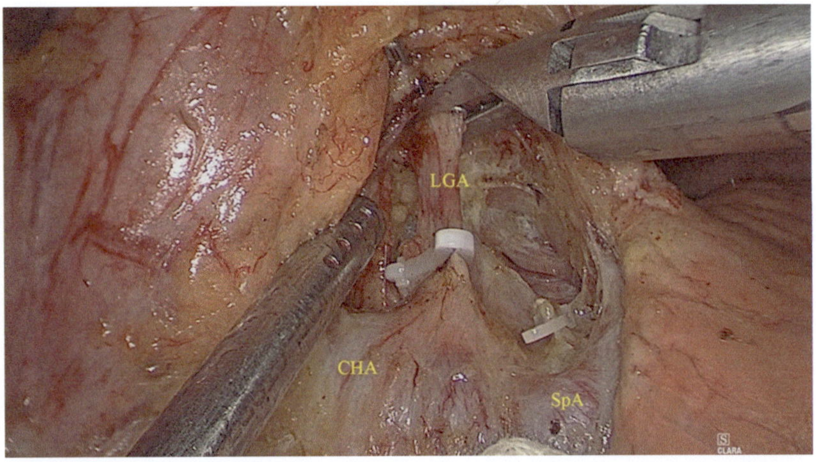

Fig. 3.23 The division of the LGA at its root

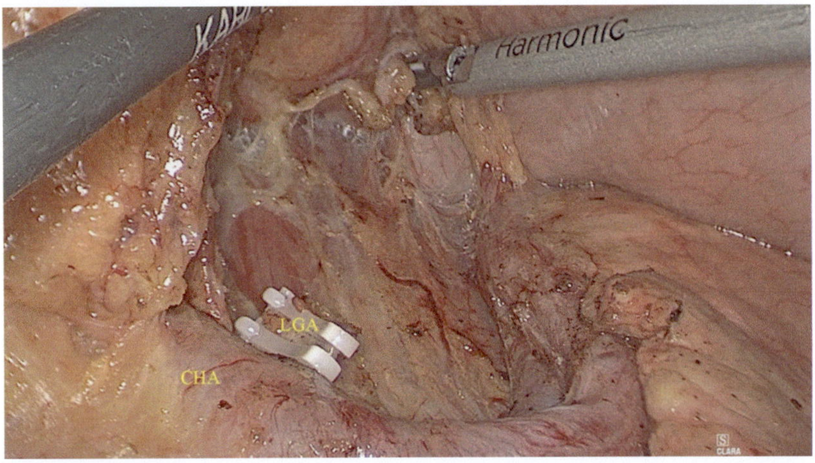

Fig. 3.24 Exposure of the CHA on the superior border of the pancreas

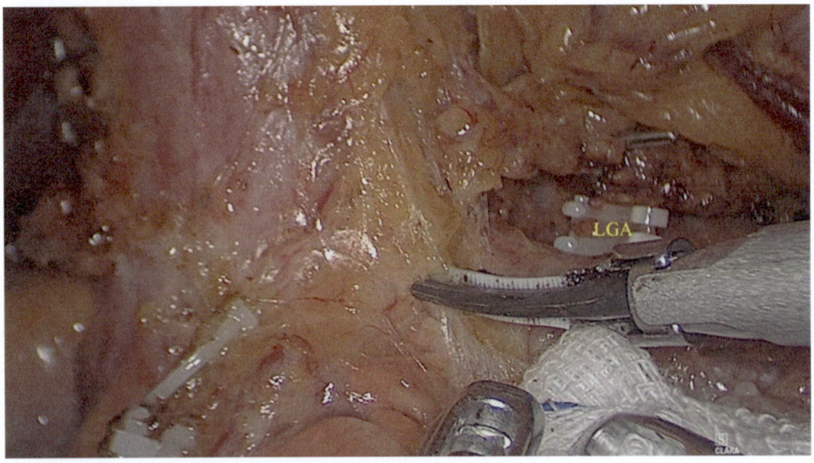

Fig. 3.25 Dissection of No. 8a LNs

CHA. The surgeon uses the ultrasonic scalpel to carefully dissect along the anatomic space on the surface of the CHA in the direction of the duodenum (Fig. 3.25) until the origin of the GDA and PHA from the CHA is reached (Fig. 3.26). The fatty lymphatic tissue in front of the CHA is completely dissected, and No. 8a LNs are completely removed.

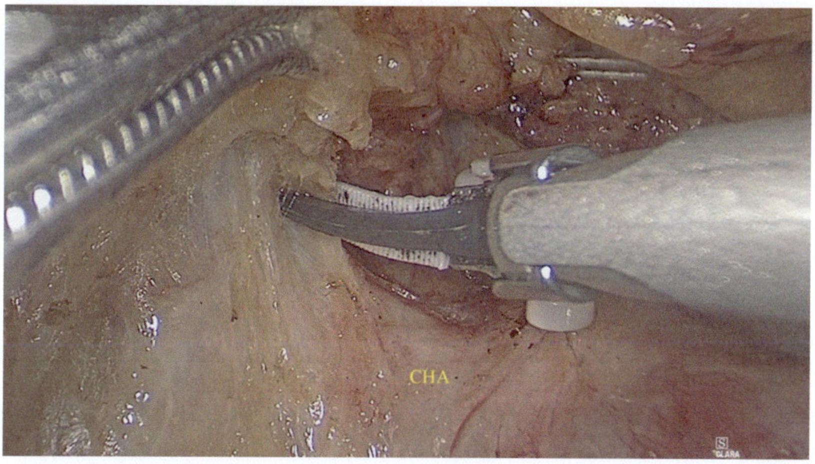

Fig. 3.26 Dissection of No. 8a LNs until furcation of the CHA

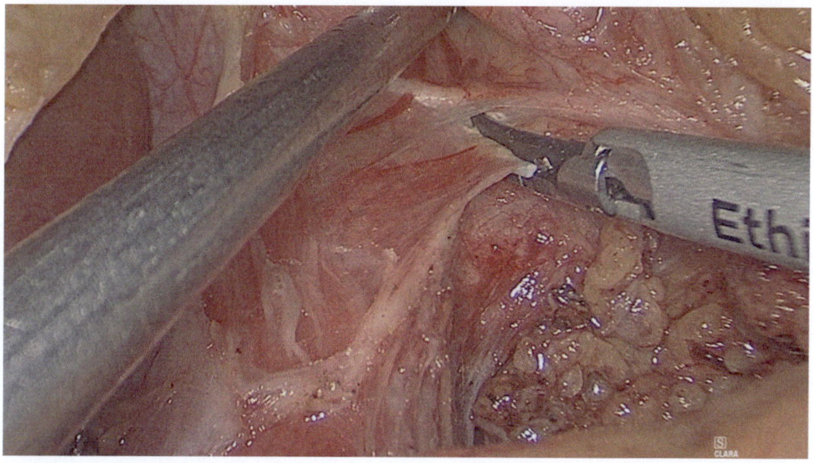

Fig. 3.27 Exposure and further separation of diaphragmatic feet and gastrophrenic ductility

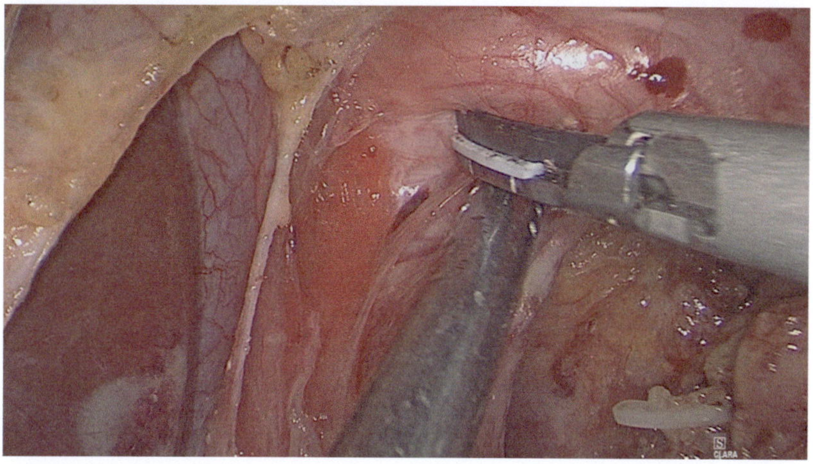

Fig. 3.28 Separation and exposure of the esophageal hiatus

The assistant's right hand gently lifts the lower edge of the left liver upwards and outwards to expose the crus of the diaphragm and the GPL (Fig. 3.27). The surgeon uses the ultrasonic scalpel along the avascular space on the surface of the left and right crura of the diaphragm to divide the GPL until the esophageal hiatus is exposed Fig. 3.28).

3.1.2 Dissection of No. 5 and No. 12a LNs

3.1.2.1 Operative Procedures

GDA: Gastroduodenal artery; PHA: Proper hepatic artery.

Dissection of No. 5 and No. 12a LNs starts from the origin of the PHA (Fig. 3.29), where the CHA divides into the GDA and the PHA. At this point, it is easy to identify and isolate the hepatic artery.

3.1.2.2 Exposure Methods

RGEV: Right gastroepiploic vessel; SpA: Splenic artery; GDA: Gastroduodenal artery.

The assistant's left hand loosens the GPF and lifts up the posterior wall of the gastric antrum, while the right hand pushes the duodenal bulb out using noninvasive grasper forceps. The surgeon gently presses down on the pancreas using a gauze pad near the fork of the CHA to keep tension on the HDL and full exposure of the suprapyloric area from the back of the stomach (Fig. 3.30).

3.1.2.3 Operation Stages

CHA: Common hepatic artery.

PHA: Proper hepatic artery; GDA: Gastroduodenal artery; RGA: Right gastric artery.

RGA: Right gastric artery.

The surgeon uses the ultrasonic scalpel along the course of the PHA, starting from the medial margin of its origin (Fig. 3.31) to open the medial

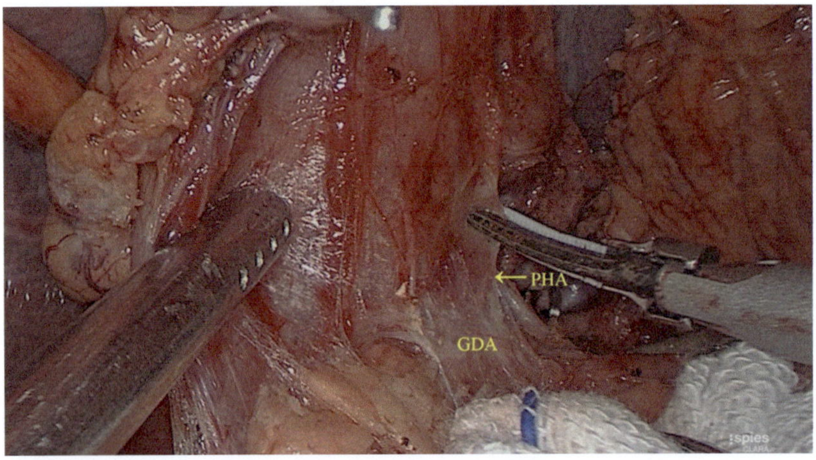

Fig. 3.29 The dissection approach starts from the origin of the PHA

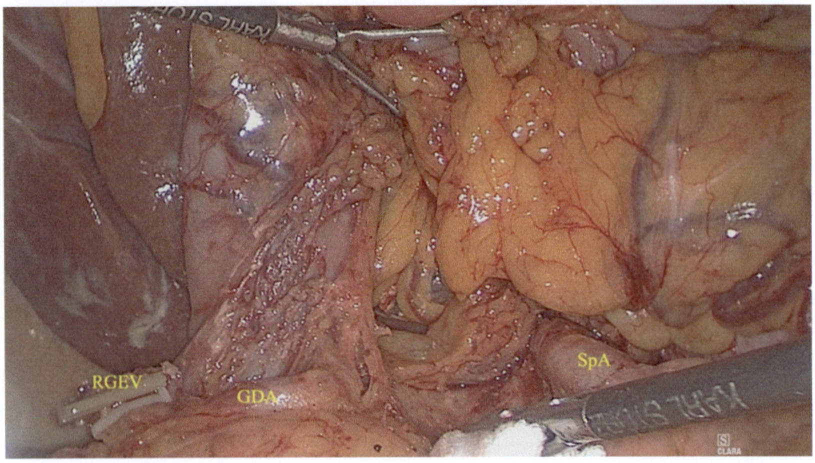

Fig. 3.30 The assistant lifts up the posterior wall of the gastric antrum, while the surgeon presses down on the pancreas to expose the suprapyloric area

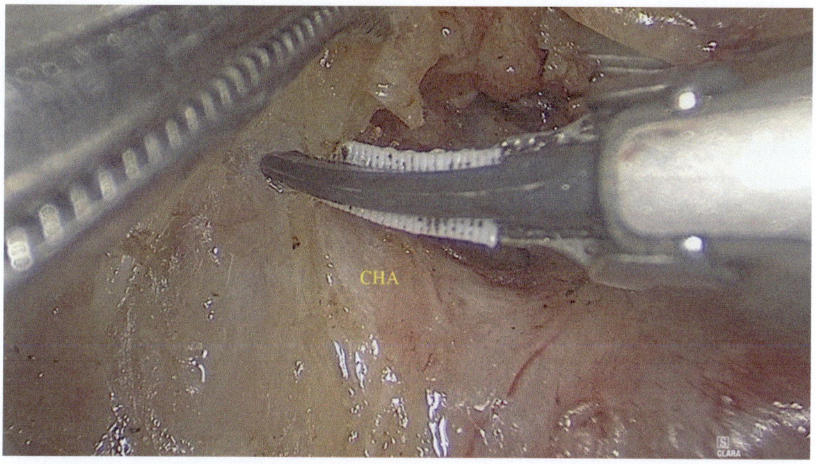

Fig. 3.31 Dissection of No. 12a LNs starts from the medial margin of the origin of the PHA

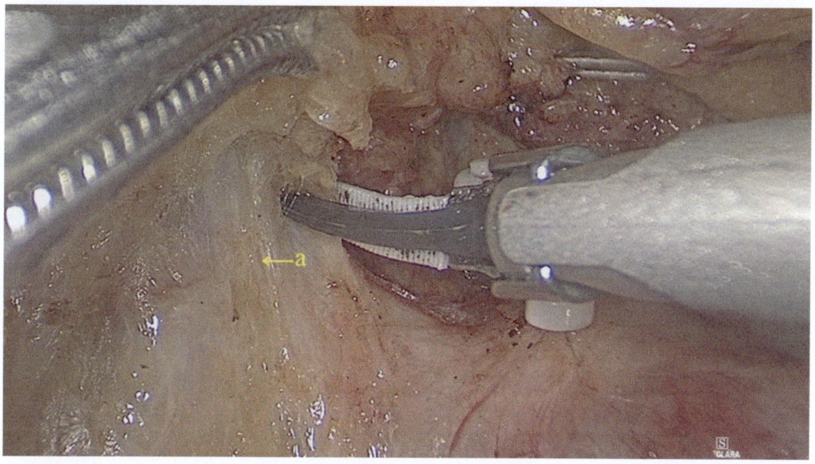

Fig. 3.32 The medial margin of the HDL is opened along the CHA (**a**)

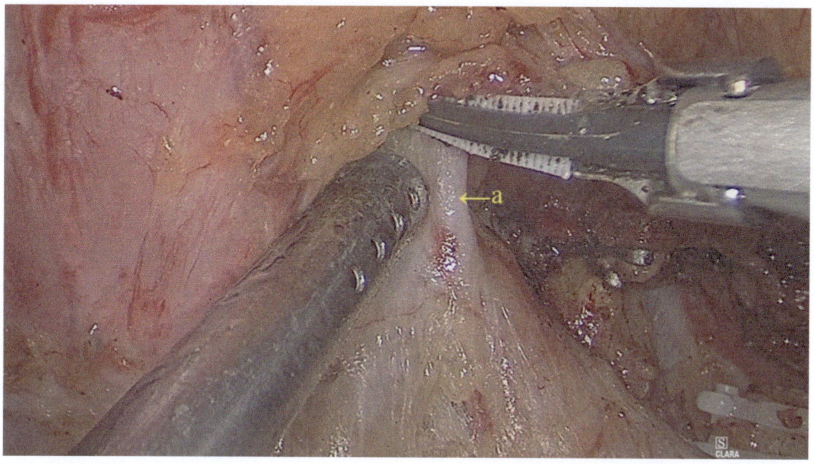

Fig. 3.33 Exposure of the root of the RGA (**a**)

margin of the HDL (Fig. 3.32). Next, the assistant's right hand pushes the duodenum up and down along its surface to help the surgeon expose the root of the RGA near the origin of the PHA (Fig. 3.33). The RGA is carefully and meticulously vascularized (Fig. 3.34), then divided at its root between the clips (Fig. 3.35) to allow complete removal of No. 5 LNs.

Fig. 3.34 The root of the RGA is vascularized

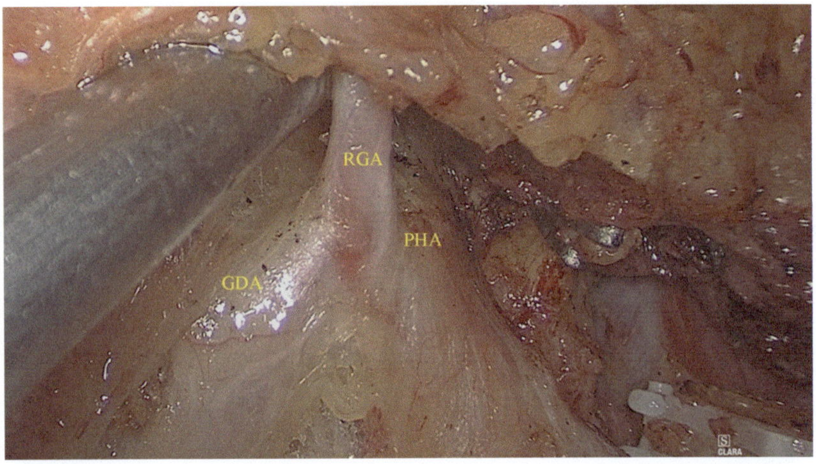

Fig. 3.35 The RGA is divided at its root

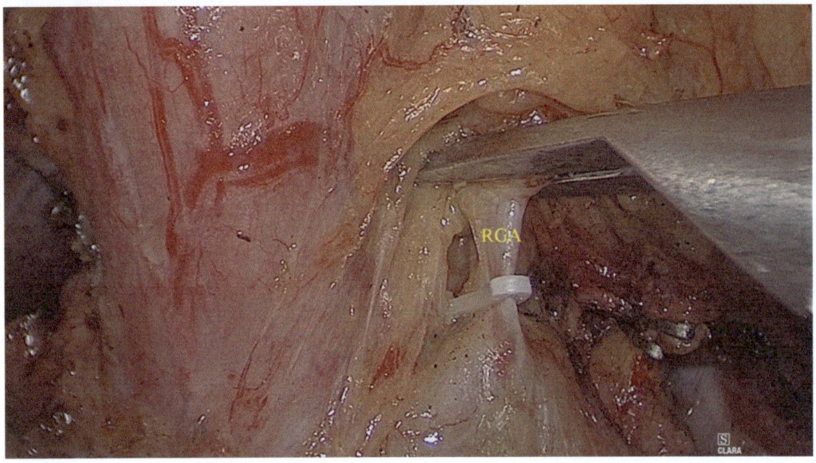

PHA: Proper hepatic artery.

PHA: Proper hepatic artery.

GDA: Gastroduodenal artery; RGA: Right gastric artery; PHA: Proper hepatic artery; CHA: Common hepatic artery; LGA: Left gastric artery.

SpA: Splenic artery; LGA: Left gastric artery; PHA: Proper hepatic artery; GDA: Gastroduodenal artery; RGA: Right gastric artery; CV: Coronary vein; CHA; Common hepatic artery.

The assistant's right non-invasive grasping forceps gently lift up the fatty lymphoid tissue on the surface of the PHA. The ultrasonic scalpel carefully dissects this tissue along the anatomical space on the vessel's surface towards the hepatic hilum until reaching the origin of the left and right hepatic arteries. The soft tissues in front of the PHA and root of the RGA are dissected and removed en bloc (Fig. 3.36), then excision of No. 12 LNs is completed. At this point, the assistant's right hand continues to protrude the upper-lateral anterior lobe of the HDL (Fig. 3.37), and the ultrasonic scalpel separates the anterior lobe of the ligament to the right. A window is opened on the right side of the anterior lobe of the HDL (Fig. 3.38), which provides an accurate entry point for the next step of amputating the hepato-gastric ligament from the front of the stomach. Further nudity of the duodenum can be made to determine if it should be cut off from the site according to the opinion of the operator (Figs. 3.39 and 3.40). This completes dissection of LNs in the suprapancreatic area (Figs. 3.41 and 3.42).

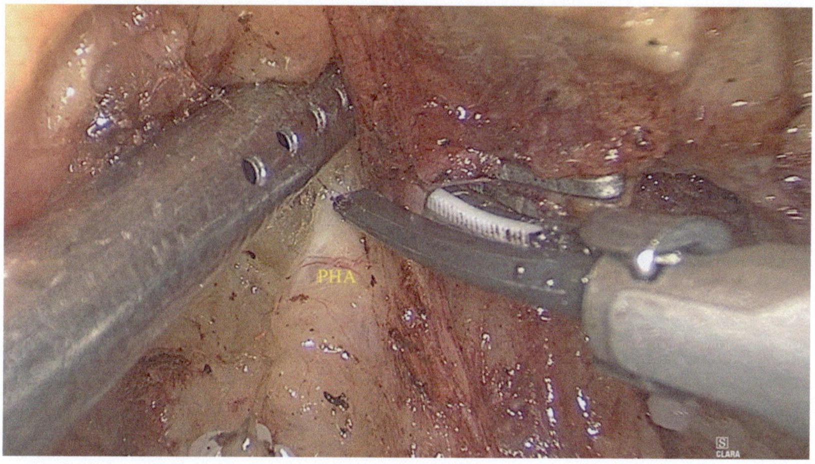

Fig. 3.36 Dissection of No. 12a LNs starts from the medial margin of the origin of the PHA

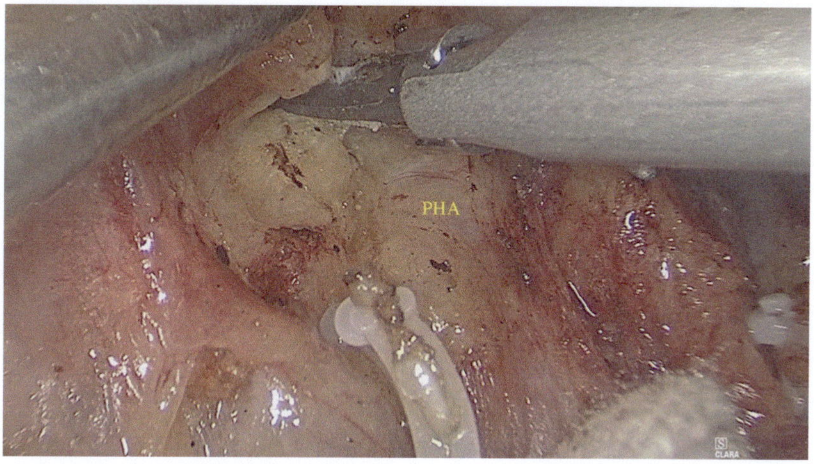

Fig. 3.37 Separation of the anterior lobe of hepatoduodenal ligament

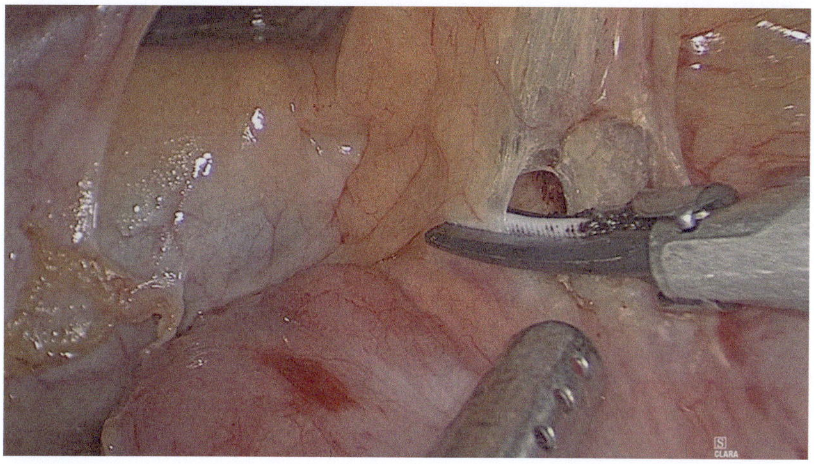

Fig. 3.38 A window opens in the lateral lobe of the HDL

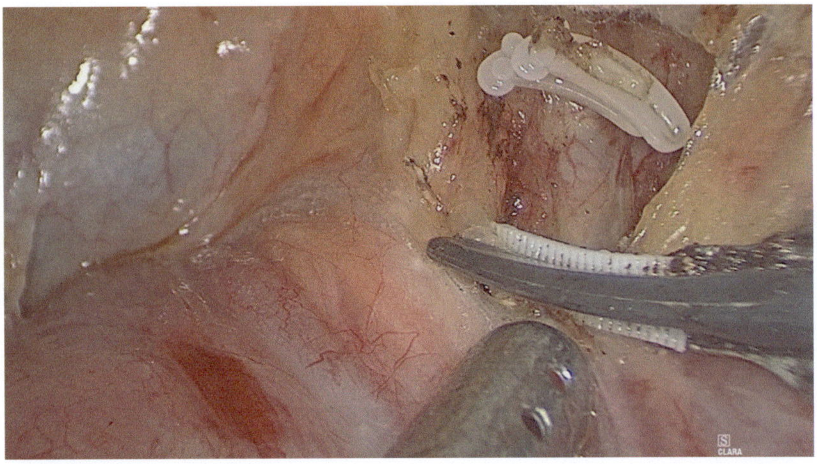

Fig. 3.39 Fully bare duodenum

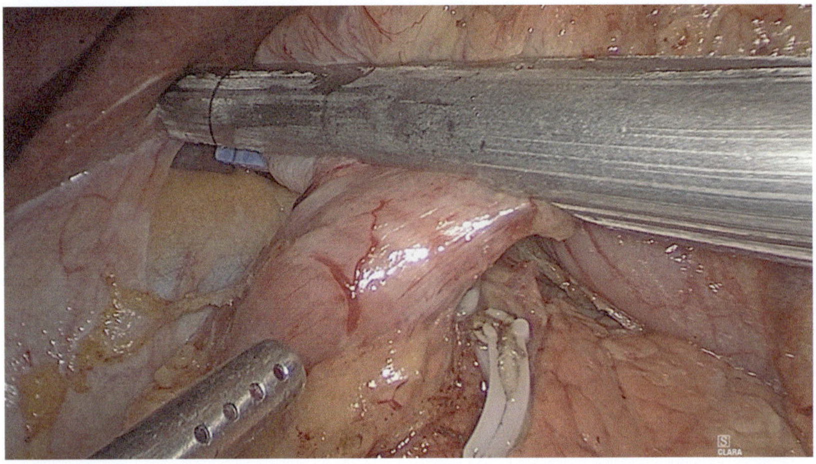

Fig. 3.40 Mutilation of the duodenum

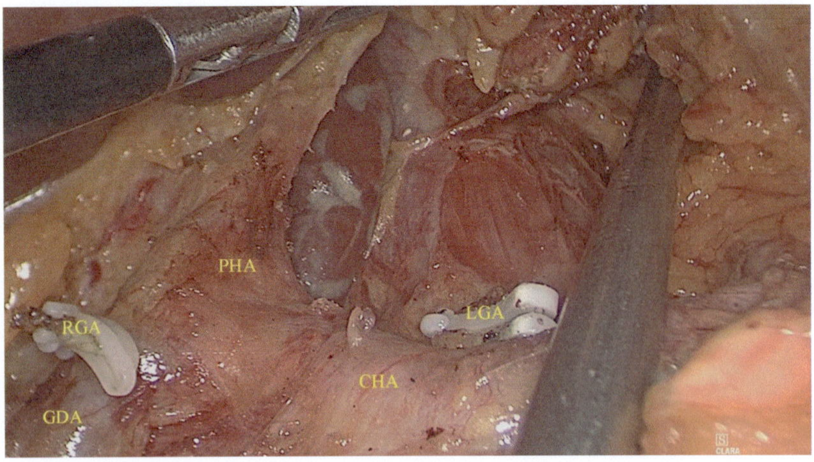

Fig. 3.41 After dissection of No. 5 and No. 12a LNs

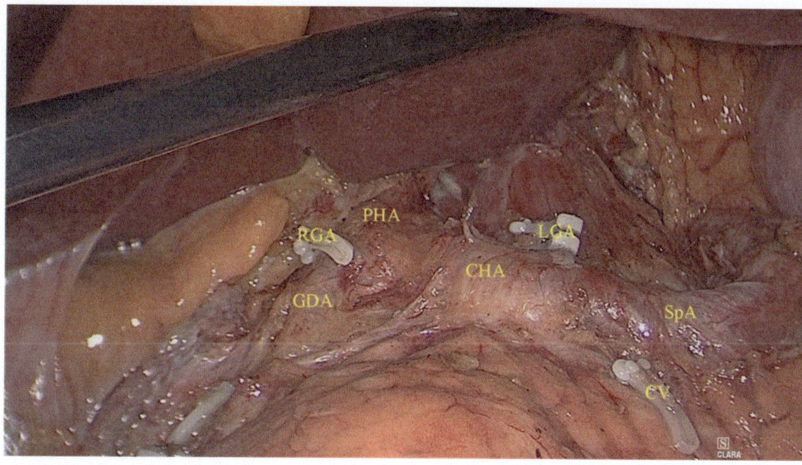

Fig. 3.42 LN dissection within the suprapancreatic area is accomplished

3.2 Operative Announcements of Laparoscopic Suprapancreatic Area LN Dissection for Gastric Cancer

3.2.1 Anatomy Associated with LN Dissection in the Suprapancreatic Area

3.2.1.1 Fascial Space Associated with LN Dissection in the Suprapancreatic Area

Anterior and Posterior Fascia of the Pancreas and its Interspace

SpA: Splenic artery.

The pancreatic fascia encompasses the pancreas, forming the anterior and posterior pancreatic fascia. A space between the anterior and posterior fascias of the pancreas (Fig. 3.43) encircles the pancreatic glands, and the vessels and branches distributed within the pancreas.

Gastropancreatic and Hepatopancreatic Folds

The section extending from the middle upper border of the pancreatic body to the posterior wall of the gastric lesser curvature is known as the gastropancreatic fold. It passes along the upper border of the pancreas and becomes continuous with the left edge of the posterior HDL to form the hepatopancreatic fold (Figs. 3.44 and 3.45).

HDL

PHA: Proper hepatic artery; LGA: Left gastric artery.

The HDL consists of two layers of peritoneum, which cover the anterior and posterior walls of the lower part of the gastric lesser curvature, the portahepatis, and the upper edge of the duodenum. A portion of the lesser omentum extends between the liver and the superior part of the duodenum (Figs. 3.46 and 3.47).

Retrogastric Space (RGS)

PHA: Proper hepatic artery.

The RGS is the space between the peritoneum of the upper margin of the pancreas and the posterior wall of the abdomen that is potentially filled with loose connective tissue. No. 9 LNs and the celiac trunk pass through this space (Fig. 3.48).

3.2.1.2 Arteries Associated with LN Dissection in the Suprapancreatic Area

CA

Also known as the celiac trunk, the CA is the first unpaired branch of the abdominal aorta. The artery of the stomach originates from the CA,

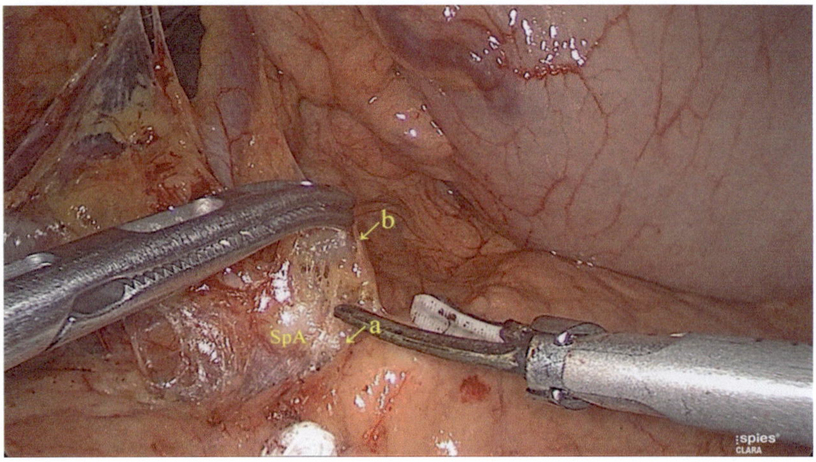

Fig. 3.43 Anterior pancreatic fascia (APF) (**a**), pancreatic anterior fascia (**b**)

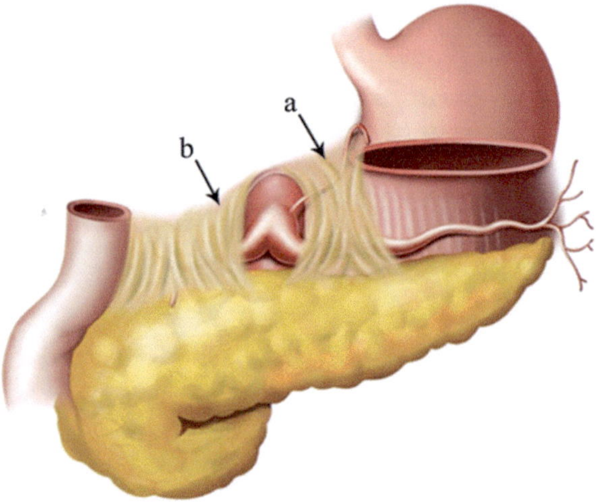

Fig. 3.44 Gastropancreatic folds (**a**), hepatopancreatic folds (**b**) (Reproduced with permission from [1])

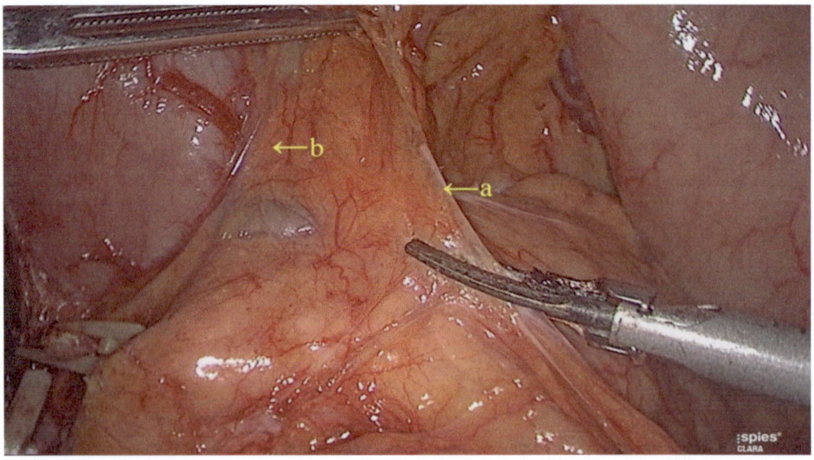

Fig. 3.45 Gastropancreatic folds (**a**), hepatopancreatic folds (**b**)

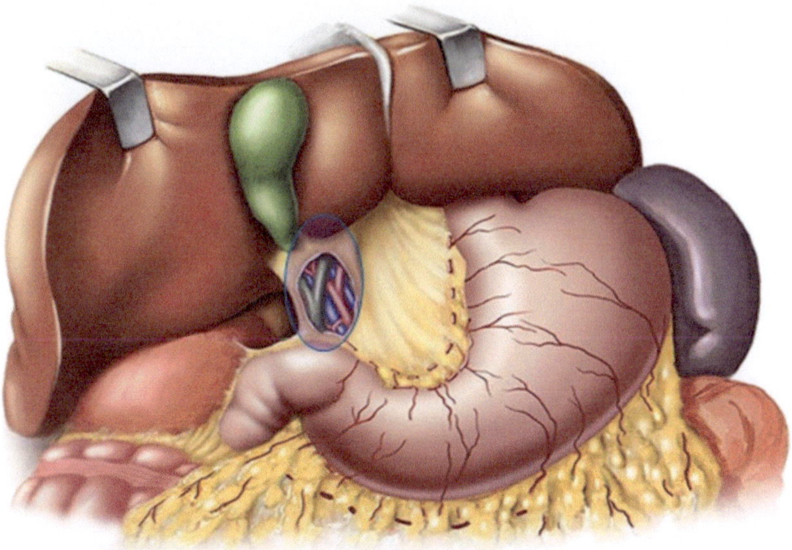

Fig. 3.46 HDL (Reproduced with permission from [1])

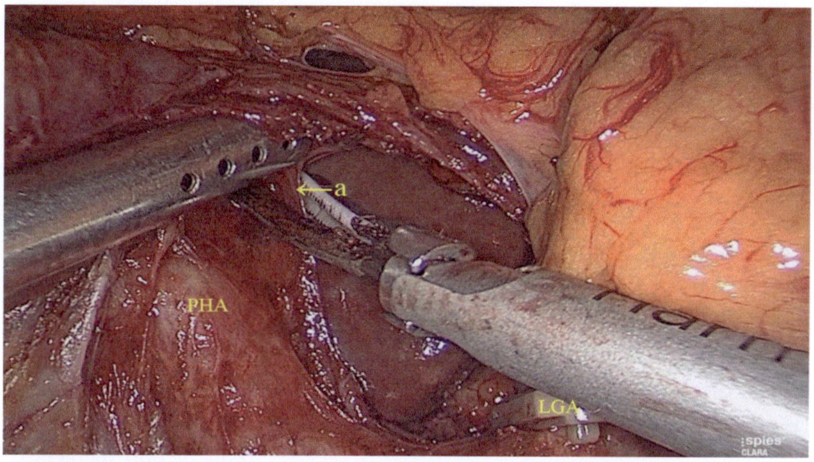

Fig. 3.47 HDL (**a**)

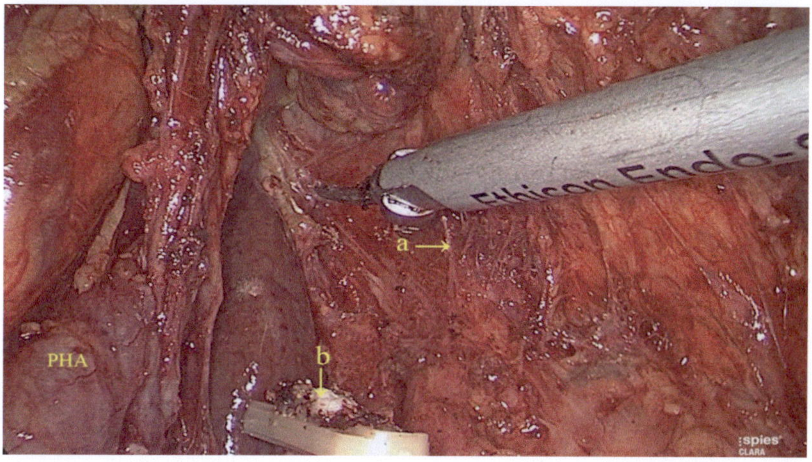

Fig. 3.48 RGS (**a**), end of the LGA (**b**)

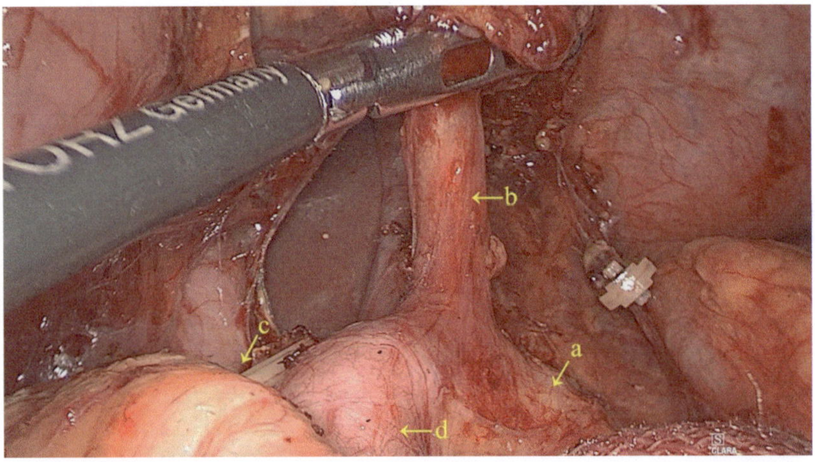

Fig. 3.49 The CA (**a**) divides into the LGA (**b**), CHA (**c**), and SpA (**d**)

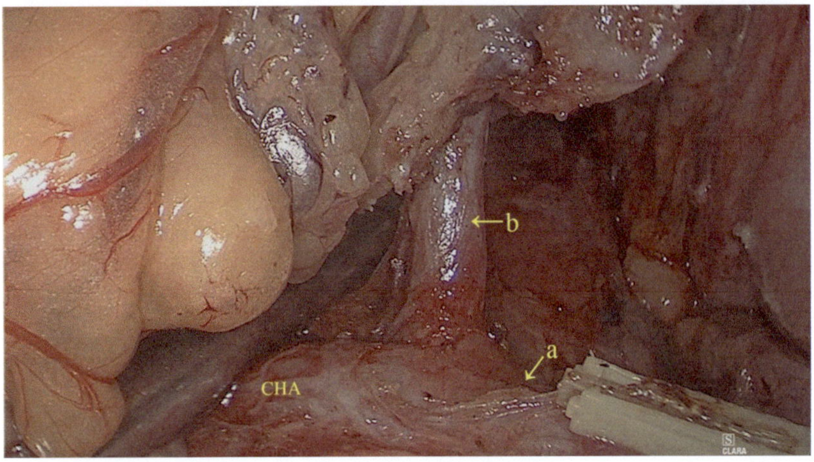

Fig. 3.50 The CA (**a**) branches off into the LGA (**b**)

which separates into the LGA, CHA, and SpA (Fig. 3.49).

LGA

CHA: Common hepatic artery.

Most of the LGA originates from the celiac trunk, with only 2.5%–7.5% separating directly from the CA (in this case, the route was not in the original position, but originated from the upper part of the celiac trunk and the posterior right side of the CA). After departing from the CA, the LGA clings to the posterior abdominal wall and runs towards the upper left side along the deep parietal peritoneum of the omental bursa to the dorsal side of the cardia. Then, it turns right and passes along the lesser curvature of the stomach between the layers of the lesser omentum to join with the RGA (Fig. 3.50).

PHA: Proper hepatic artery.

Around 1.0%–23.0% of the LHA or PHA branches off the accessory ALGA (Fig. 3.51).

The incidence of an ALHA has been reported to be 5.0%–11.5%. Of our 1173 patients who underwent radical gastrectomy for gastric cancer, 135 (11.5%) had an ALHA [2] (Fig. 3.52).

CHA

RHA: Right hepatic artery; LHA: Left hepatic artery; LGA: Left gastric artery; SpA: Splenic artery; CV: Coronary vein.

The CHA, which arises from the celiac trunk, passes to the right side and runs forwards along the upper border of the pancreatic head. It then enters the HDL and branches off to give the GDA and PHA above the duodenum (Fig. 3.53). There is little variation in the CHA, and it is occasionally absent

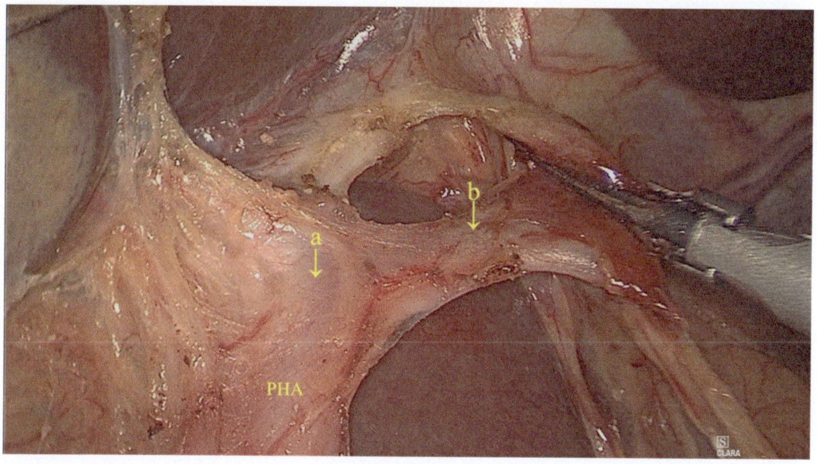

Fig. 3.51 The LHA (**a**) branches off the accessory left gastric artery (ALGA) (**b**)

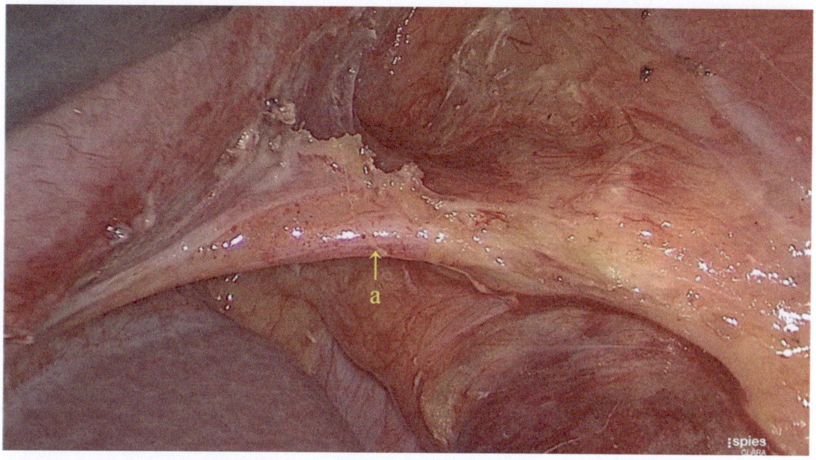

Fig. 3.52 LGA branches off the ALHA (**a**)

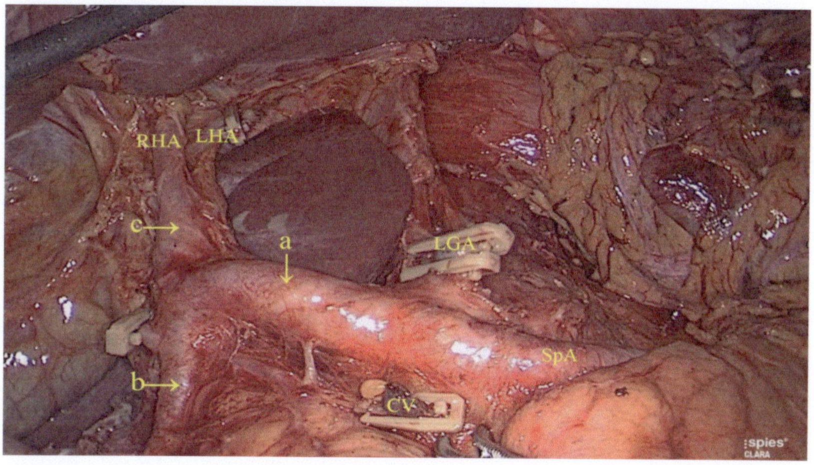

Fig. 3.53 The CHA (**a**) branches off the GDA (**b**) and the PHA (**c**)

(range, 1.4%–6.2% of cases). Based on the statistics of 2170 patients with gastric cancer, the CHA was absent in 38 cases, with an incidence of 1.8%.

GDA

RGA: Right gastric artery; PHA: Proper hepatic artery.

The GDA stems from the CHA and descends behind the first part of the duodenum. Upon reaching the lower border of the pylorus, it splits into the right gastroepiploic and anterior superior pancreaticoduodenal arteries (Fig. 3.54).

PHA

RGA: Right gastric artery; CHA: Common hepatic artery; LGA: Left gastric artery.

The PHA is a direct continuation of the CHA and is located in the upper right part of the hepatoduodenum. The PHA is separated from the CHA by bifurcation of the GDA, known as the T-shape intersection. The PHA is distal to the division, while the CHA is proximal to it (Fig. 3.55).

RGA

The RGA most frequently arises from the PHA above the first part of the duodenum. It runs upwards between the two layers of the HDL to the pylorus, then passes from right to left along the lesser curvature of the stomach, supplying both of its surfaces with branches, and joins with the LGA (Fig. 3.56).

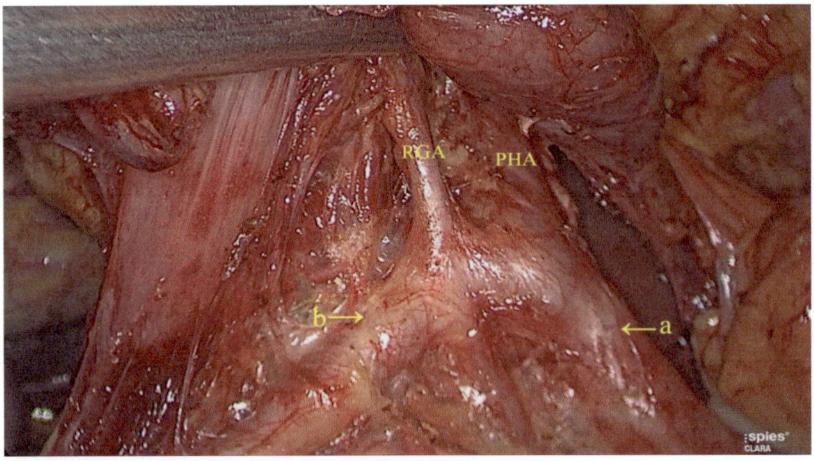

Fig. 3.54 The CHA (**a**) branches off the GDA (**b**)

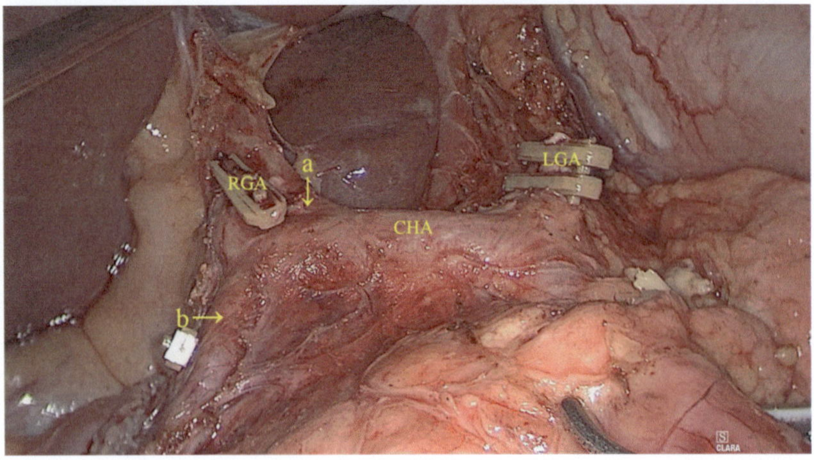

Fig. 3.55 The PHA (**a**) starts at the beginning of the GDA (**b**)

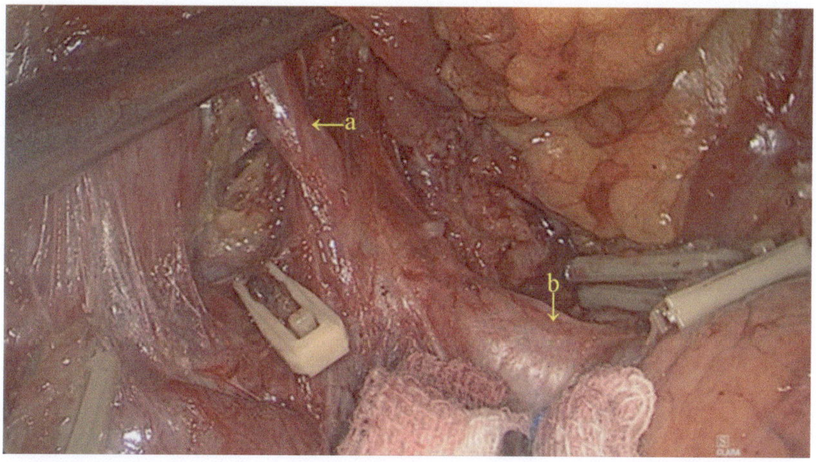

Fig. 3.56 The RGA (**a**) originating from the PHA (**b**)

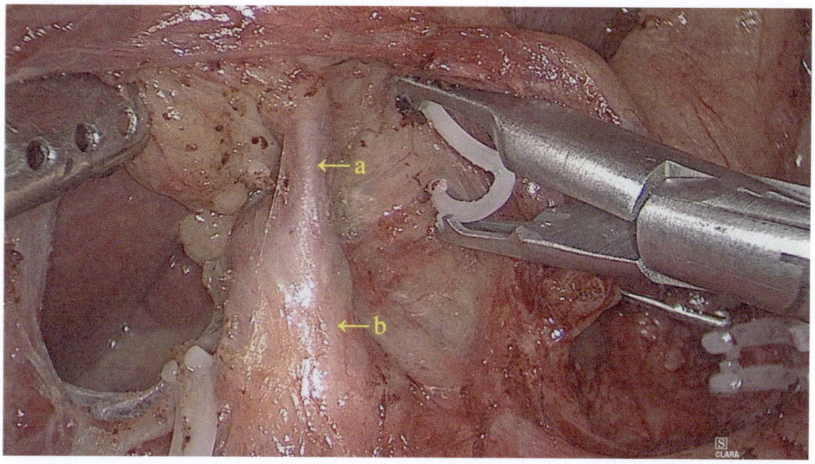

Fig. 3.57 The RGA (**a**) arising from the PHA (**b**)

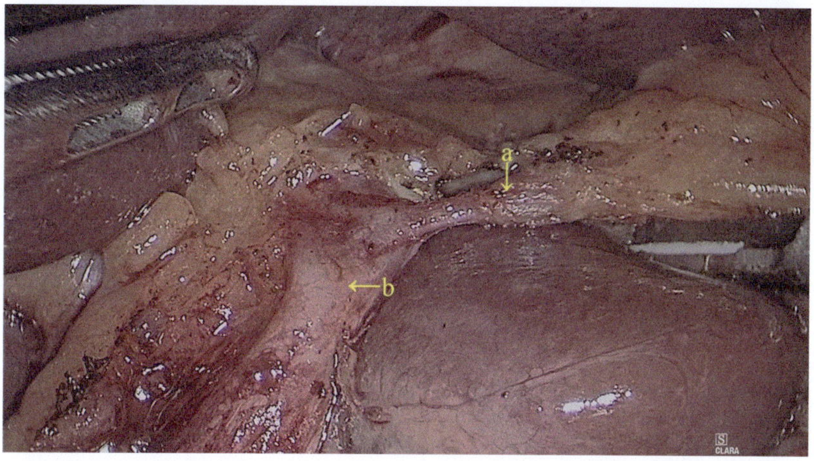

Fig. 3.58 The RGA (**a**) arising from the LHA (**b**)

The anatomic location of the RGA can often differ. According to a study of 191 cases by Adachi [3], the RGA emanated from the PHA in 93 cases (48.7%) (Fig. 3.57).

In 38 cases (19.9%), the RGA emanated from the LHA (Fig. 3.58).

CHA: Common hepatic artery; PHA: Proper hepatic artery.

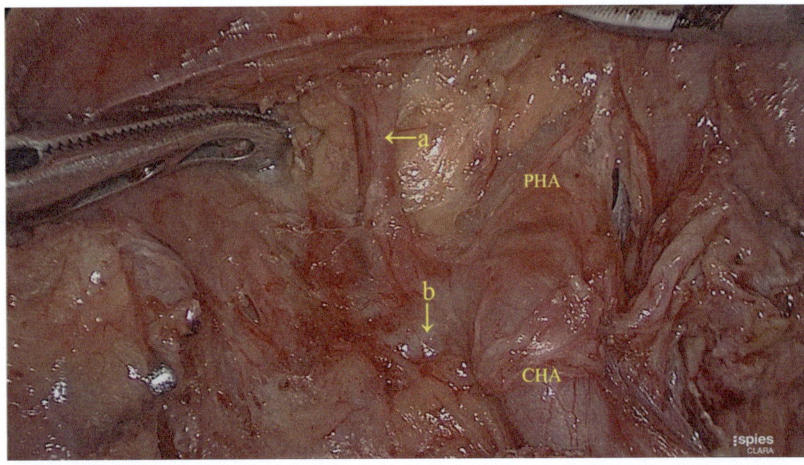

Fig. 3.59 The RGA (**a**) arising from the GDA (**b**)

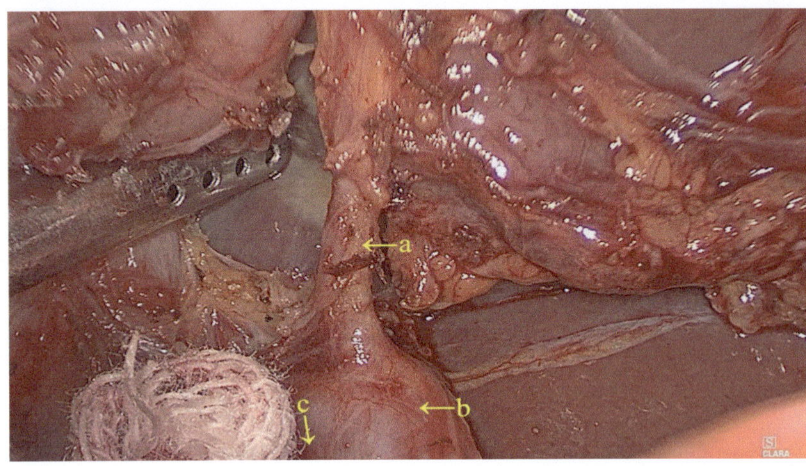

Fig. 3.60 The RGA (**a**) originating near the bifurcation of the PHA (**b**) and GDA (**c**)

In 28 cases (14.7%), the RGA emanated from the GDA (Fig. 3.59).

The RGA originated near the T-shape intersection of the CHA, PHA, and GDA in 17 patients (8.9%) (Fig. 3.60).

PHA: Proper hepatic artery; GDA: Gastroduodenal artery.

The RGA originated from the CHA in three patients (1.6%) (Fig. 3.61).

SpA

The SpA, which originates from the celiac trunk and traverses the superior edge of the pancreas, gives off blood vessels supplying the pancreas and the stomach wall and is the blood supply vessel of the spleen. Further details are provided in chap. IV, sect. II).

3.2.1.3 Veins Associated with LN Dissection in the Suprapancreatic Area

LGV

The LGV, also known as the coronary vein, drains venous blood from the region of the LGA (Figs. 3.62 and 3.63).

About 1.6% of the LGV is not accompanied by the artery of the same name in the GPF, but runs independently in the hepatogastric ligament and flows into the portal vein at the hilar part of the liver, also known as the intrahepatic LGV (Fig. 3.64).

In about 0.5% of cases, the LGV is absent, and the RGV is enlarged to compensate (Figs. 3.65 and 3.66).

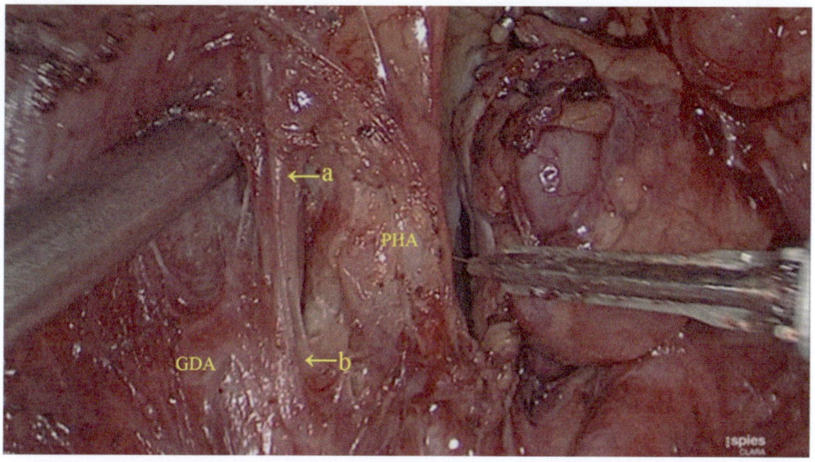

Fig. 3.61 The RGA (**a**) arising from the PHA (**b**)

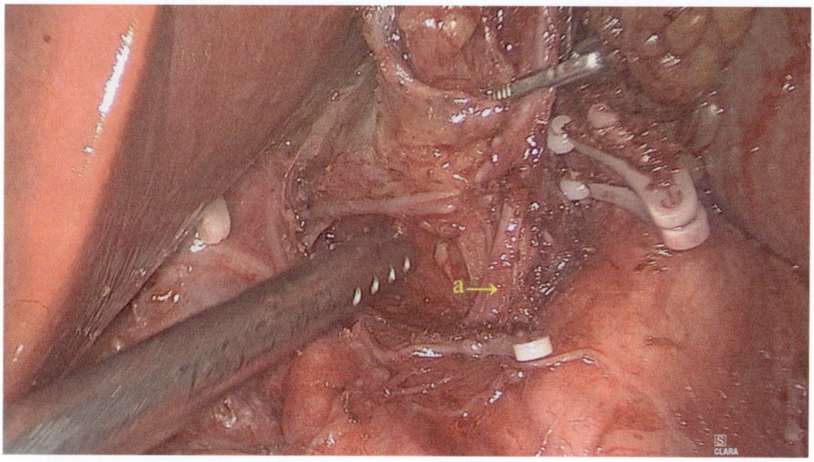

Fig. 3.62 The LGV (**a**) ends in the PV

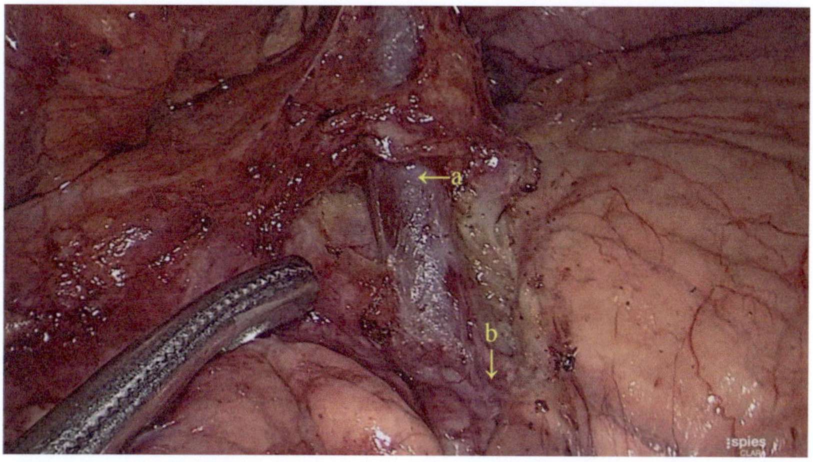

Fig. 3.63 The LGV (**a**) drains into the SpV (**b**)

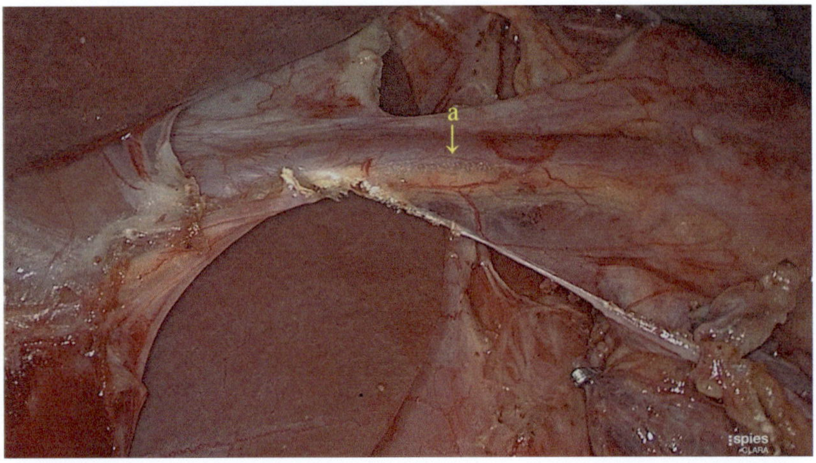

Fig. 3.64 The intrahepatic LGV (**a**)

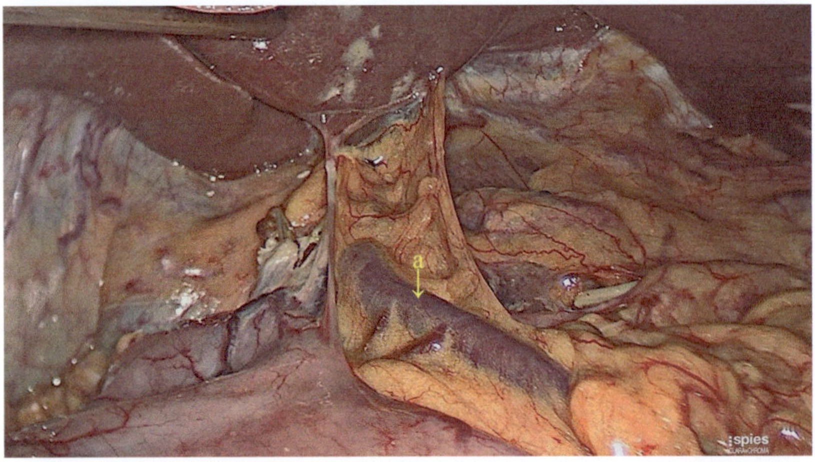

Fig. 3.65 Absence of LGV and compensatory thickening of the right gastric vein (RGV) (**a**) (frontal view)

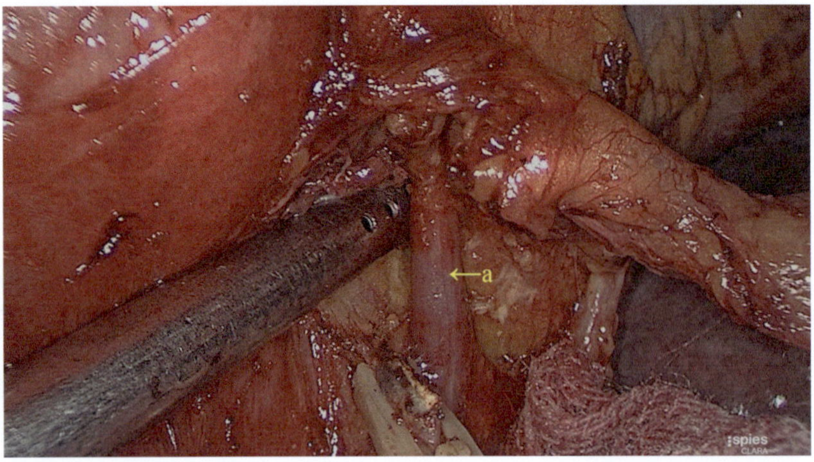

Fig. 3.66 Absence of LGV and compensatory thickening of RGV (**a**) (rear view)

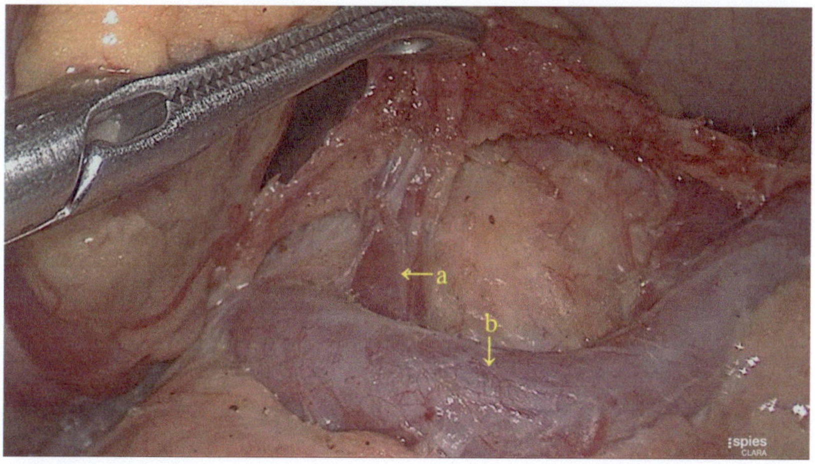

Fig. 3.67 The LGV (**a**) runs across the dorsal side of the SpA (**b**)

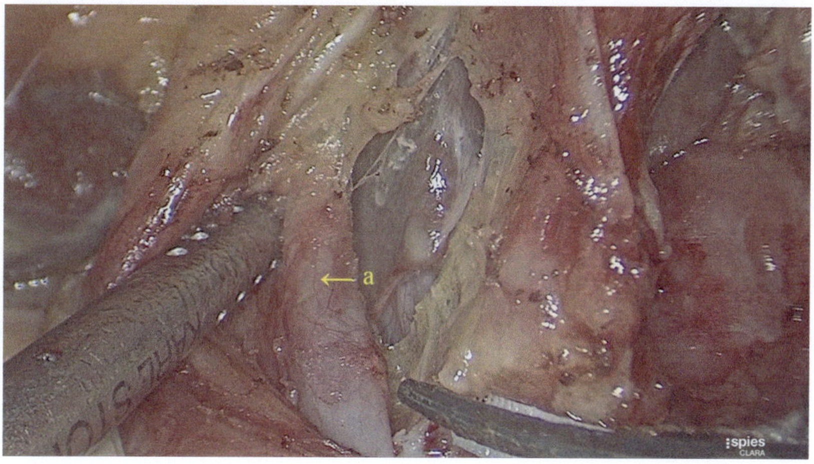

Fig. 3.68 The PV (**a**) is an important component of the tubular system in the hepatoduodenal ligament

In about 0.3% of cases, the LGV runs across the dorsal side of the SpA.

SpV

The SpV is formed by the confluence of the splenic lobar veins in the portal area of the spleen, and also receives blood from the splenic polar vein, the branch of the pancreatic vein, the short gastric vein, the left gastric omentum vein, as well as the inferior mesenteric vein during the journey (see chap. IV, sect. II, for further details).

PV

The PV is a short, thick vein trunk, about 6–8 cm long and 1. 4 ± 1. 8 cm in diameter. In the hepatoduodenal ligament, the PV is an important component of the tubular system in the ligaments of the liver and duodenum, behind the HPA and the common bile duct (Fig. 3.68).

RGV

The RGV is small, at approximately 1.0–4.5 mm in diameter (average: 2.18 mm). Usually, two or three RGVs are present. The left one passes from left to right along the lesser curvature of the stomach within the lesser omentum, receiving small veins from the gastric walls. A tributary of the RGV called the prepyloric vein passes vertically anterior to the pylorus in the subserosa (Fig. 3.69). The RGV runs continually towards the right and ultimately empties into the PV (Fig. 3.70).

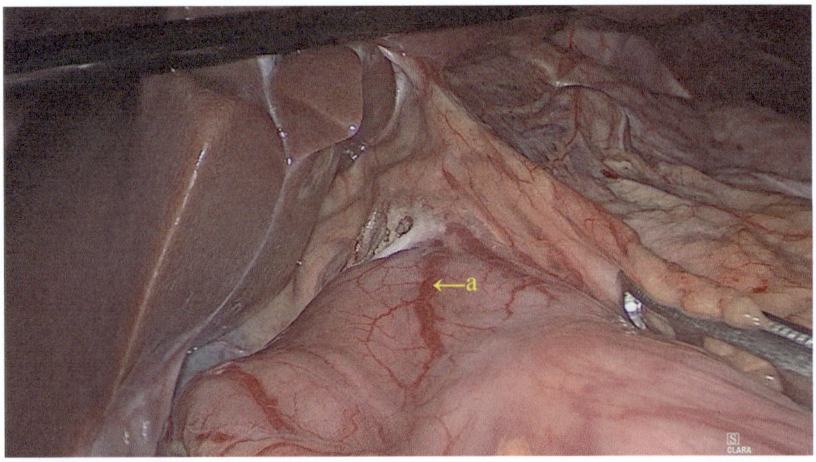

Fig. 3.69 Prepyloric vein (**a**)

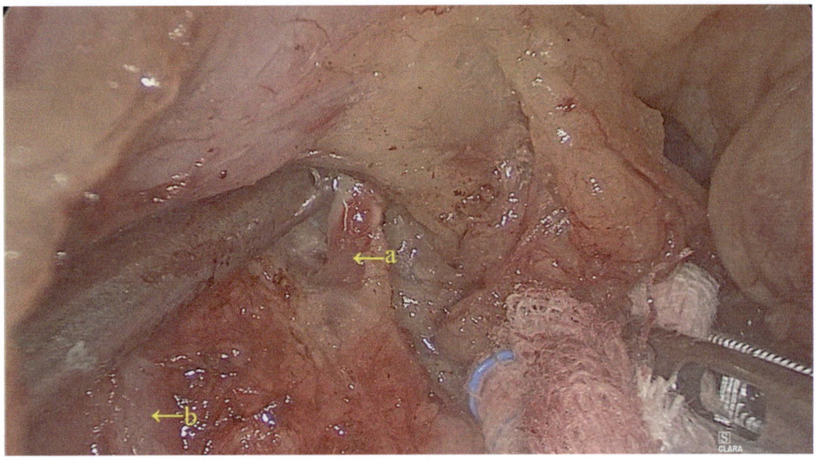

Fig. 3.70 The RGV (**a**) enters the HDL before draining into the PV (**b**)

3.2.1.4 LN Anatomy of the Suprapancreatic Area

No. 9 LNs (LNs Around the CA)

Definition of No. 9 LNs.

LGA: Left gastric artery; CHA: Common hepatic artery; SpA: Splenic artery.

No. 9 LNs are located at the root of the LGA, the CHA, and the SpA, adjacent to the surrounding LNs of the CA (Fig. 3.71).

Cases of No. 9 LNM are shown in Figs. 3.72 and 3.73.

LGA: Left gastric artery.

LGA: Left gastric artery; CHA: Common hepatic artery; SpA: Splenic artery.

Visualization of No. 9 LNs by ICG is shown in Figs. 3.74 and 3.75.

No. 7 LNs (LNs Around the LGA)

Definition of No. 7 LNs.

CHA: Common hepatic artery; LGA: Left gastric artery.

No. 7 LNs lie around the left gastric vessels in the GPF outside the lesser omentum. They are distributed from the root of the LGA to the bifurcation of the ascending branch (Fig. 3.76).

Cases of No. 7 LNM are shown in Figs. 3.77 and 3.78.

CHA: Common hepatic artery; CA: Celiac artery.

An ICG display of No. 7 LNs is seen in Figs. 3.79 and 3.80.

No. 8 LNs (LNs Around the CHA)

Definition of No. 8 LNs.

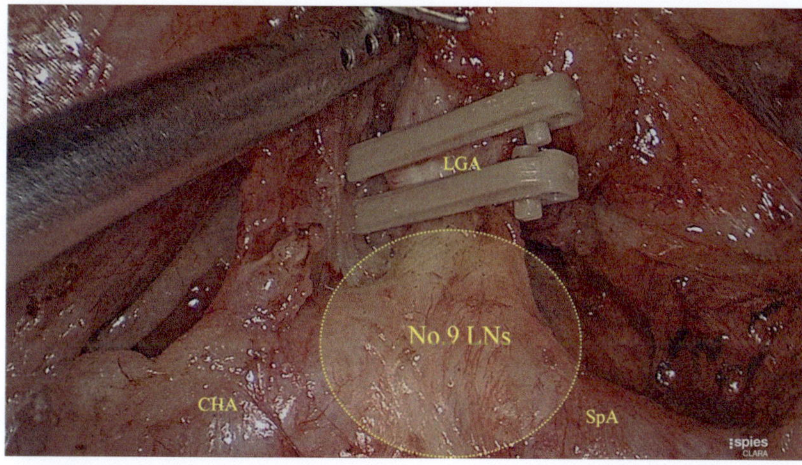

Fig. 3.71 Scope of No.9 LNs

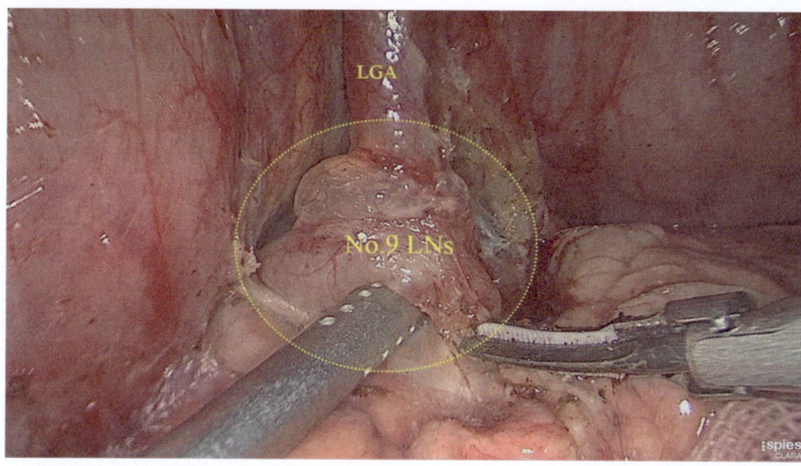

Fig. 3.72 No. 9 LNs before dissection

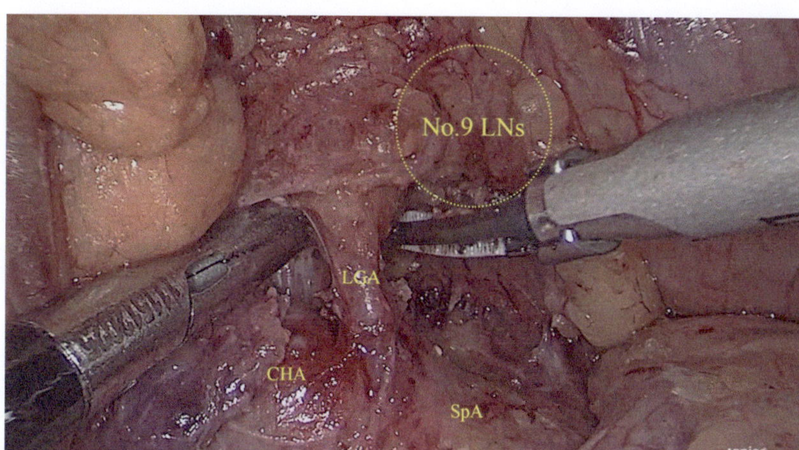

Fig. 3.73 No. 9 LNs after dissection

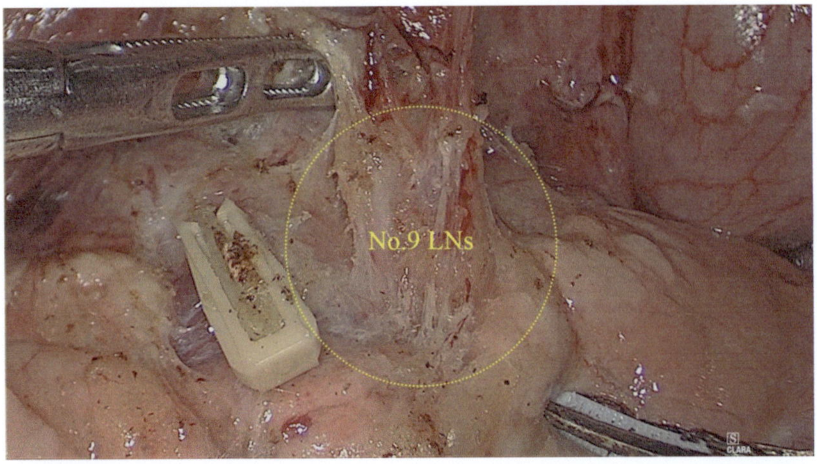

Fig. 3.74 No. 9 LNs

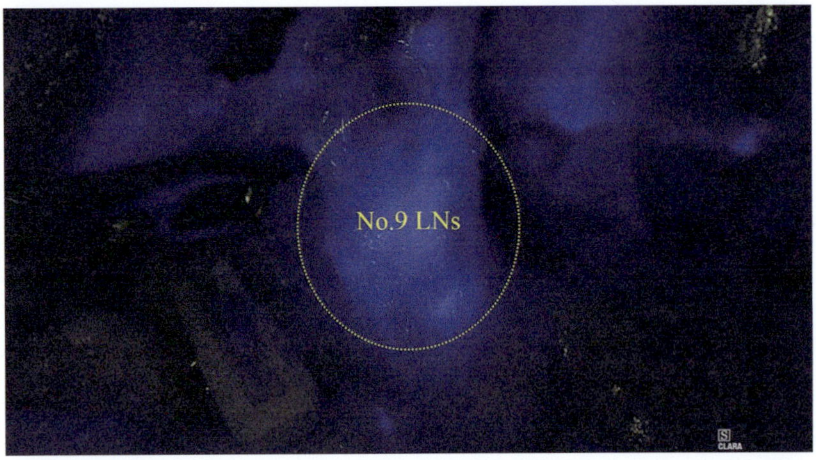

Fig. 3.75 ICG display of No. 9 LNs

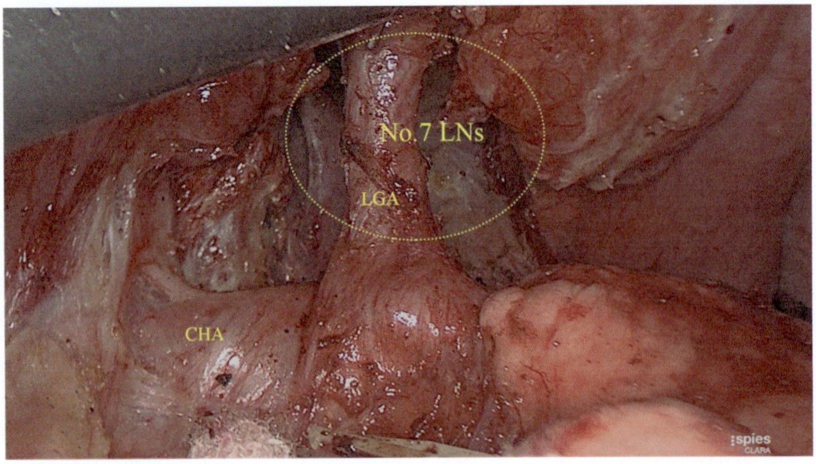

Fig. 3.76 The scope of No. 7 LNs

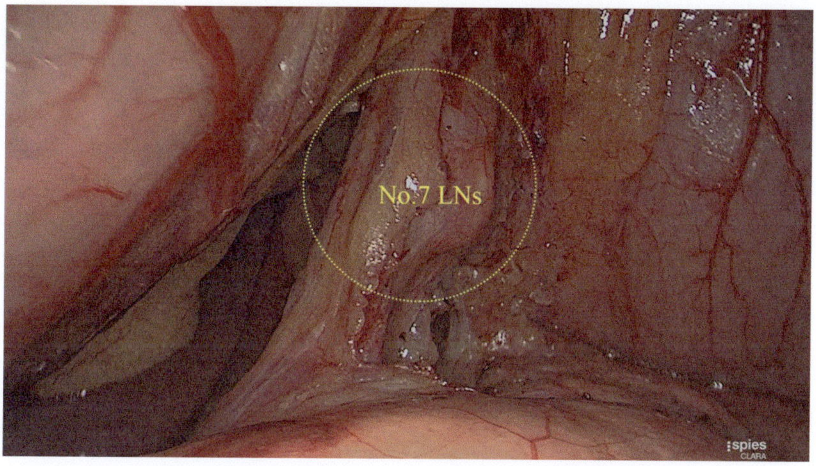

Fig. 3.77 No. 7 LNs before dissection

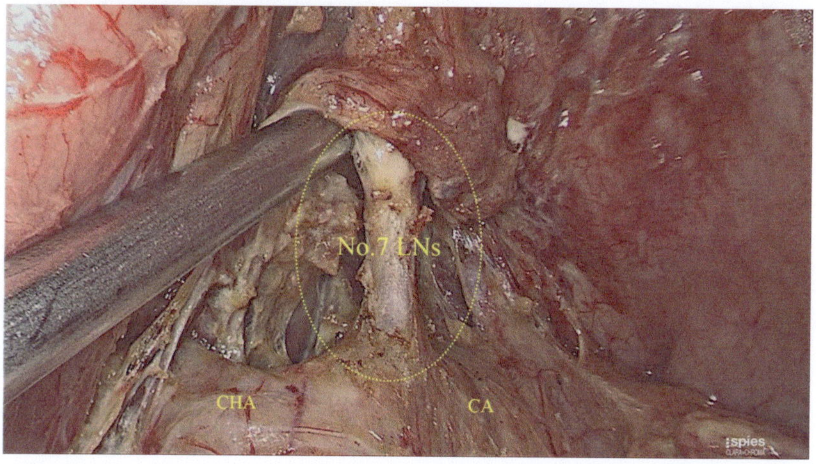

Fig. 3.78 No. 7 LNs after dissection

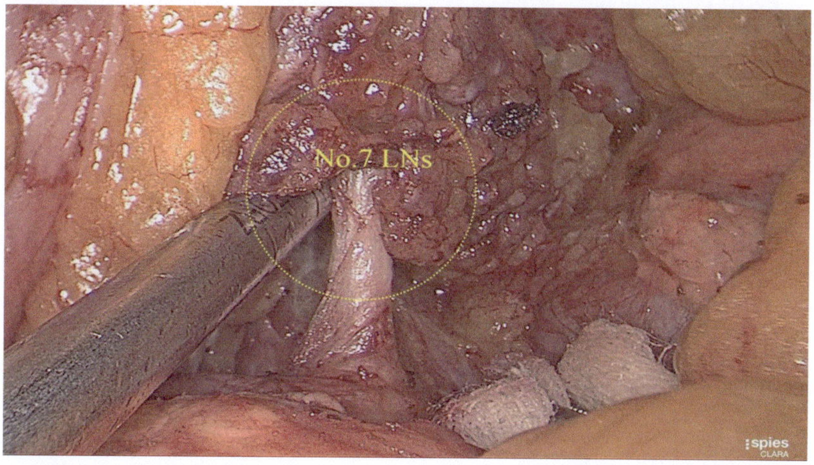

Fig. 3.79 No. 7 LNs

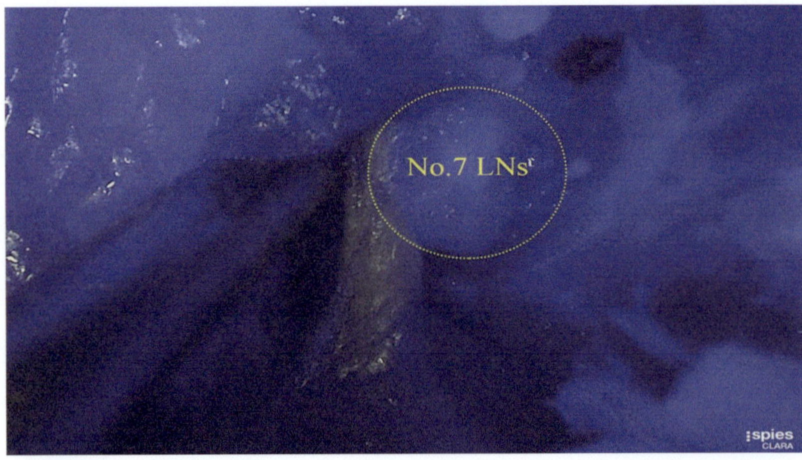

Fig. 3.80 ICG display of No. LNs

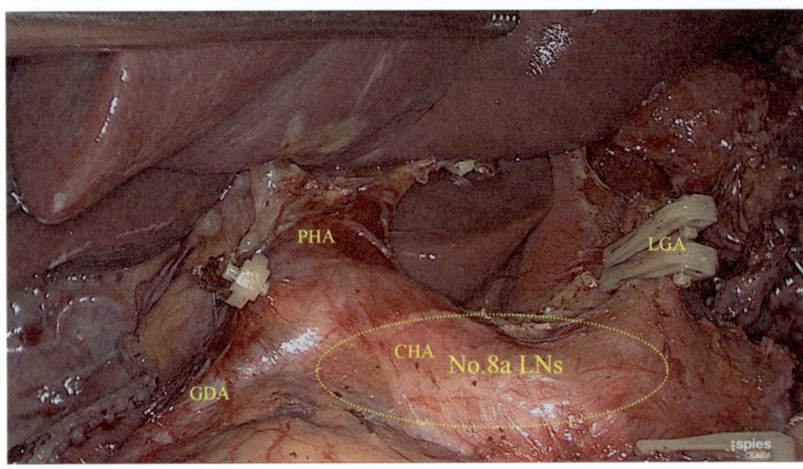

Fig. 3.81 The scope of No. 8a LNs

PHA: Proper hepatic artery; LGA: Left gastric artery; GDA: Gastroduodenal artery; CHA: Common hepatic artery.

No. 8 LNs are located at the origin of the CHA to the anterior and posterior CHA of the GDA. Anterior and superior CHA LNs are also known as No. 8a LNs, while posterior CHA LNs are known as No. 8p LNs (Fig. 3.81).

Cases of No. 8 LNM are shown in Figs. 3.82, 3.83, 3.84, and 3.85.

CHA: Common hepatic artery; LGA: Left gastric artery; GDA: Gastroduodenal artery; RGA: Right gastric artery.

RGA: Right gastric artery; LGA: Left gastric artery; PHA: Proper hepatic artery.

The ICG display of No. 8 LNs is seen in Figs. 3.86 and 3.87.

CHA: Common hepatic artery; LGA: Left gastric artery; SpA: Splenic artery.

No. 12 LNs (LNs in the HDL)

Definition of No. 12 LNs.

RHA: Right hepatic artery; LHA: Left hepatic artery; ALGA: Accessory left gastric artery; CHA: Common hepatic artery; GDA: Gastroduodenal artery.

RGA: Right gastric artery.

No. 12 LNs are located in the HDL alongside the hepatic artery, bile duct, and PV. They are divided into the following five substations

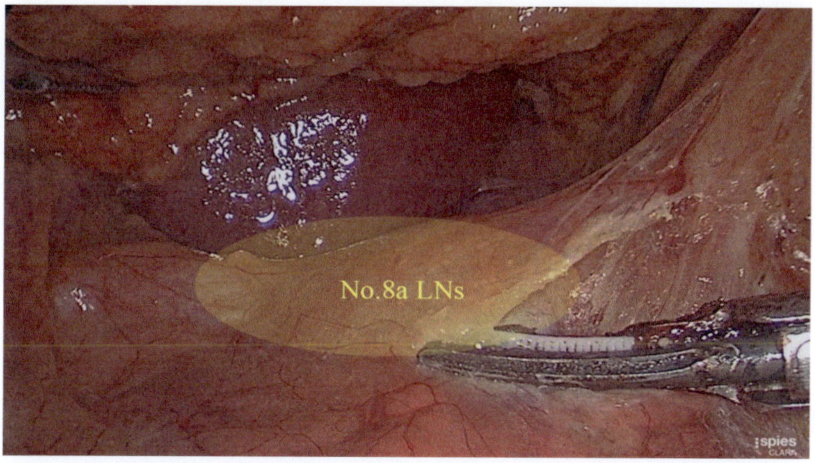

Fig. 3.82 No. 8 LNs before dissection

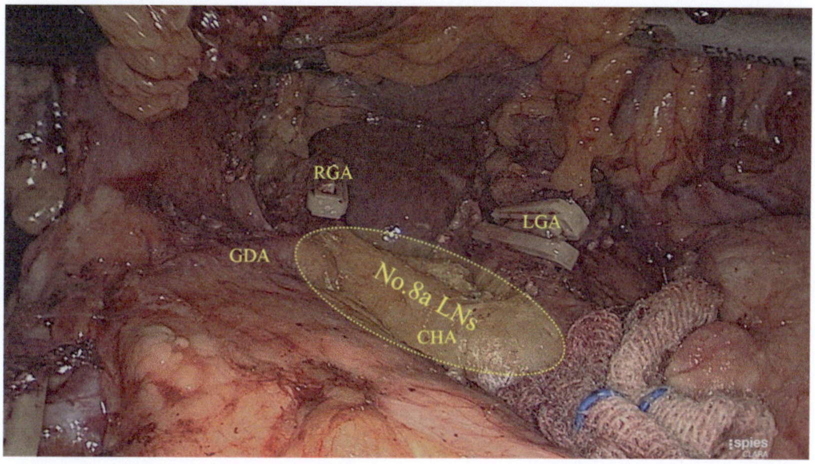

Fig. 3.83 No. 7 LNs after dissection

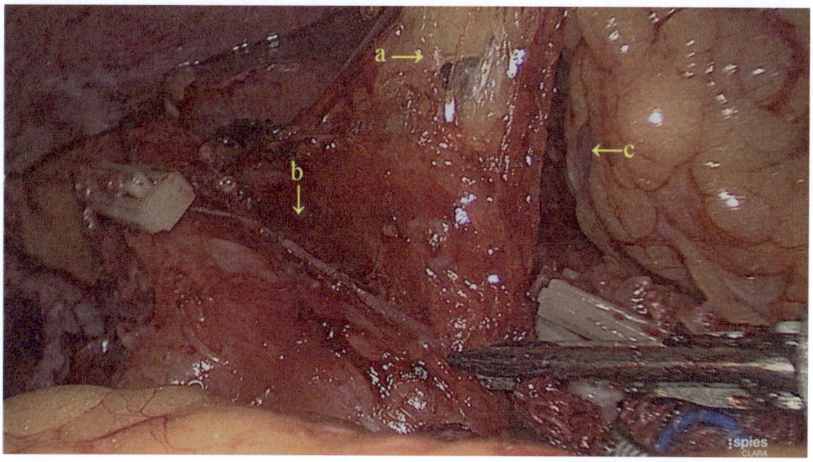

Fig. 3.84 No. 8p LNM (**a**), PV (**b**), RGV (**c**)

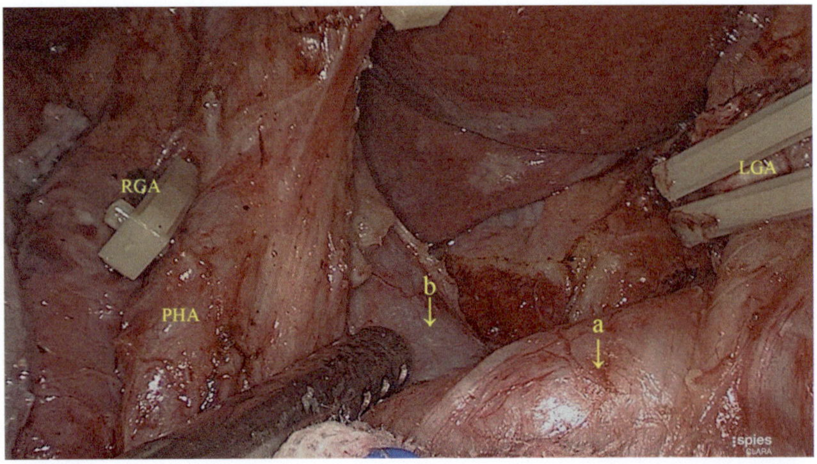

Fig. 3.85 No. 8p LNs after dissection, CHA (**a**), PV (**b**)

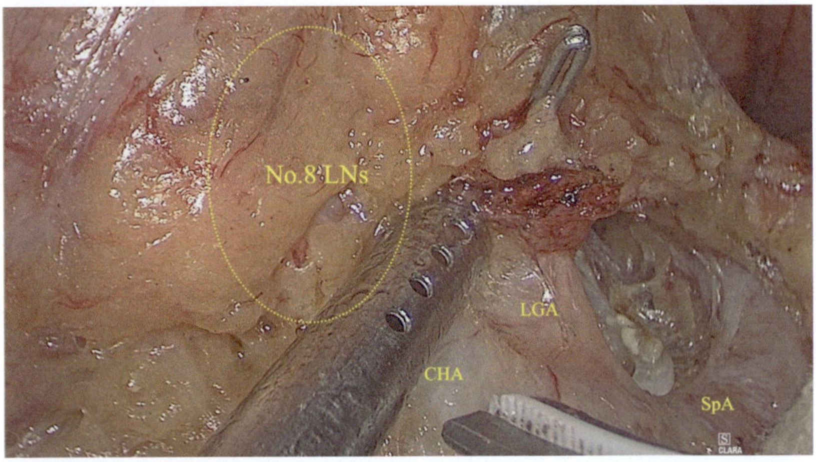

Fig. 3.86 No. 8 LNs

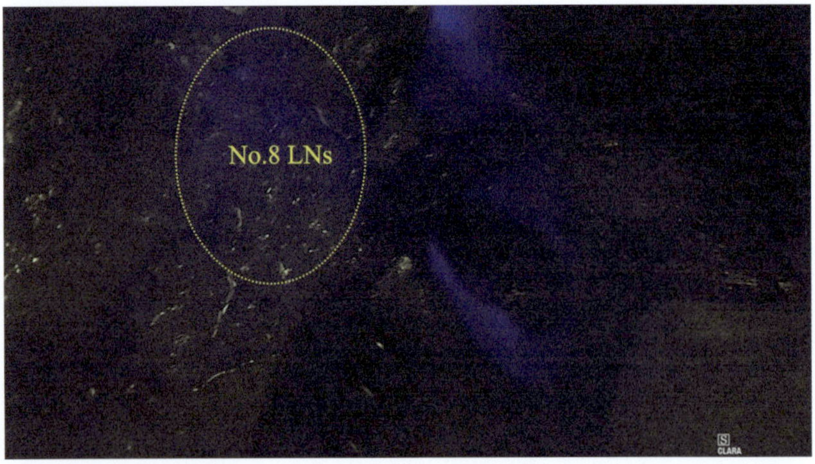

Fig. 3.87 ICG display of No. 8 LNs

based on studies of bile duct cancer (Fig. 3.88): No. 12a, beside the hepatic artery and along the CHA; No. 12b, beside the bile duct; No. 12p, behind the PV; No. 12 h, hepatic hilar LNs at the porta hepatis; and No. 12c, beside the cystic duct.

Cases of No. 12 LNM are shown in Figs. 3.89 and 3.90.

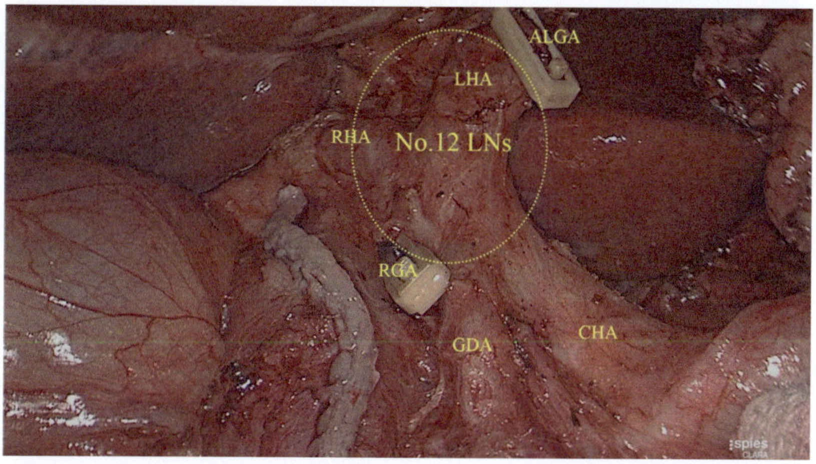

Fig. 3.88 The scope of No. 12 LNs

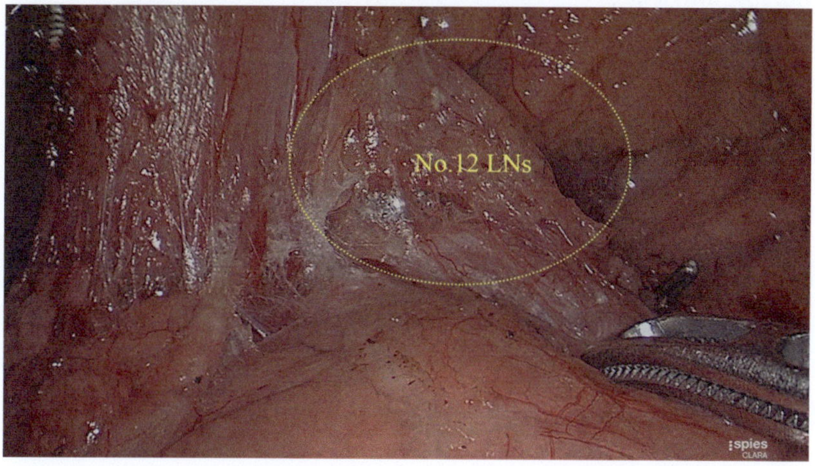

Fig. 3.89 No. 12 LNs before dissection

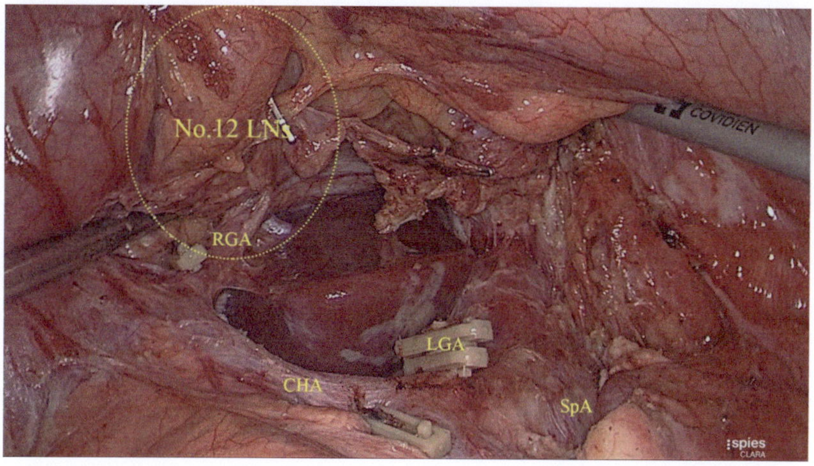

Fig. 3.90 No. 12 LNs after dissection

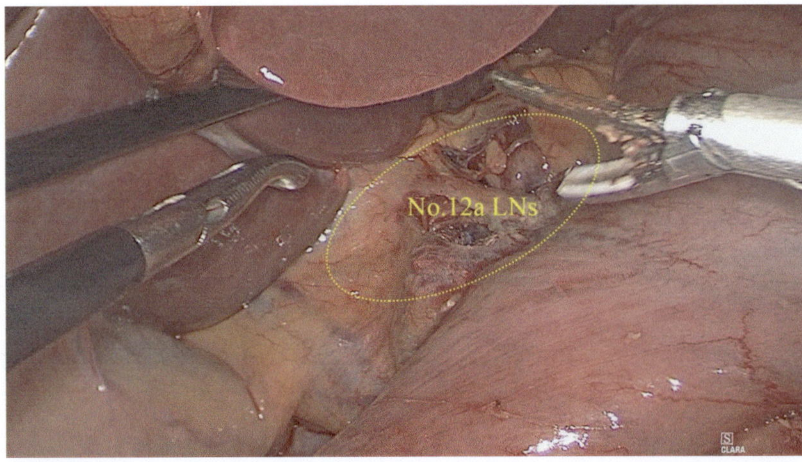

Fig. 3.91 No. 12a LNs

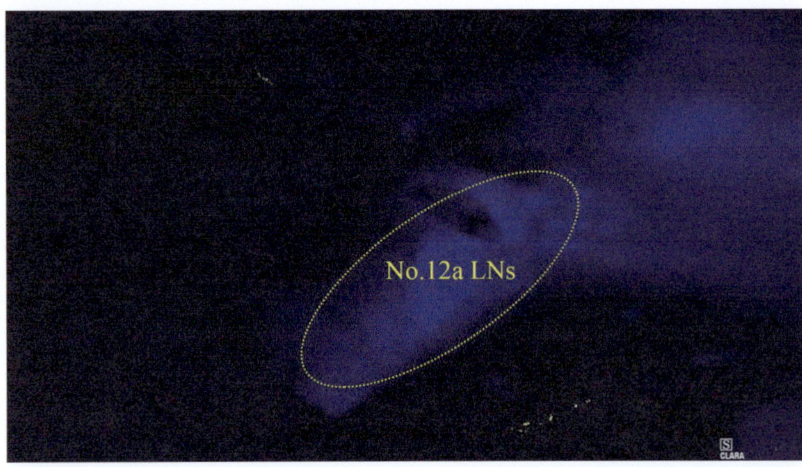

Fig. 3.92 ICG display of No. 12a LNs

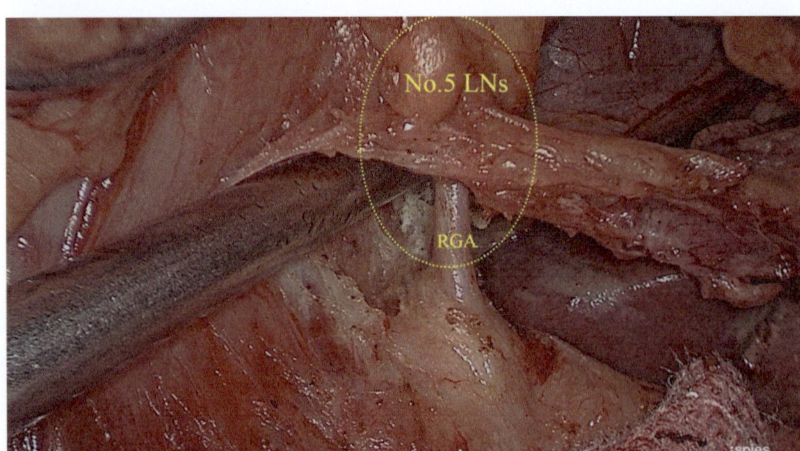

Fig. 3.93 The scope of No. 5 LNs

RGA: Right gastric artery; LGA: Left gastric artery; SpA: Splenic artery; CHA: Common hepatic artery.

ICG display of No. 12a LNs is seen in Figs. 3.91 and 3.92.

No. 5 LNs (Suprapyloric LNs)

Definition of No. 5 LNs.

RGA: Right gastric artery.

No. 5 LNs are distributed in the first branch of the gastric wall along the right gastric artery

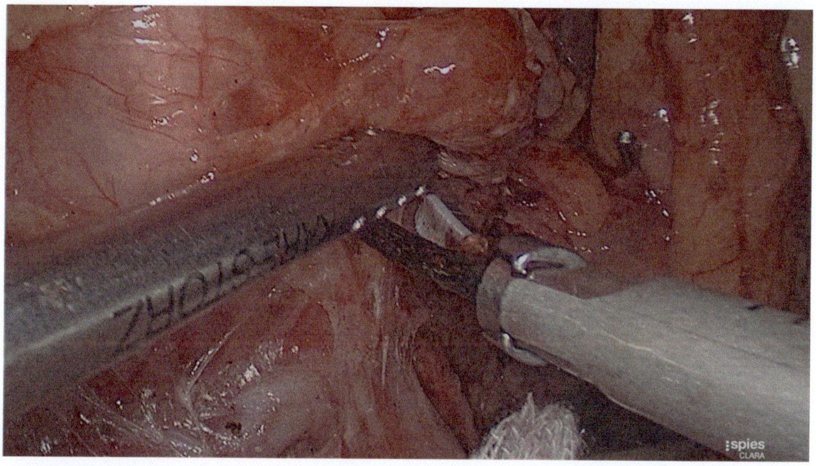

Fig. 3.94 No. 5 LNs before dissection

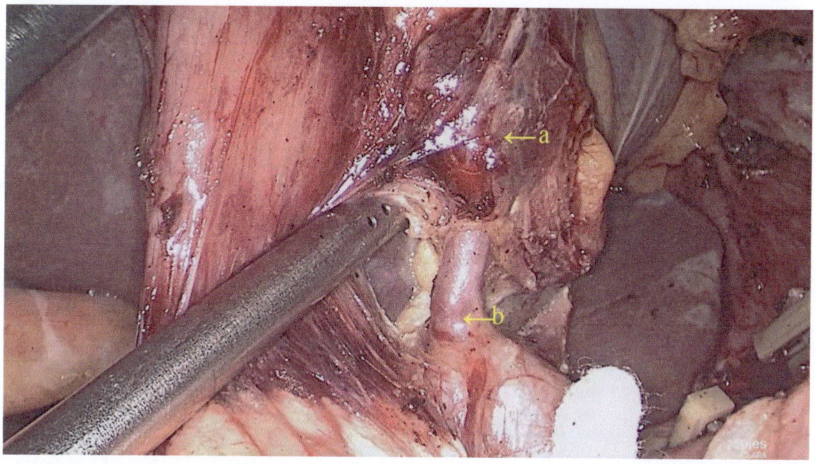

Fig. 3.95 No. 5 LNs (**a**) after dissection, RGA (**b**)

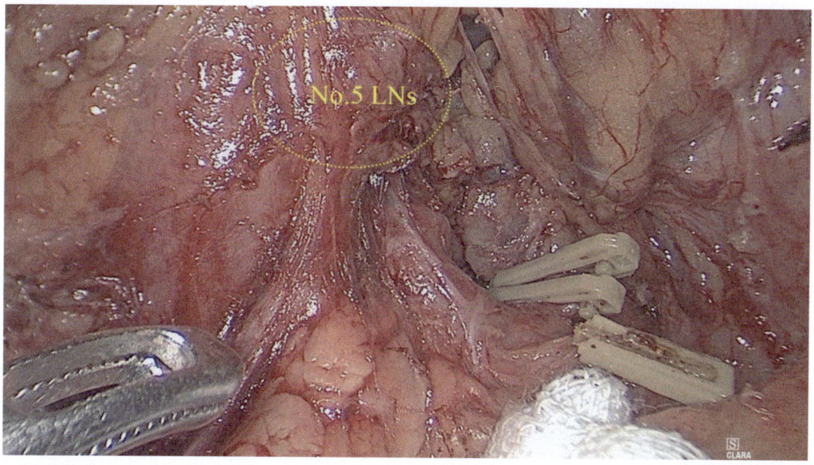

Fig. 3.96 No. 5 LNs

(including the root LNs of the right gastric artery) and are located in the superior pyloric region of the hepatoduodenal ligament. No. 12 LNs border the root of the right gastric artery; LNs below are No. 12, and those above are No. 5 (Fig. 3.93).

Cases of No. 12 LNM are shown in Figs. 3.94 and 3.95.

An ICG display of No. 5 LNs is seen in Figs. 3.96 and 3.97.

Fig. 3.97 ICG display of No. 5 LNs

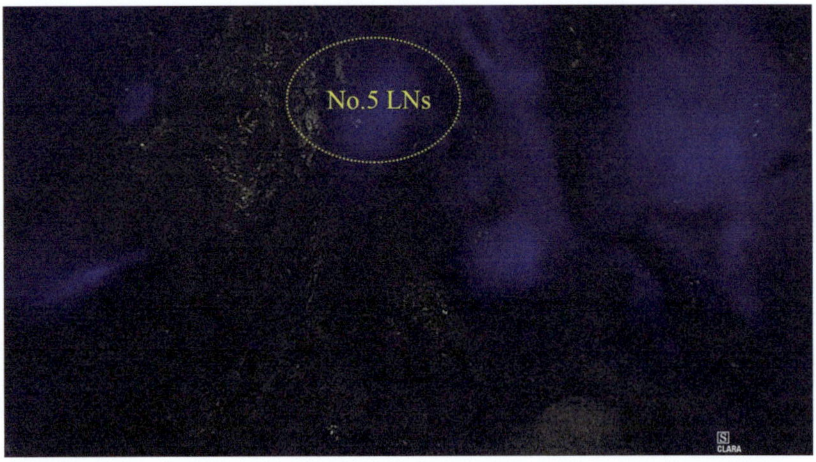

3.2.2 Intraoperative Announcements of Laparoscopic Suprapancreatic Area LN Dissection for Gastric Cancer

3.2.2.1 Points of Attention in the Dissection of No. 7, 8a, 9, and 11p LNs

Before LN dissection in the suprapancreatic area, it is necessary to fully separate the transverse mesenteric membrane and the adhesion of the pancreatic capsule to the posterior wall of the stomach (Fig. 3.98).

The assistant clamps the GPF upwards and forwards to provide tension and to block the stomach and the greater omentum. This avoids ptosis affecting exposure of the surgical field (Fig. 3.99).

When the GPF is invaded by advanced gastric body cancer or with obviously enlarged LNs in the suprapancreatic area, it is difficult to grasp and pull the fold. Gastric forceps are therefore used to hold the GPF and lift it up to reveal the visual field (Fig. 3.100).

LGA: Left gastric artery; RGA: Right gastric artery.

During LN dissection in this area, the left splenic artery of the GPF is usually selected as the operative approach. In some patients, the CHA runs far from the superior margin of the pancreas (Fig. 3.101), so if it is used as the surgical approach for LN dissection, the dividing plane may be too deep to prevent damage to the PV during exploration of this artery. Alternatively, incorrect identification of the CHA as swollen LNs may result.

The GDA is a more suitable approach for LN dissection in the suprapancreatic area when the surgeon is located on the right side of the patient. However, when the superior edge of the pancreas is not exposed, the area between the posterior wall of the duodenum and the head of the pancreas is narrow and the field of vision is difficult to expose. The duodenum is limited by the left and right gastric vessels, and the assistant cannot lift the duodenum to create proper tension (Fig. 3.102).

Small vessels distributed around the posterior wall of the duodenum are easy to injure and it is difficult to achieve hemostasis once bleeding occurs (Fig. 3.103).

To avoid skidding and reduce pancreatic injury, the surgeon should hold a piece of small gauze with the radiopaque marker as a pad to press the pancreas (Fig. 3.104).

The assistant's right hand should flexibly and gently apply different techniques such as lifting, pulling, holding, pushing, picking, and peeling to

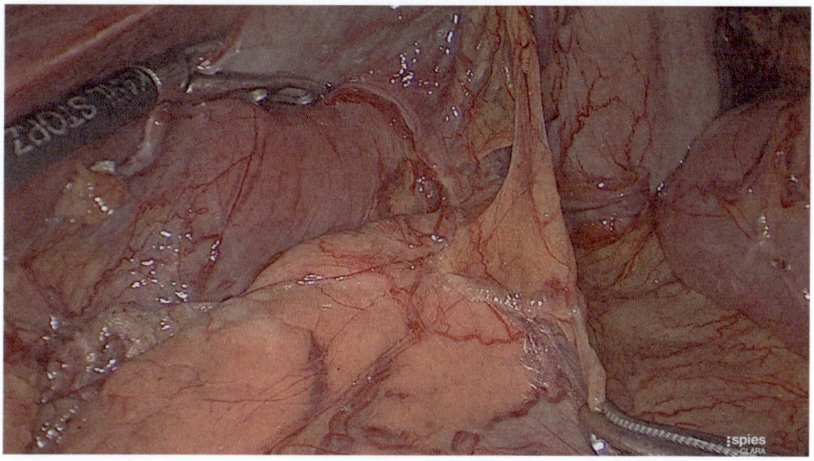

Fig. 3.98 The adhesion of the transverse mesentery and pancreatic capsule to the posterior wall of the stomach should be separated fully

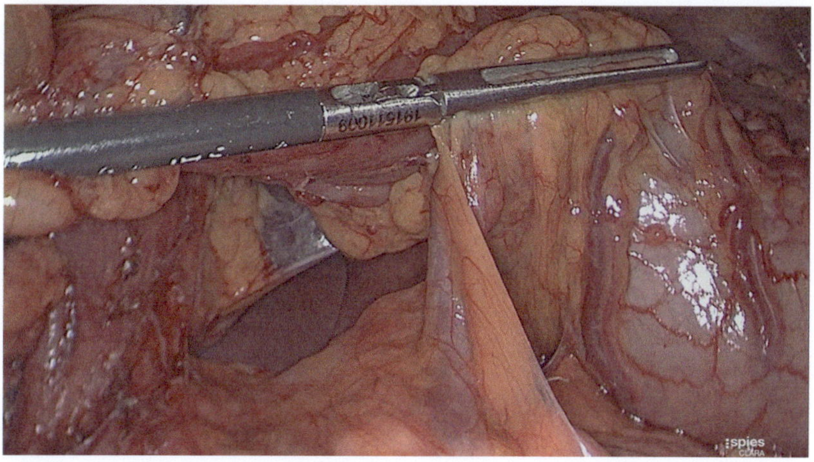

Fig. 3.99 The assistant's left hand lifts up the GPF by clamping the junction of its upper and middle segments

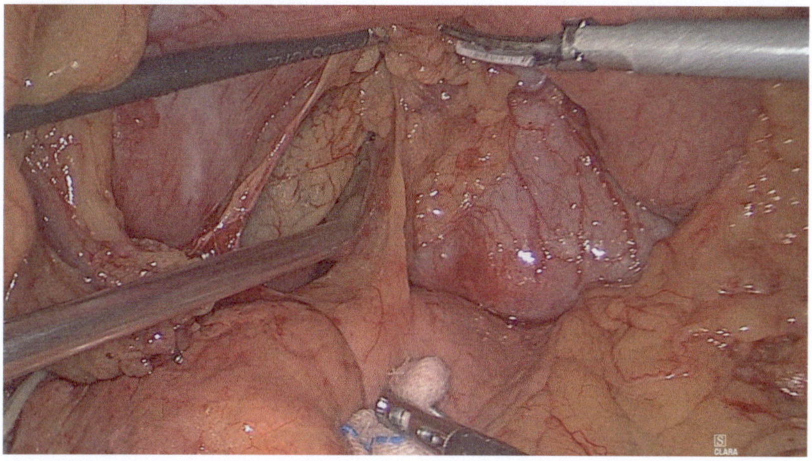

Fig. 3.100 When the LN is enlarged, non-invasive intestinal forceps lift the GPF to the large curved side and tighten to reveal the field of view

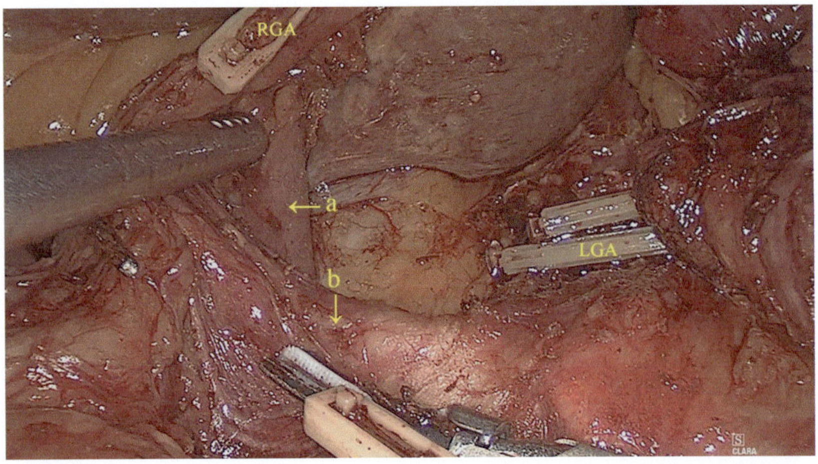

Fig. 3.101 The PV (**a**) may be injured during exploratory procedures if the CHA (**b**) is located far from the superior margin of the pancreas

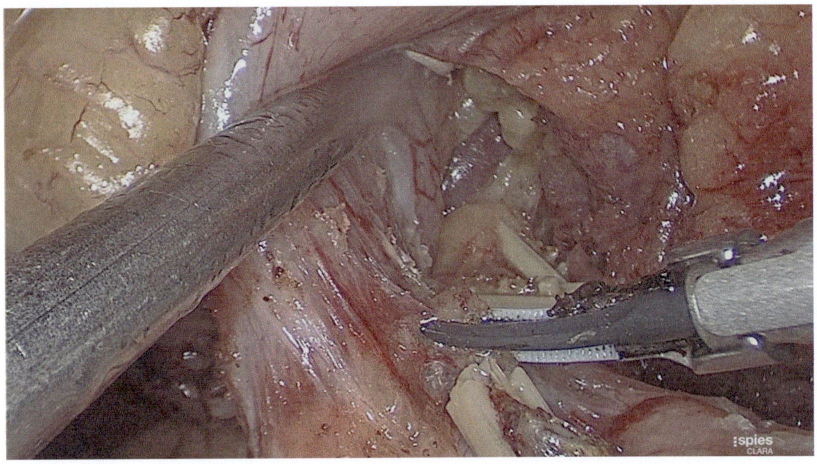

Fig. 3.102 The space of the duodenal approach is small and the operation field is difficult to expose

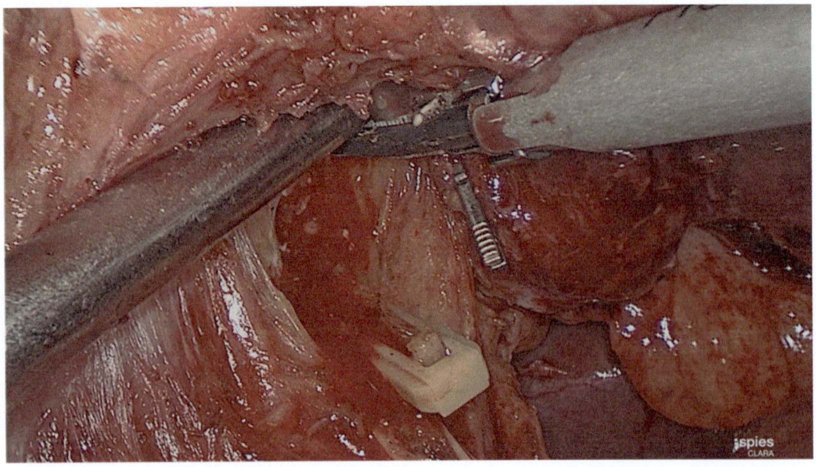

Fig. 3.103 The posterior wall of the duodenum is often supplied with small branches of blood vessels that are prone to bleeding and difficult to stop

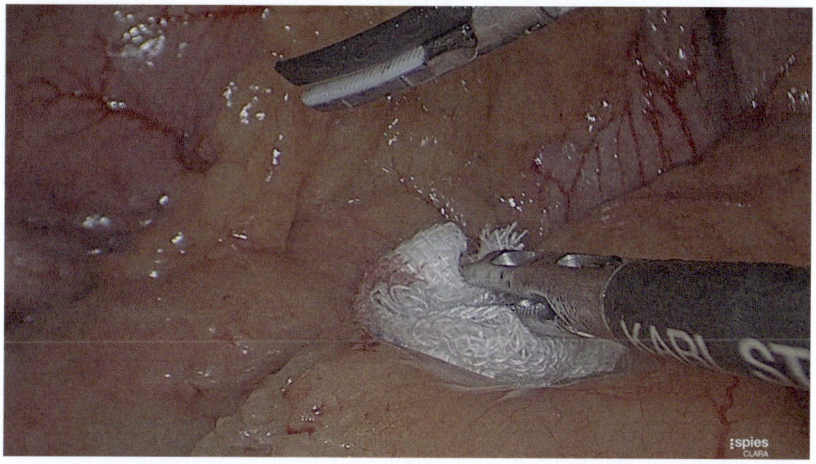

Fig. 3.104 The surgeon should hold a piece of small gauze with the radiopaque marker as a pad

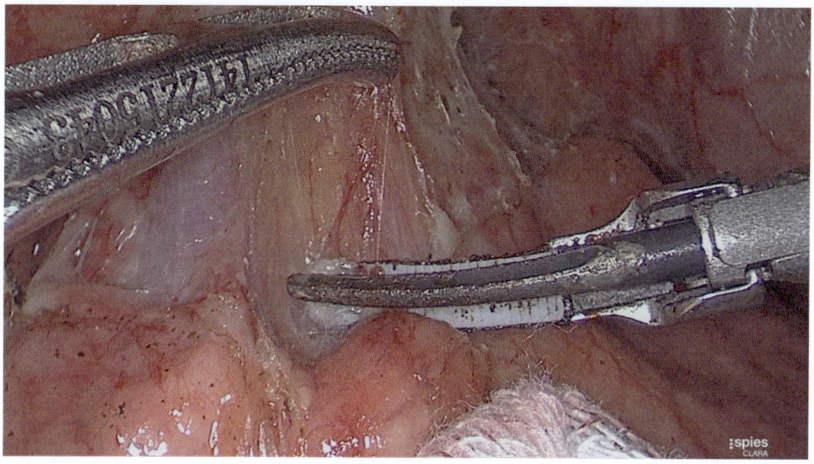

Fig. 3.105 "Lifting"

assist the surgeon in maintaining appropriate tension (Figs. 3.105 and 3.106).

If lens contamination results in unclear vision, the lens should be removed quickly after wiping with iodophor gauze, then wiped with dry gauze to remove oil stains (Fig. 3.107).

Laparoscopic dissection of the pancreatic capsule is an anatomic approach for the upper margin of the pancreas. Because of its brittle nature, it is easy to damage the pancreatic surface and cause bleeding during separation of the pancreatic capsule. Therefore, gauze compression or electrocoagulation can be used to stop the bleeding. If the ultrasound scalpel is used to do this, it is not only difficult to clamp the bleeding point, but also easy to further damage the pancreas and lead to more serious bleeding (Fig. 3.108). The nonfunctional surface of the ultrasonic scalpel should always be close to the pancreas to prevent damage to the pancreatic tissue (Fig. 3.109).

Efferent lymphatic vessels along the LGA, SpA, and CHA and its branches are thick, and drain into LNs around the CA. It is therefore better to sever them with ultrasonic scalpels set at minimum speed, or to ligature them with clips if necessary (Fig. 3.110).

SpA: Splenic artery; PV: Portal vein; LGA: Left gastric artery.

After the CV is exposed, the operator should disconnect the CV first, then dissect the LNs

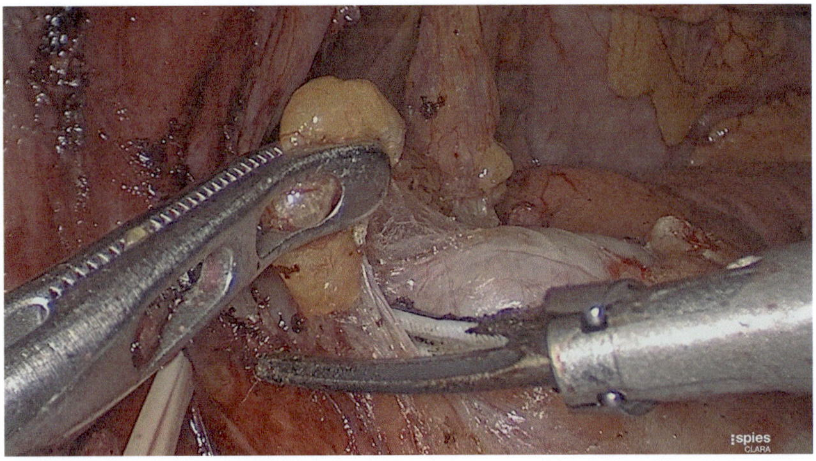

Fig. 3.106 "Holding"

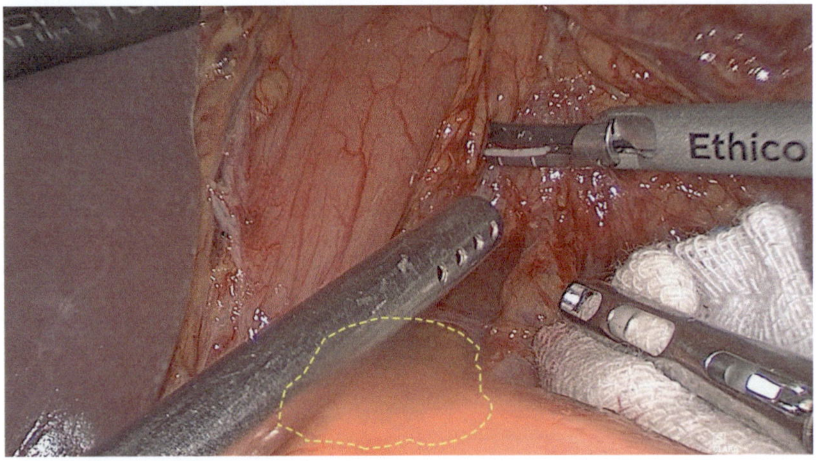

Fig. 3.107 Lens contamination leads to a unclear view

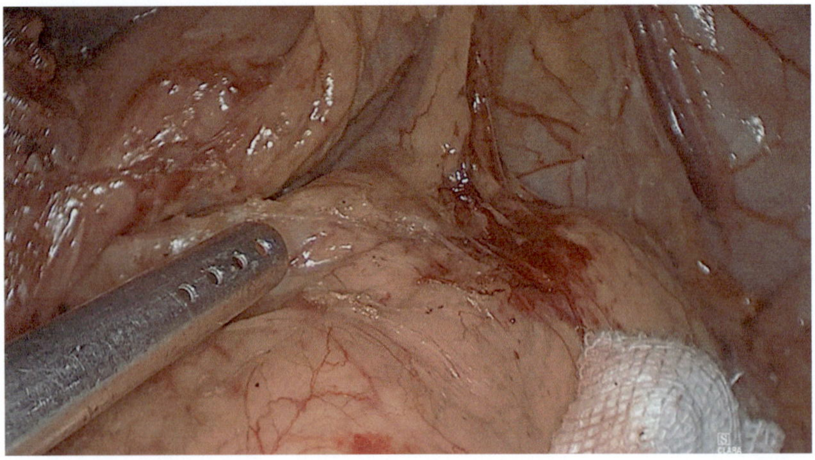

Fig. 3.108 Using a gauze to control small infiltration of blood from the pancreas

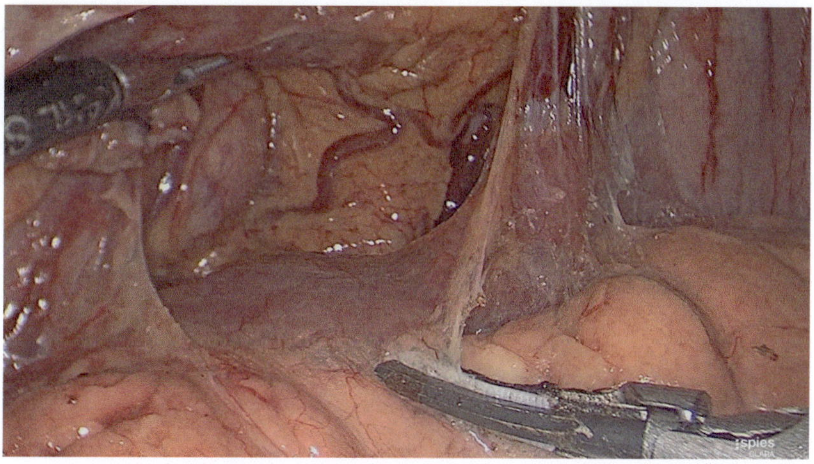

Fig. 3.109 The nonfunctional surface of the ultrasonic scalpel operates in pancreatic tissue

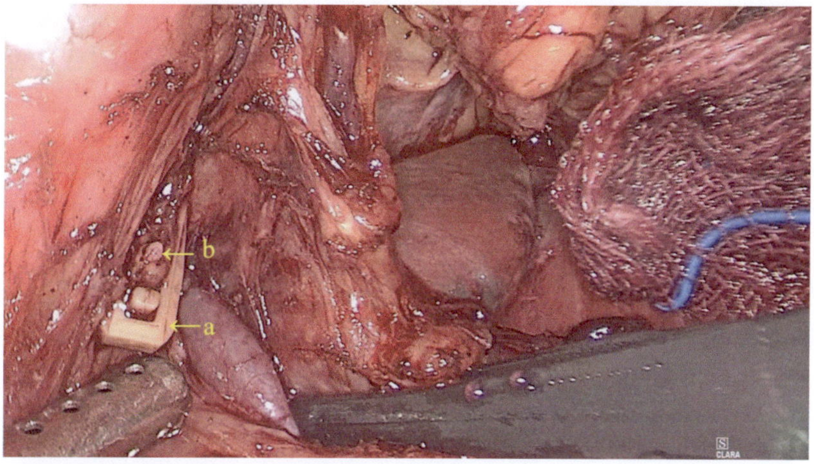

Fig. 3.110 A clip (**a**) is used to ligate the lymphatic vessel at the root of the CHA; the stump of the lymphatic vessel (**b**)

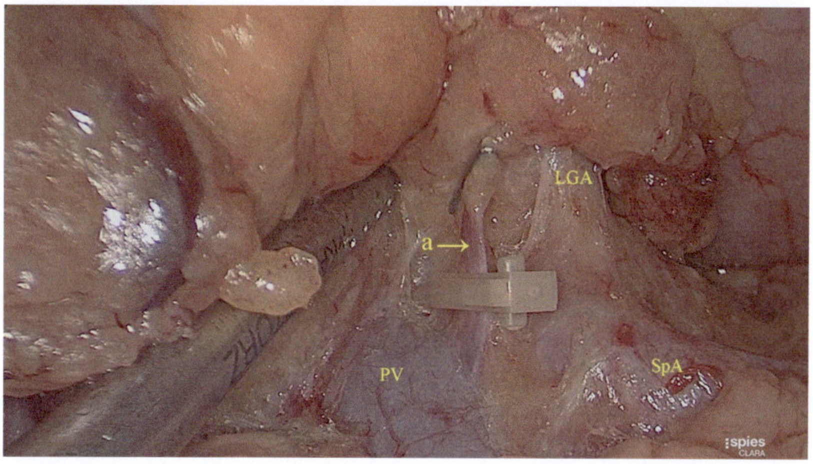

Fig. 3.111 The operator should disconnect the CV (**a**) first when LNs are enlarged around the LGA

around the LGA to prevent injury of the CV (Fig. 3.111).

CV: Coronary vein.

Branches of small veins can drain into the CV. In the process of CV vascularized this can cause hemorrhage, so the CV should be cut off below the branch of the small vein after full exposure (Fig. 3.112).

In a small number of patients, the CV is located far from the LGA. Such situations should

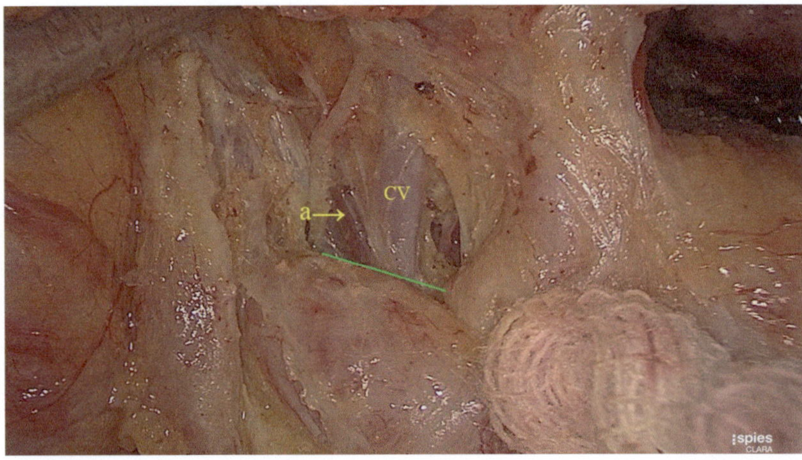

Fig. 3.112 The small branch of CV (**a**) should be separated from the CV at the green dotted line level

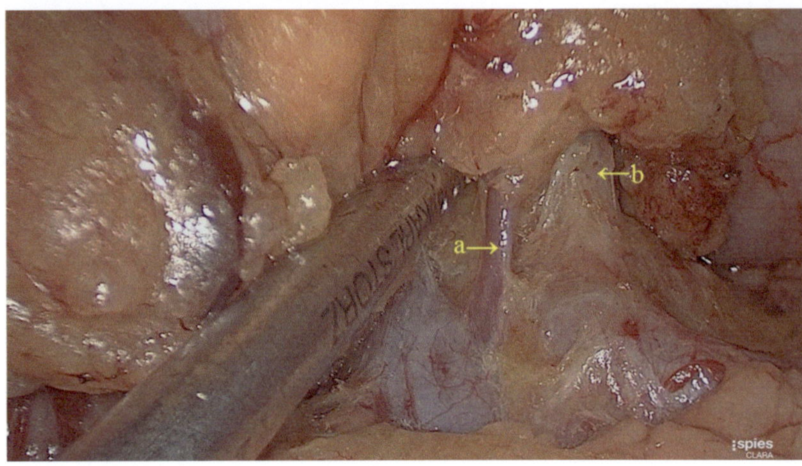

Fig. 3.113 The CV (**a**) located far from the LGA (**b**)

be carefully monitored to prevent damage to the CV (Fig. 3.113).

If accidental injury occurs to the LGV, the surgeon should rapidly clamp the LGV in the GPF with the left hand, and use a titanium clip to ligature the distal end of the vein with the right hand to reduce venous blood reflux. Using a low-volume aspirator, the assistant should then compress the hemorrhagic area and suck up the blood intermittently (Fig. 3.114).

CHA: Common hepatic artery; GDA: Gastroduodenal artery; SpA: Splenic artery.

In some patients, the LGA originates from the abdominal aorta. In these cases, the LGA is located above the posterior right side of the CA, and may not be found near the initial segment of the SpA. Therefore, lymphatic adipose tissue of the area should be dissected along the plane of the CA to the right rear to expose the root of the LGA (Fig. 3.115).

LGA: Left gastric artery; CHA: Common hepatic artery.

If the LGA is accidentally injured, the operation team should first remain calm because of severe short-term bleeding. The assistant's left hand should remain in the same position as the pull, and the right hand should immediately use an attractor to locate the bleeding area. Appropriate compression of the bleeding point wall should be used to control bleeding (Fig. 3.116).

LGA: Left gastric artery.

The clamp should be kept away from the root of the LGA to avoid injury to the proximal end of the LGA by the ultrasonic scalpel and unnecessary bleeding (Fig. 3.117).

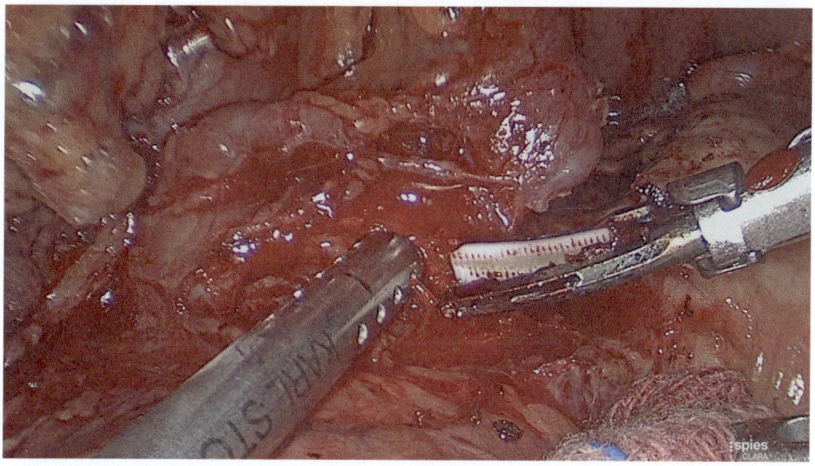

Fig. 3.114 A low-volume aspirator is used to intermittently suck up the blood and expose the hemorrhagic area

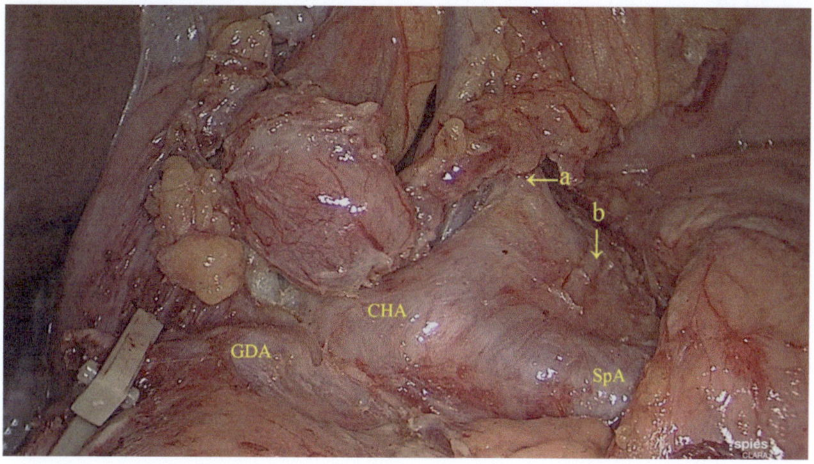

Fig. 3.115 The LGA (**a**) originates from the abdominal aorta, and is located above the CA (**b**) at the right posterior aspect

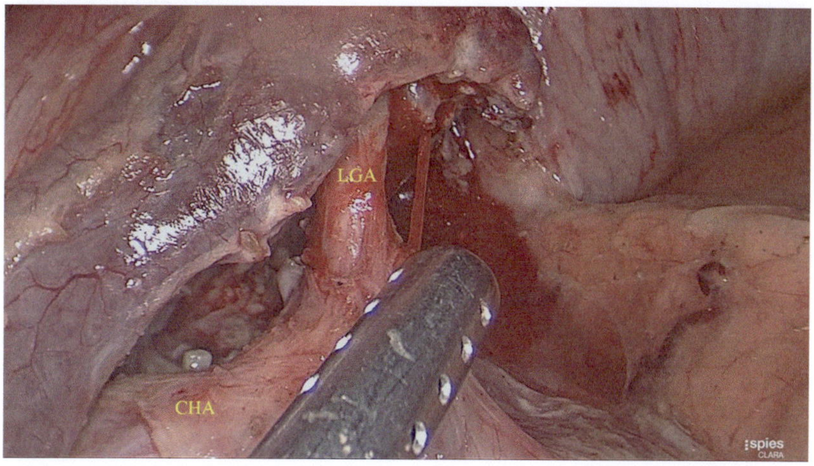

Fig. 3.116 The assistant immediately uses an attractor to locate the bleeding area after injury to the LGA

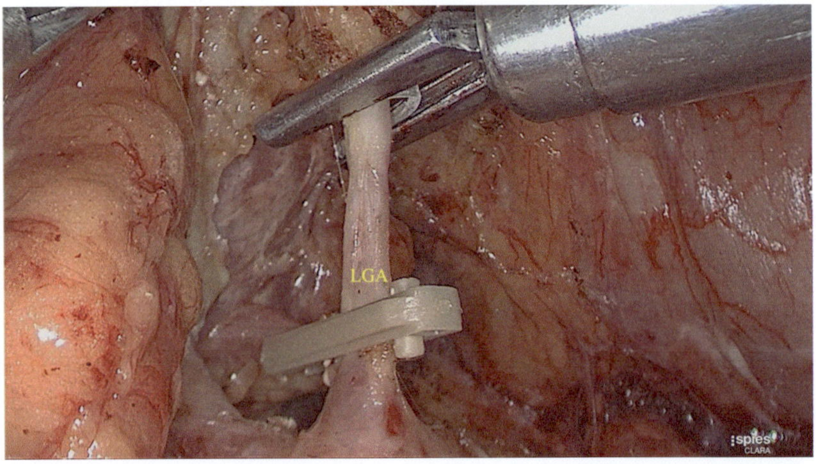

Fig. 3.117 When the surgeon clamps at the distal end of the LGA, this should be as far away as possible from the root

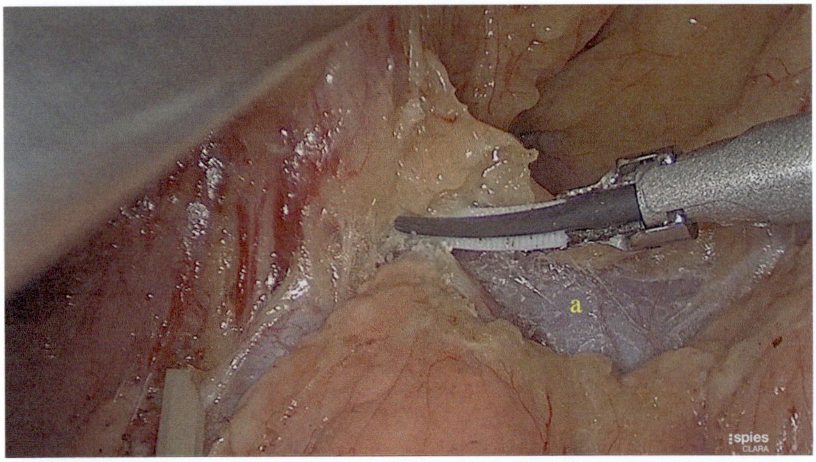

Fig. 3.118 The fascia on the ventral side of the vein should be peeled to expose the PV (**a**)

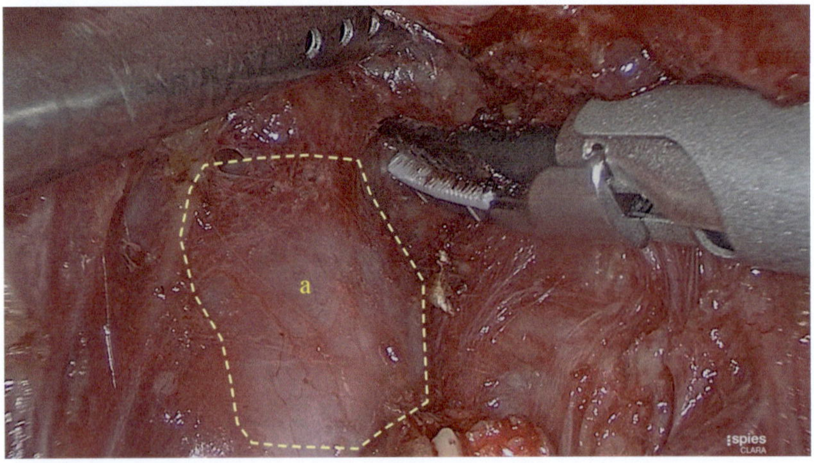

Fig. 3.119 Surgery directly on the surface of the PV (**a**) because of the absence of a CHA

LN dissection in patients without a CHA will be done directly on the surface of the PV or SpV. The surgeon should directly shear with ultrasonic scalpels and gently rather than bluntly dissect to avoid injuring the PV and causing bleeding (Figs. 3.118 and 3.119).

The surgeon should meticulously detect the anatomic space between the LNs and the CHA

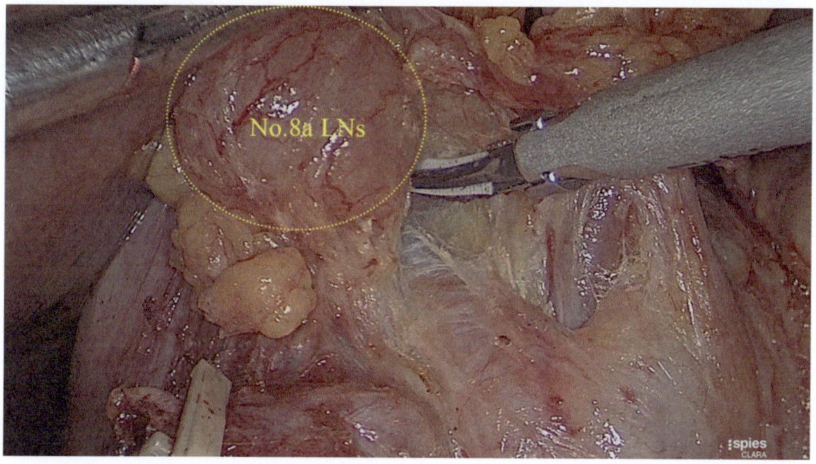

Fig. 3.120 The gap between the base of the LN and the surface of the vessel should be carefully searched when No. 8a LNs are enlarged

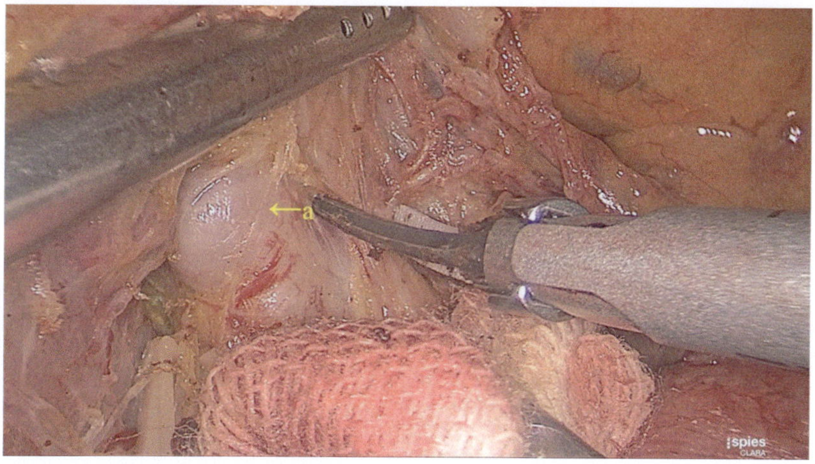

Fig. 3.121 The CHA (**a**) can be tortuous and should be distinguished from enlarged LNs

when No. 8a LNs are obviously enlarged. The assistant can remove the base of the LNs to facilitate exposure. The surgeon fastens the non-functional surface of the ultrasound scalpel to the blood vessels, dissecting the swollen LNs from the surface of the CHA (Fig. 3.120).

In some patients, the CHA is relatively long and tortuous, and is easily confused with enlarged LNs. To prevent this, the arterial pulse can be identified to confirm the CHA (Fig. 3.121).

During LN dissection in this area, the focal distance of the lens should be set to the close view, and the best focal length can be determined by imaging the surrounding tissue. When reflected light appears in the view, or tissue capillaries or the nonfunctional face of the ultrasonic scalpel become distinct, the focal distance can be demonstrated to be optimal (Figs. 3.122, 3.123, and 3.124).

3.2.2.2 Points for Attention in No. 12a, 5 LN Dissection

No. 5 LNs can be dissected to the right along the surface of the CHA. The assistant lifts the posterior wall of the gastric antrum right upwards with the forceps in the left hand, and pushes the duodenum outwards with the other hand to expose the CHA, the GDA, and the partially vascularized PHA (Fig. 3.125).

CHA: Common hepatic artery; GDA: Gastroduodenal artery.

At this point, the assistant may use an attractor or grab forceps to bluntly dissect the posterior wall of the duodenum up and down, assisting the surgeon in separating and exposing of the course of the RGA. Dissection of No. 5 LNs is completed after vascularizing and severing the vessel at the root (Fig. 3.126).

RGA: Right gastric artery.

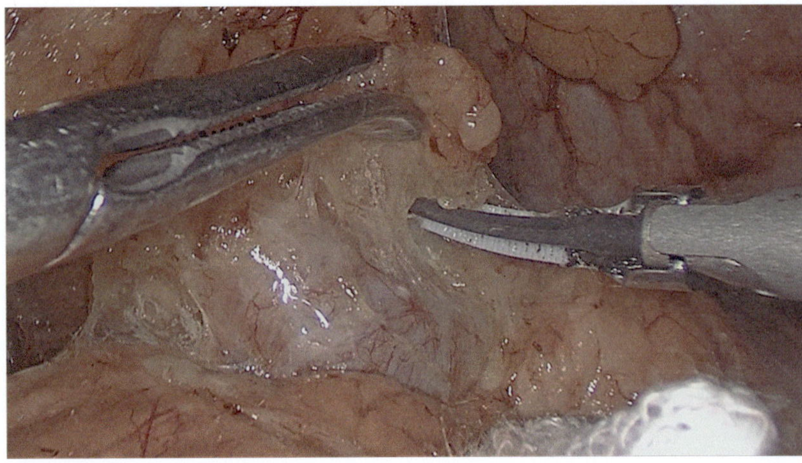

Fig. 3.122 Reflection of light in the view

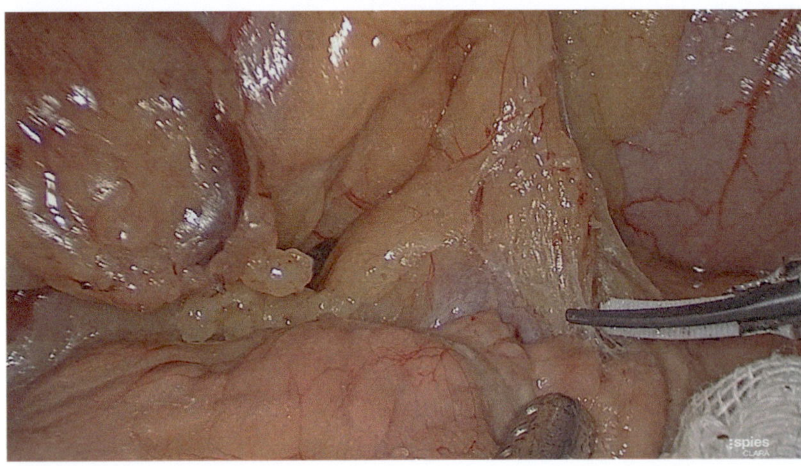

Fig. 3.123 Capillaries becoming distinct

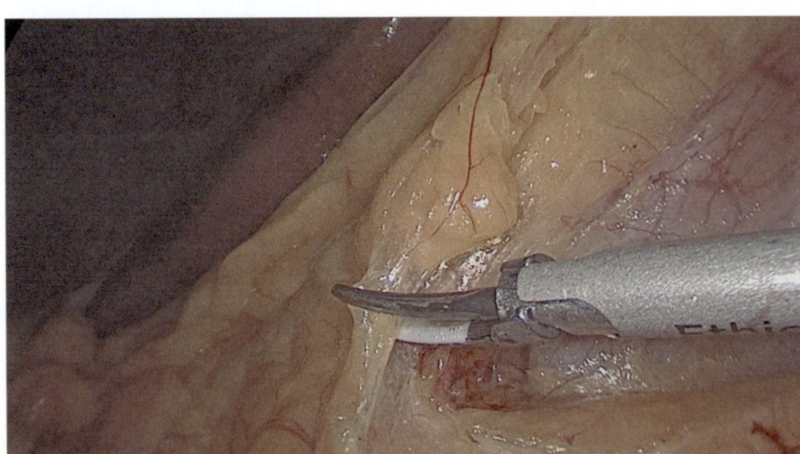

Fig. 3.124 The non-functional face of the ultrasonic scalpel is distinct

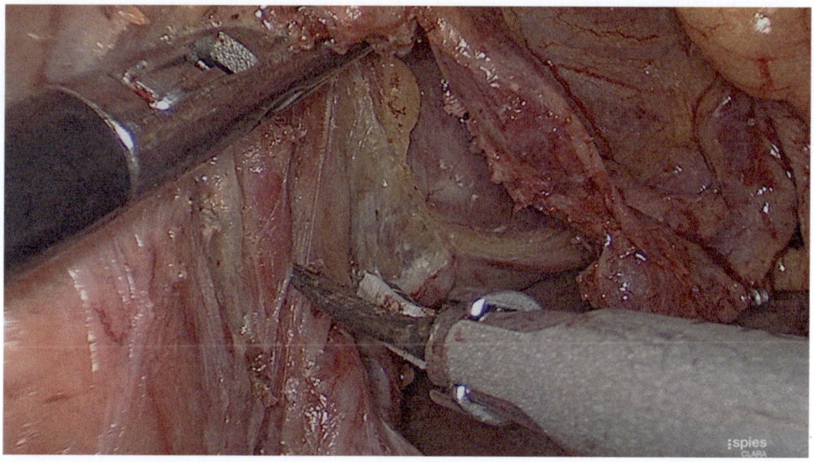

Fig. 3.125 The assistant lifts the posterior wall of the gastric antrum right upwards with the forceps in the left hand, and pushes the duodenum outwards with the other hand to expose the CHA, the GDA, and the partially vascularized PHA

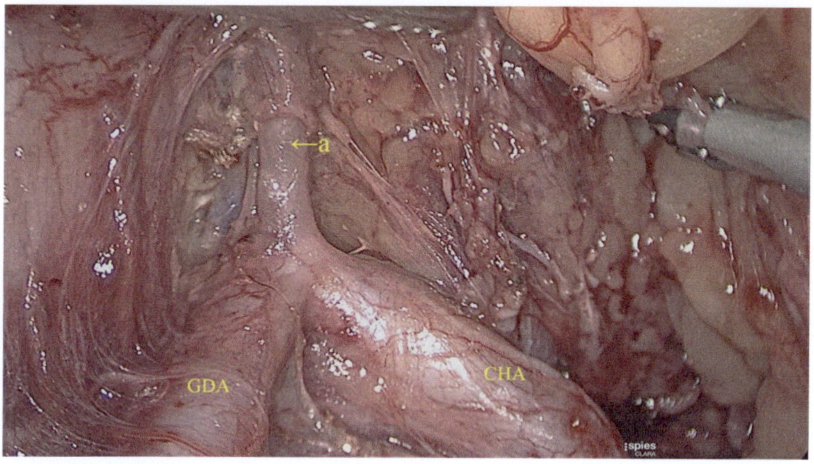

Fig. 3.126 The RGA (**a**) along the vertical path with the pull of the gastric antrum

When the RGA is severed, the anterior lobe of the HLD can be completely dissociated by continuing along the surface of the PHA. Opening a window on the right side of the free HLD serves as a landmark to separate the dissociated ligament from the ventral side later (Figs. 3.127 and 3.128).

It is difficult to open a window in patients with partial obesity or inflammatory adhesions on the right edge of the hepatogastric ligament. In such cases, a gauze can be placed in front of the PHA to mark the ligaments of the liver and stomach, and avoid damage from separating the common bile duct (Figs. 3.129 and 3.130).

Because of the deep position and the small operating space, the camera assistant should adjust the direction of the optical fiber to prevent it being blocked by other instruments (Fig. 3.131).

RGA: Right gastric artery; CHA: Common hepatic artery.

RGA: Right gastric artery; PHA: Proper hepatic artery; SpA: Splenic artery; LGA: Left gastric artery.

The PHA is the main anatomic marker for the dissection of No. 12a LNs. After vascularizing the CHA, the initial segment of the PHA can be exposed by continuing to the right side. No. 12a LN dissection is achieved after the PHA has been

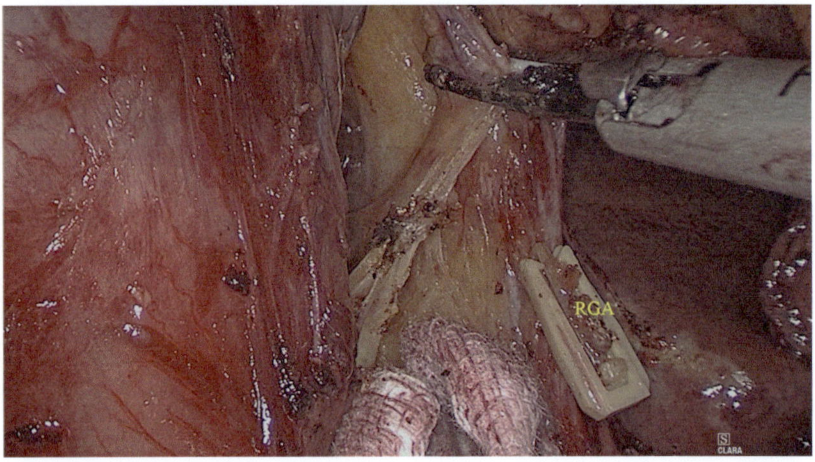

Fig. 3.127 Open a window on the right side of the dissociated anterior lobe of the HDL

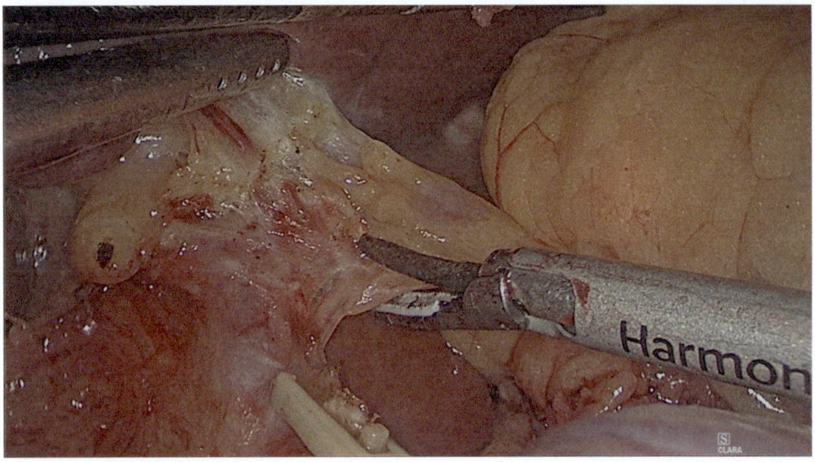

Fig. 3.128 The anterior lobe of the HDL is divided through the window

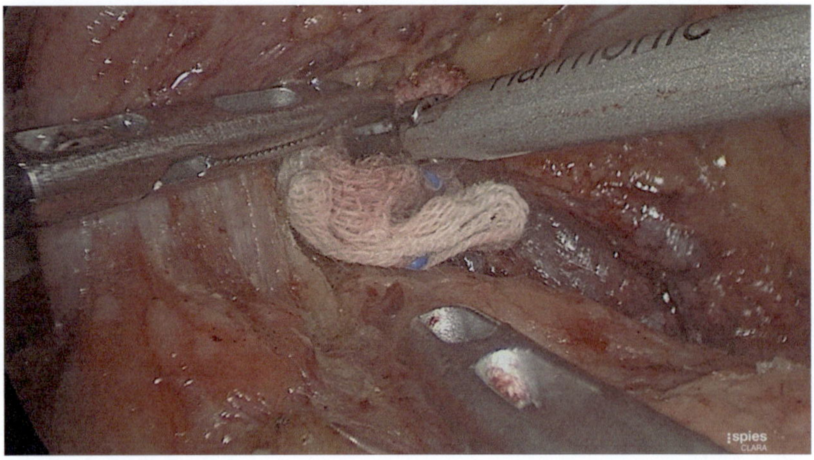

Fig. 3.129 A gauze is stuffed in front of the PHA as a landmark to separate the HDL

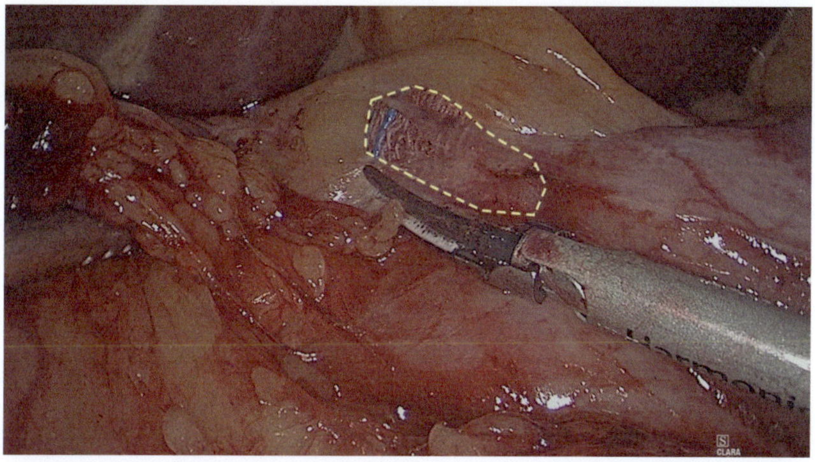

Fig. 3.130 Placing a gauze in front of the PHA can prevent the separation plane from being too deep

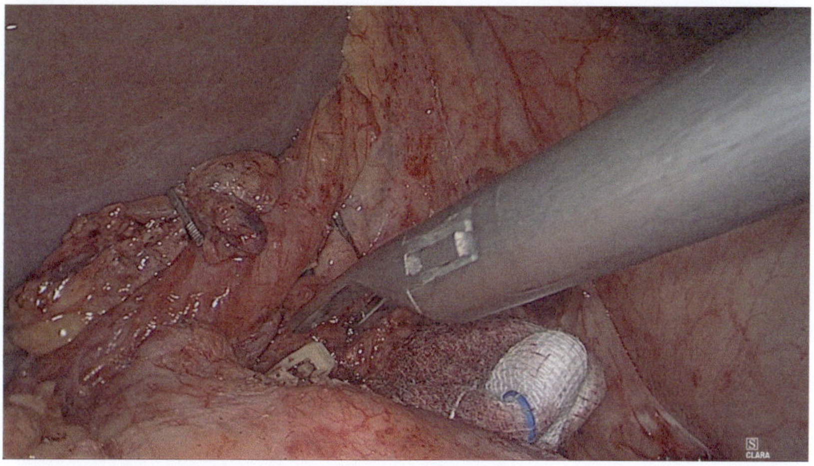

Fig. 3.131 The camera assistant should adjust the orientation of the optical fiber to avoid obscuring with a titanium clip applier

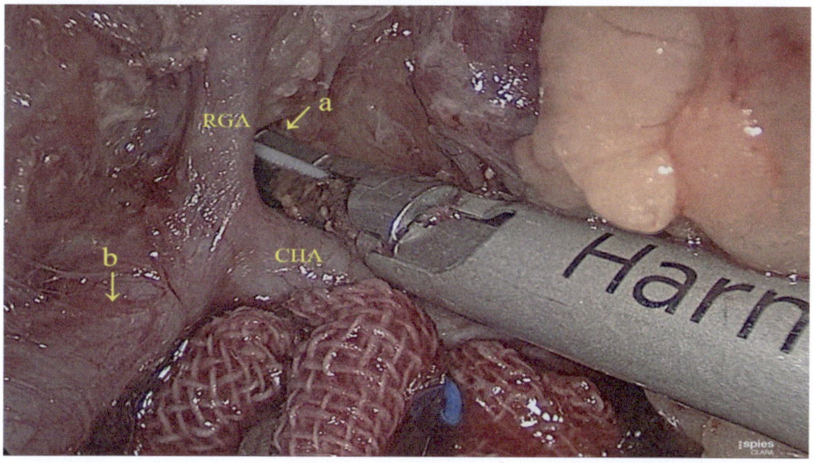

Fig. 3.132 The RGA originates from the angle between the PHA (**a**) and the GDA (**b**)

vascularized from the origin to the porta hepatis (Figs. 3.132 and 3.133).

When denuding the duodenum, the small vessels that branch off from the GDA and supply the posterior wall of the duodenum should be divided carefully. These vessels should be occluded sufficiently with ultrasonic scalpels and then severed with minimum speed (Fig. 3.134).

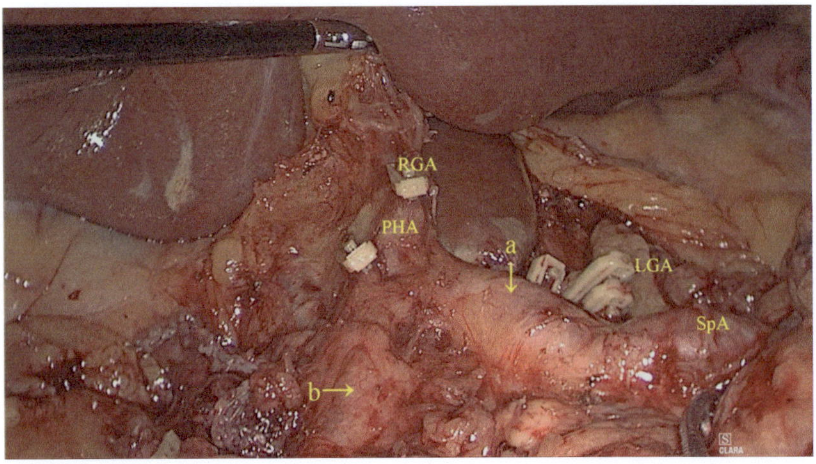

Fig. 3.133 After exposure of the origin of the GDA (**b**) from the CHA (**a**), the PHA is exposed

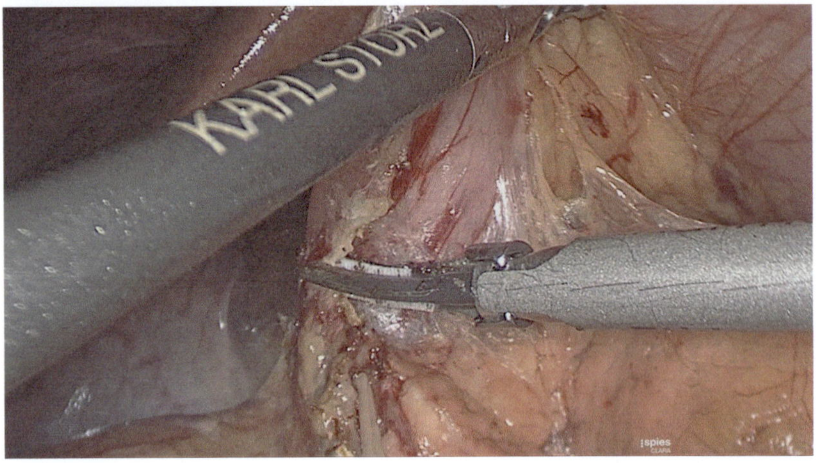

Fig. 3.134 Denuding the posterior wall of the duodenum, and the complete clamping of small vessels with an ultrasonic scalpel

When the assistant elevates the gastric antrum, the thin and long PHA may be incorrectly identified as the RGA (Fig. 3.135).

The hepatic branch of the vagus nerve is relatively enlarged in some patients. In such cases, it should be cut off first to facilitate exposure of the RGA (Fig. 3.136).

RGA: Right gastric artery; RGV: Right gastric vein.

Most RGVs are accompanied by RGAs so can be clipped together (Fig. 3.137). Sometimes the RGA (a) and RGV (b) are located far from each other, so should be separately ligated (Fig. 3.138).

LHA: Left hepatic artery.

When separating the HDL, attention should be paid to whether there are ALGAs or ALHAs. ALGAs can be cut off at the initial segment of origin (Figs. 3.139 and 3.140).

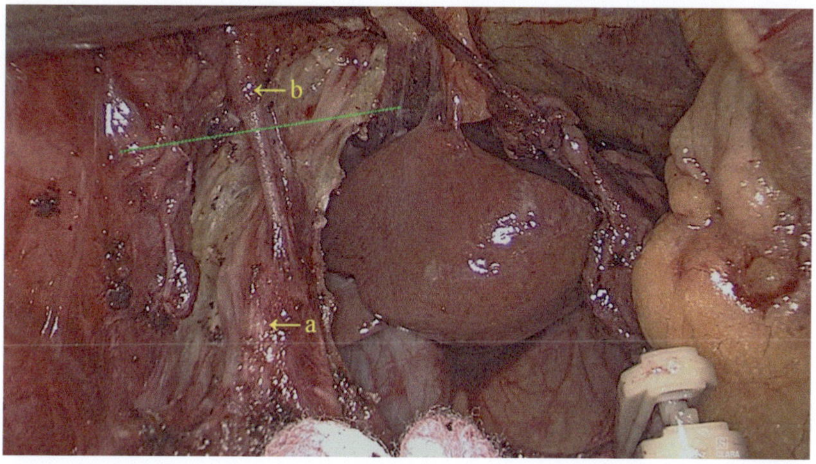

Fig. 3.135 The PHA (**a**) will form an angle with the elevation of the RGA (**b**), and the RGA should be severed at the plane of the green dotted line

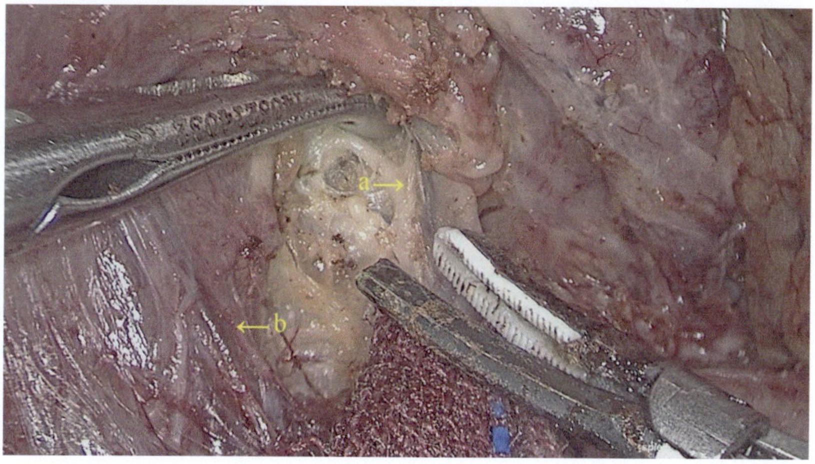

Fig. 3.136 The enlarged hepatic branches of the vagus nerve (**a**) are difficult to distinguish from the RGA (**b**)

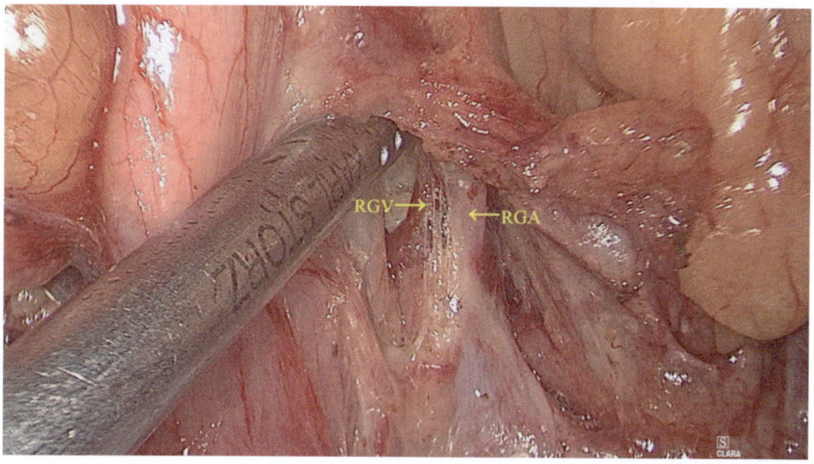

Fig. 3.137 The RGV accompanies the RGA

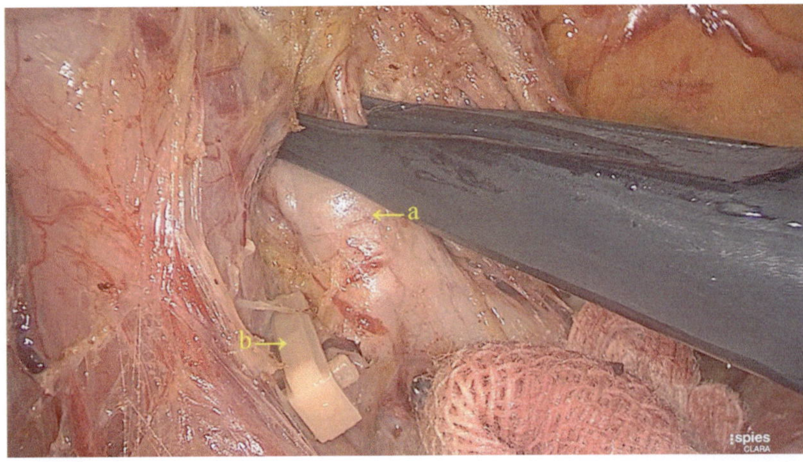

Fig. 3.138 The RGA (**a**) and RGV (**b**) can be located far from each other, so should be separately ligated

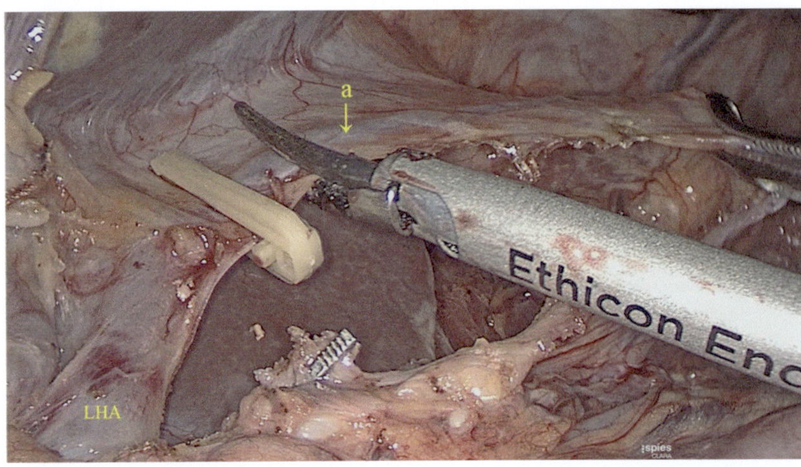

Fig. 3.139 The ALGA (**a**) is severed at its segment of origin

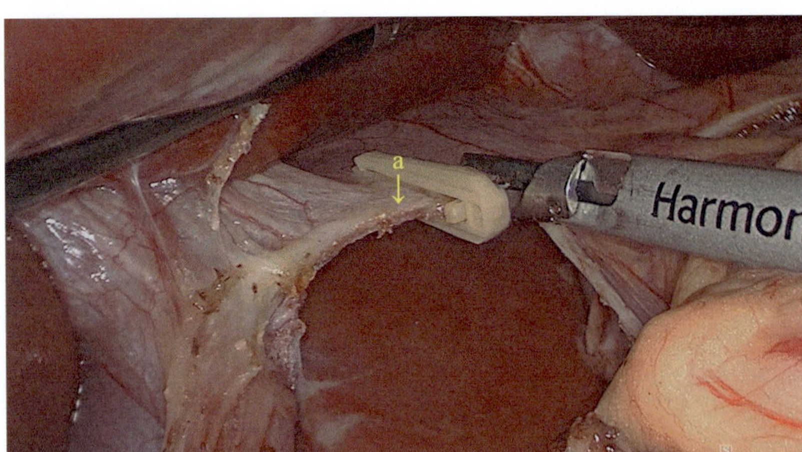

Fig. 3.140 A thin ALHA (**a**) can be severed at the inferior margin of the liver

Clarification

All images of the chapter come from FuJian Medical University gastric surgery database and video database.

References

1. Huang C-M, Zheng C-H, editors. Laparoscopic gastrectomy for gastric cancer: Springer; 2015.
2. Huang CM, Chen QY, Lin JX, et al. Short-term clinical implications of the accessory left hepatic artery in patients undergoing radical gastrectomy for gastric cancer. PLoS One. 2013;8(5):e64300.
3. Adachi B. Das Arteriensyste m der Japaner. Suppl To Acta Sch Med Univ Kyoto; 1928.

4 Laparoscopic Splenic Hilar Area LN Dissection for Gastric Cancer

4.1 Operative Steps for LN Dissection in the Splenic Hilar Area

LNs in the splenic hilar area (Fig. 4.1) consist of No. 4sb, 10, and 11d LNs. In clinical practice, we summarize a set of effective operative steps known as 'Huang's three-step maneuver' for laparoscopic spleen-preserving splenic hilar lymphadenectomy [2]. The first step is LN dissection in the inferior part of the spleen; the second step is LN dissection in the trunk of the SpA region; and the third step is LN dissection in the superior part of the spleen.

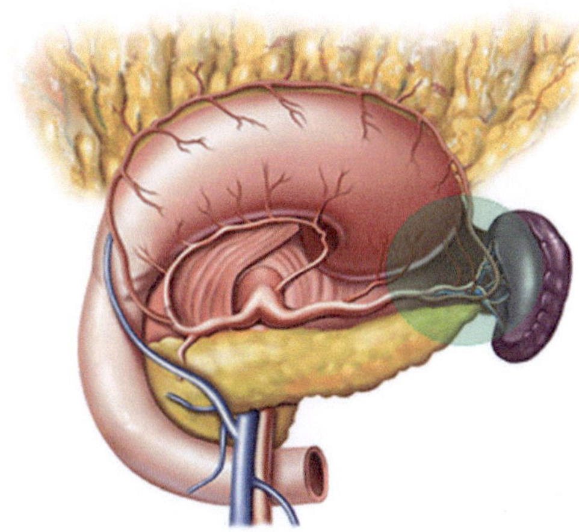

Fig. 4.1 Splenic hilar area (Reproduced with permission from [1])

4.1.1 Operative Approach

For splenic hilar LN dissection, we use the left-side approach [2, 3], which involves separating the membrane of the pancreas from the upper margin of the pancreas tail into the posterior space of the pancreas to expose the end of the splenic vessel trunk (Fig. 4.2) [4, 5]. During LN dissection in the splenic hilar, we do not first cut off the GSL, which has the advantage of allowing the assistant to fully pull the GSL to expose the splenic hilar [6] and to maintain good tension. It is advantageous for the surgeon to dissect the splenic portal vessels and to stop bleeding quickly once the splenic vessels are damaged or splenic hemorrhage occurs.

4.1.2 Exposure Methods

Corresponding to the operative procedure 'Huang's three-step maneuver' for LN dissection in the splenic hilar area, the assistant's exposure mode is mainly divided into three steps. The first

C.-M. Huang et al., *Atlas of Laparoscopic Gastrectomy for Gastric Cancer*,
https://doi.org/10.1007/978-981-13-2862-6_4

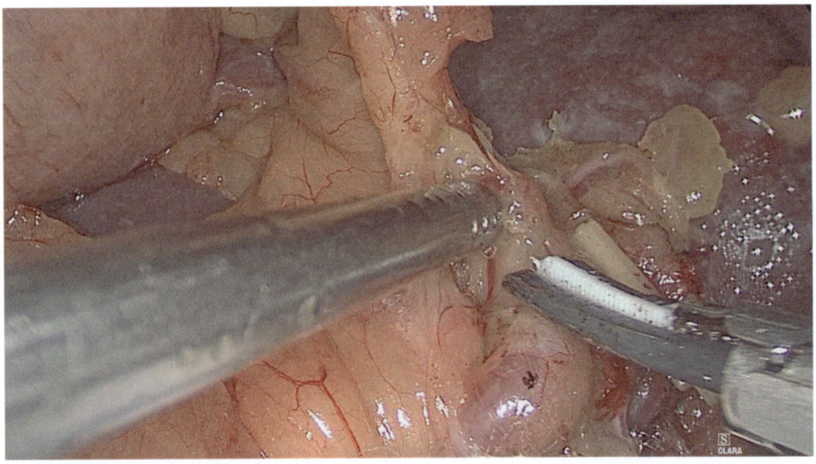

Fig. 4.2 The end of the splenic vessel trunk is exposed at the superior margin of the pancreas tail via the left-side approach

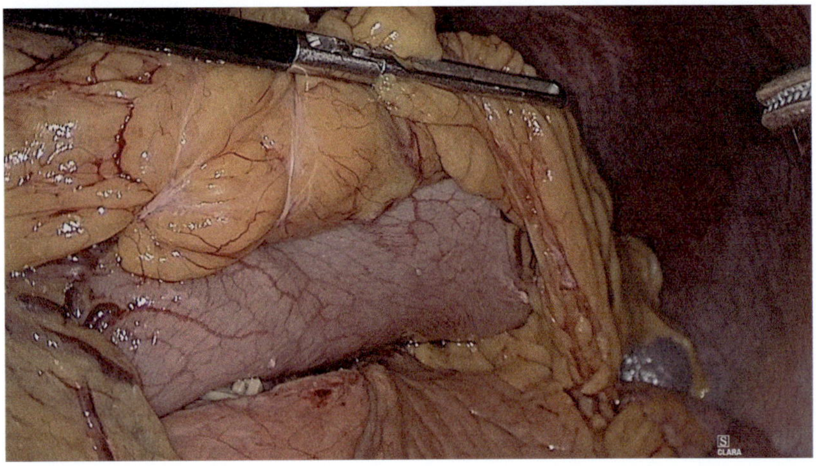

Fig. 4.3 First step: exposure of the inferior pole region of the spleen

step is to dissect LNs in the inferior pole region of the spleen: the assistant places the free omentum tissue on the right upper abdomen and the anterior wall of the stomach, and the left hand lifts up the initial segment of the GSL. The surgeon gently presses the lower margin of the body and tail of the pancreas to reveal the region of the inferior pole of the spleen with a small gauze (Fig. 4.3).

The second step is to dissect the LNs in the trunk of the splenic artery: the assistant places the free omentum and part of the GSL between the anterior wall of the stomach and the inferior margin of the liver, and their left hand pulls the posterior wall of the great curvature of the fundus of the stomach to the upper right to turn and tighten the remaining GSL. The SpA region of the retropancreatic space is further exposed by pressure of the surgeon's left hand on the body of the pancreas (Fig. 4.4).

The third step is to dissect the LNs of the superior pole region of the spleen: the assistant clamps the great curvature of the stomach fundus and pulls to the lower right with their left hand. The surgeon compresses the vessels of the splenic hilar with their left hand to fully reveal the superior pole region of the spleen. During the operative procedure, the right hand of the assistant can use different methods, including picking, lifting, holding, pushing, and peeling, to assist the surgeon in completing the splenic hilar LN dissection.

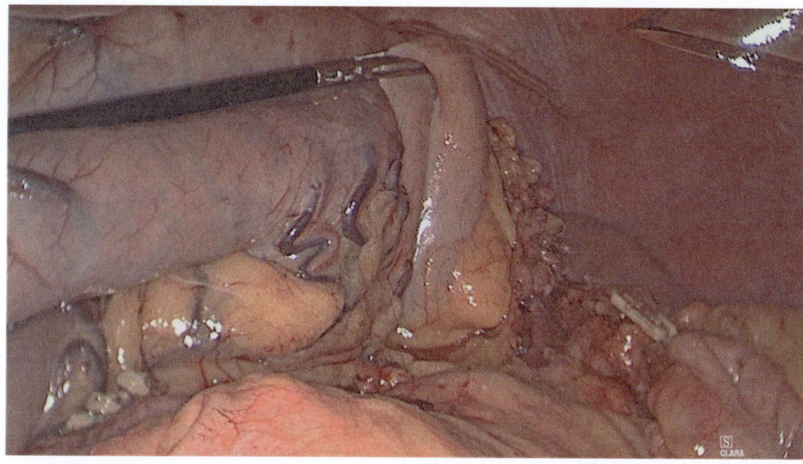

Fig. 4.4 Second step: exposure of the SpAT region

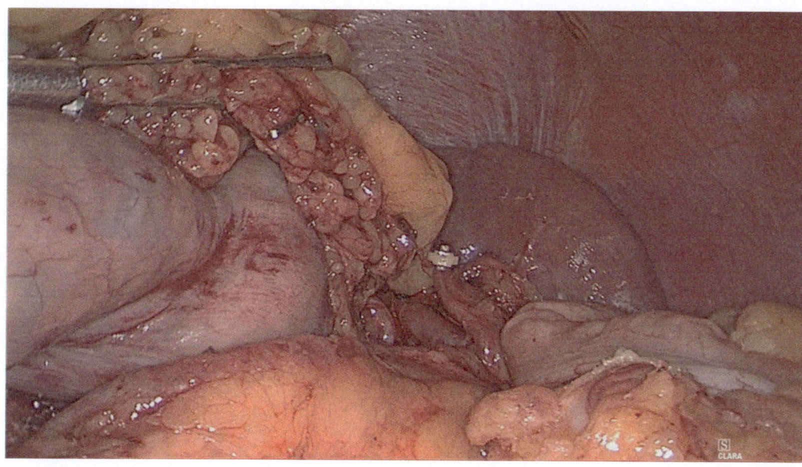

Fig. 4.5 Third step: exposure of the superior pole region of the spleen

4.1.3 Operative Procedures

In the first step, LNs are dissected in the inferior pole region of the spleen: the greater omentum is separated to the left by an ultrasound scalpel along the upper margin of the transverse colon until the splenic curvature of the colon (Fig. 4.6). Then the pancreatic capsule is removed to the superior margin of the pancreas tail in the direction of the anterior inherent pancreatic fascia (Figs. 4.7 and 4.8).

SpV: Splenic vessel.

LLVS: Lower lobar vessels of the spleen.

The APF is opened by the surgeon's ultrasonic scalpel along the continuation of the fascia, and the space is entered between the splenorenal ligament (SRL) and the GSL along the RPS. The end of the SpV trunk is exposed at the first segment of the GSL (Fig. 4.9). Further exposure of the LLVSs or the lower pole vessels of the spleen (LPVSs) is followed by the end of the splenic vessels (Fig. 4.10).

During the dissection, the roots of the LGEVs are generally exposed at the splenic lobar artery (SLA) or the splenic lower pole artery (SLPA) near the lower pole of the spleen (Fig. 4.11).

LGEV: Left gastroepiploic vessel.

LGEV: Left gastroepiploic vessel.

LGEV: Left gastroepiploic vessel.

The assistant lifts the fatty lymphatic tissue around the root of the LGEVs, and the surgeon's ultrasound scalpel vascularizes it along

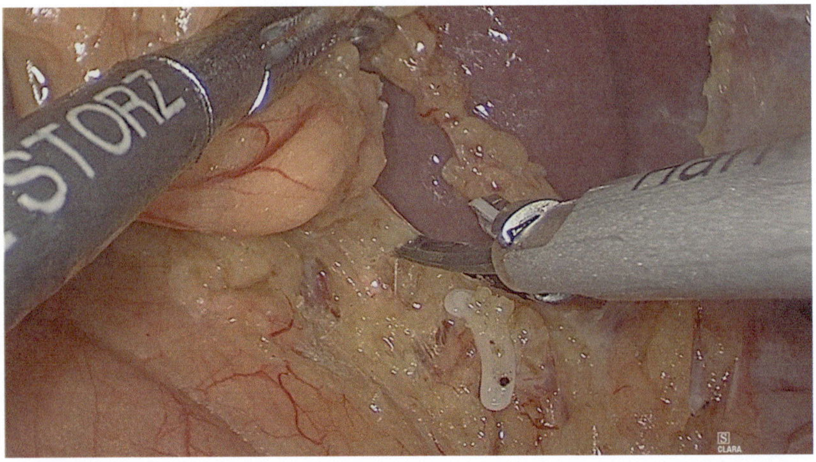

Fig. 4.6 Separation of the greater omentum to the splenic flexure of the colon

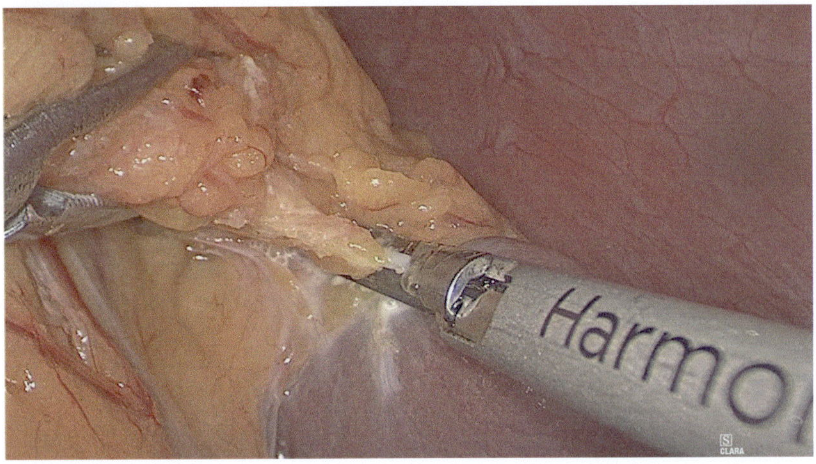

Fig. 4.7 Separation of adhesions in the splenic region

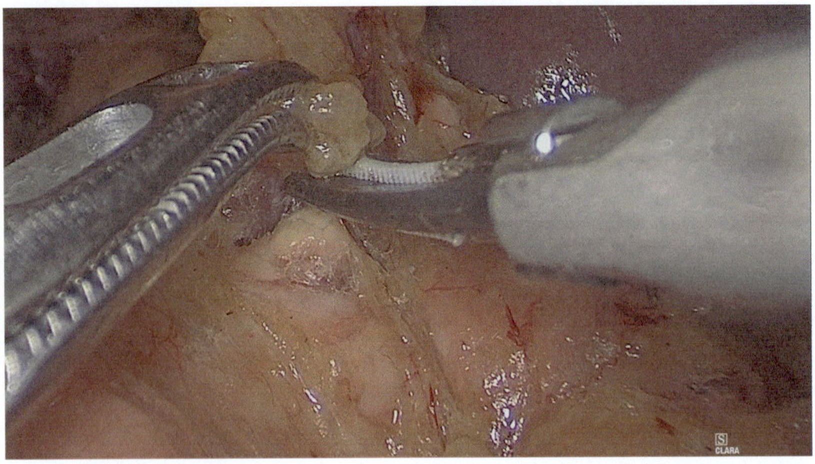

Fig. 4.8 Dissecting the posterior pancreatic fascia to the superior margin of the pancreas tail

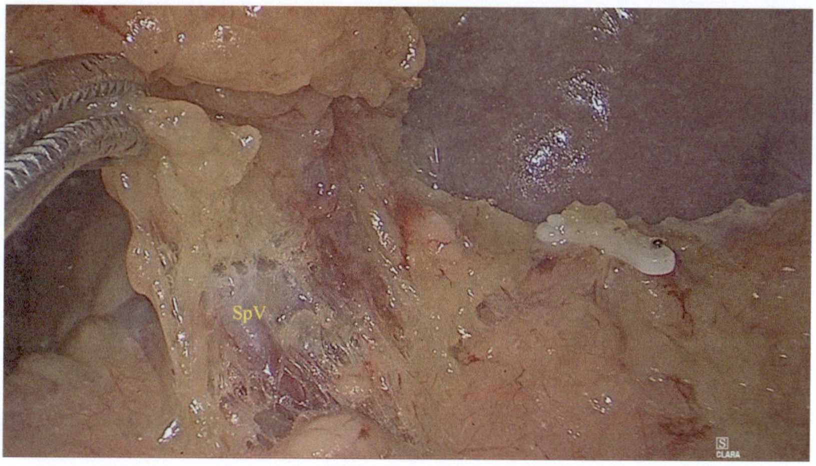

Fig. 4.9 Exposure of the end of the SpV trunk in the RPS

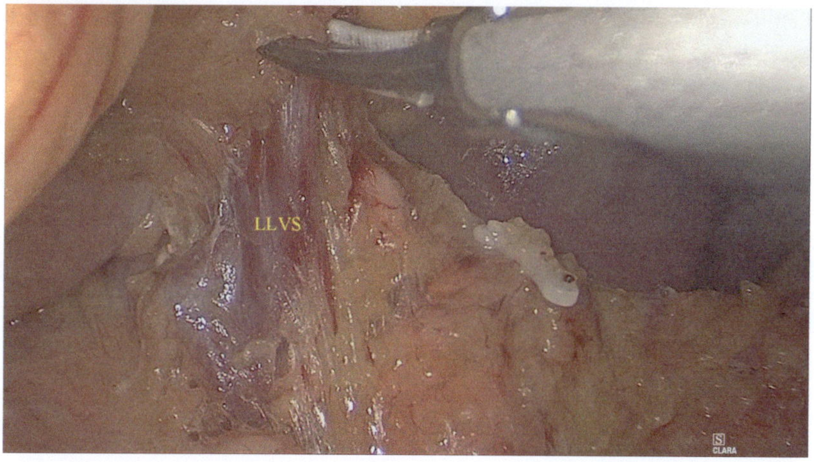

Fig. 4.10 Exposure of the LLVS

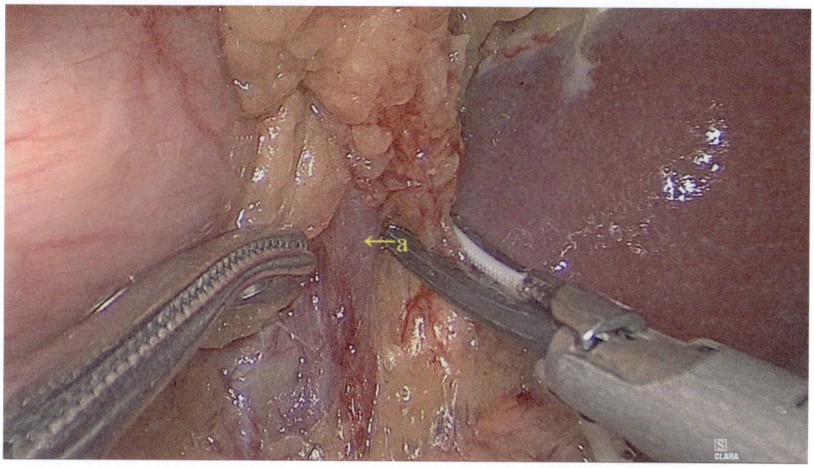

Fig. 4.11 Exposure of the root of the left gastroepiploic vessel (LGEV) (**a**)

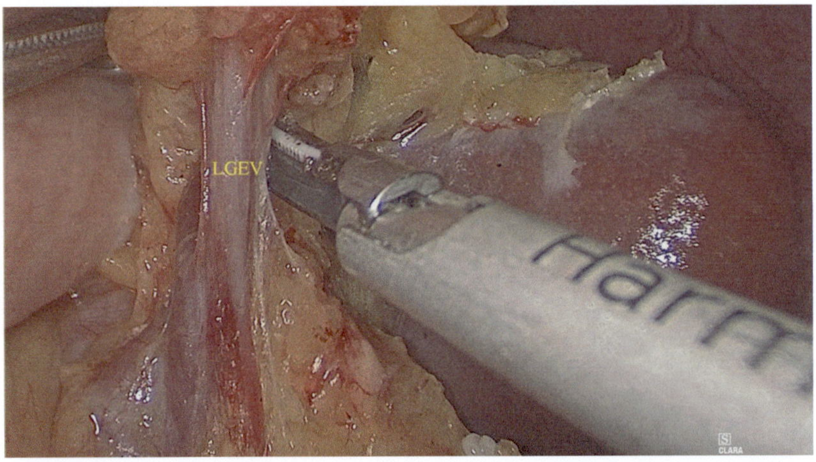

Fig. 4.12 The LGEVs are exposed along the anatomic space at the surface of the vessel

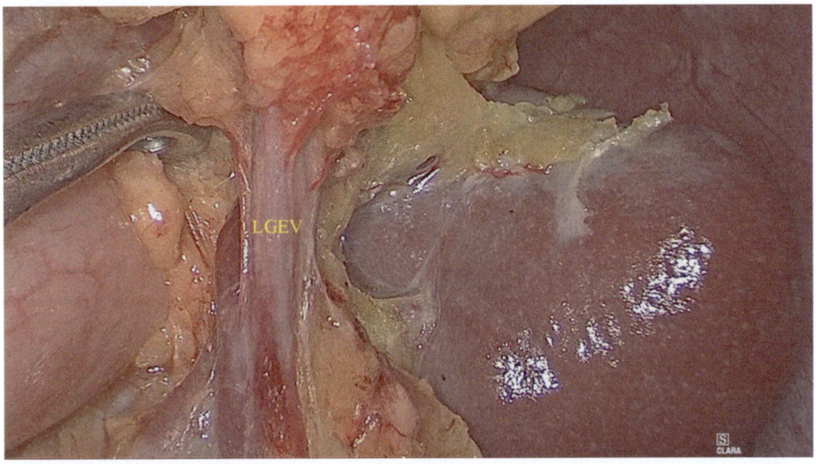

Fig. 4.13 The isolated LGEVs are lifted by the assistant

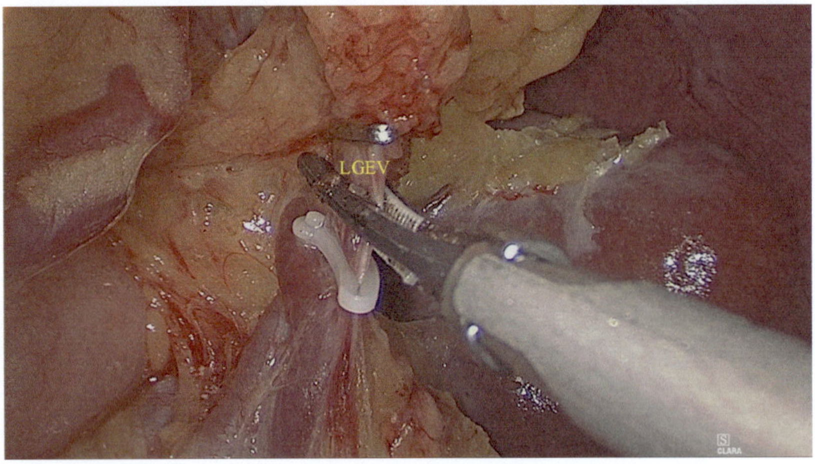

Fig. 4.14 The LGEVs are severed at their roots

the anatomic space of the vascular surface (Figs. 4.12 and 4.13). Then, the vessel at the root of the LGEVs is dissected (Fig. 4.14) to complete the dissection of No. 4sb LNs.

SGV: Short gastric vessel.

The assistant lifts the fatty lymphatic tissue on the surface of the LLVSs, and the surgeon's ultrasonic scalpel continues along the anatomic space of the surface of the LLVSs to carefully and meticulously blunt and sharply separate towards

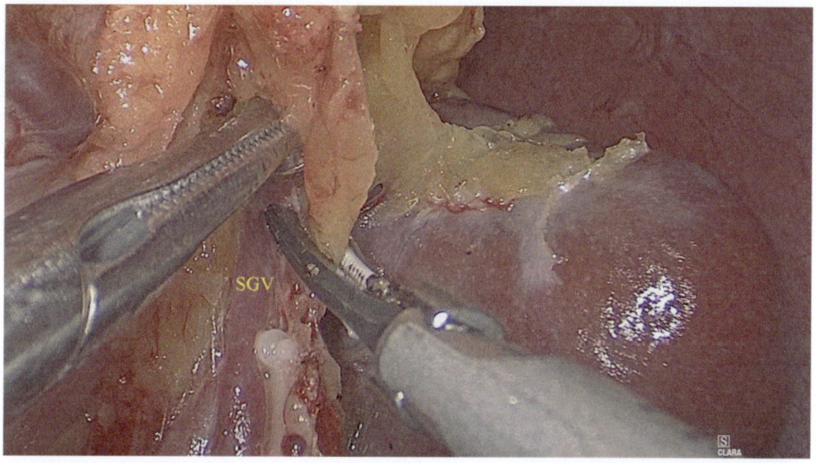

Fig. 4.15 Exposure of the first branch of the SGVs

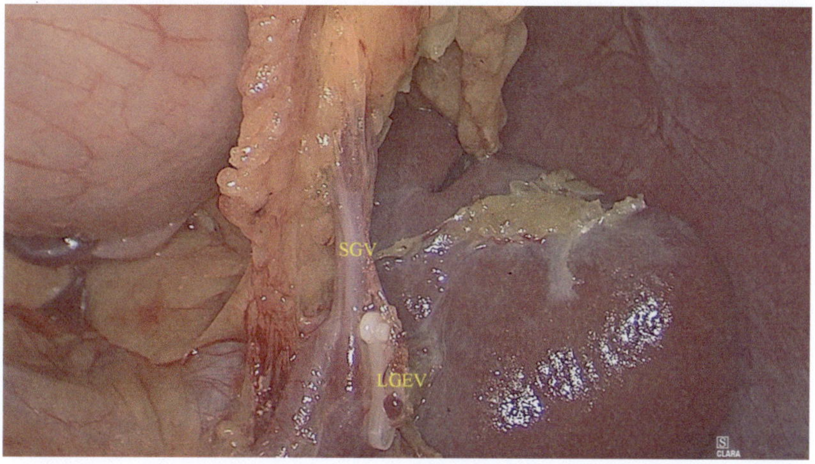

Fig. 4.16 The first branch of the SGVs is bare

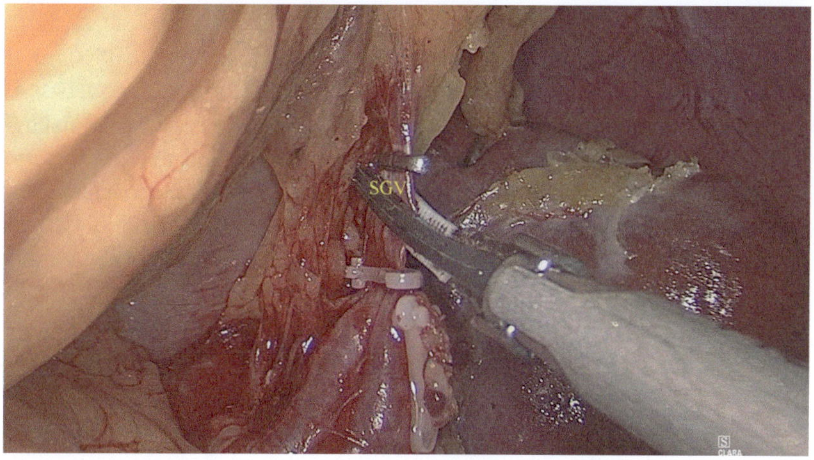

Fig. 4.17 The first branch of the SGVs is severed

the splenic hilar. During the dissection, one to three branches of the SGVs may be encountered from the inferior lobar artery of the spleen (ISLA) (Fig. 4.15).

SGV: Short gastric vessel; LGEV: Left gastroepiploic vessel.

SGV: Short gastric vessel.

The assistant gently lifts the SGVs, and the surgeon's ultrasound scalpel carefully separates the fatty lymphatic tissue around the SGVs. After this (Fig. 4.16), the vessels are severed at their roots with vascular clamps (Fig. 4.17).

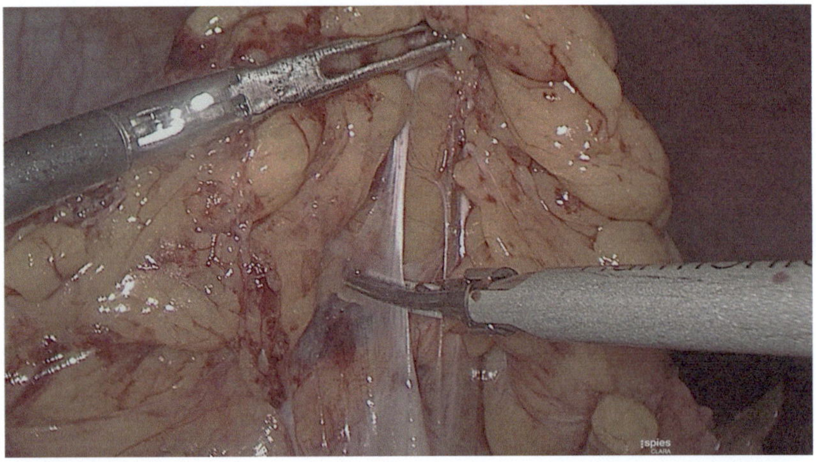

Fig. 4.18 The greater omentum is tensioned and opened by the surgeon's ultrasonic scalpel in the vascularized area

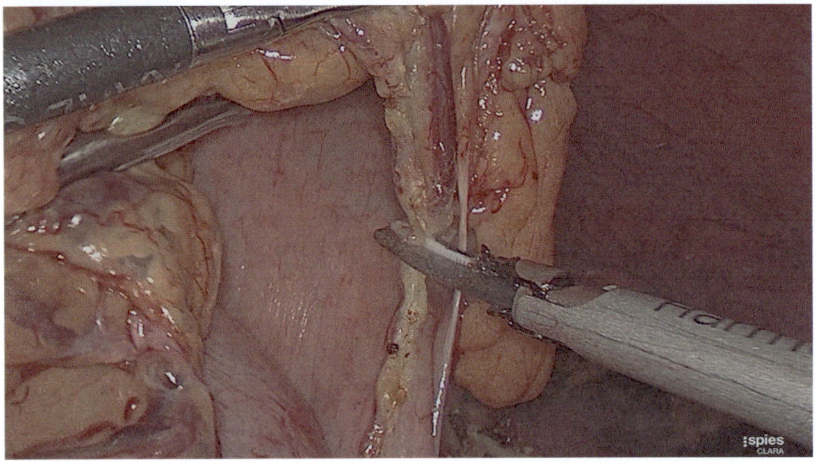

Fig. 4.19 Baring of the gastric great curvature is against the wall of the stomach

LGEV: Left gastroepiploic vein.

For patients undergoing distal subtotal gastrectomy, just one or two branches of the SGVs should continue to be disconnected from the LGEVs. Then the stomach should be returned to its natural position. The assistant lifts up the greater omentum tissue at the middle part of the greater curvature of the gastric body. The surgeon pulls the posterior wall of the stomach down to tighten the greater omentum. The surgeon's ultrasound scalpel opens the greater omentum of the great curvature of the stomach in the avascular area (Fig. 4.18). Next, the greater omentum, the vessels, and their branches are separated close to the gastric wall along the greater curvature of the stomach (Fig. 4.19). At this point, the great curvature of the stomach is exposed (Fig. 4.20).

SpA: Splenic artery.

In the second step, LNs in the region of trunk of the SpAT are dissected: the assistant's right hand pulls the isolated lymphatic tissue on the surface of the SpA. The surgeon's ultrasonic scalpel vascularizes the trunk of the SpA along the latent anatomic space of the SpA surface to the fork of the splenic lobar arteries. Then, the fatty lymphatic tissue around the end of the SpA is cleared (Fig. 4.21).

PGV: Posterior gastric vessel; SpA: Splenic artery.

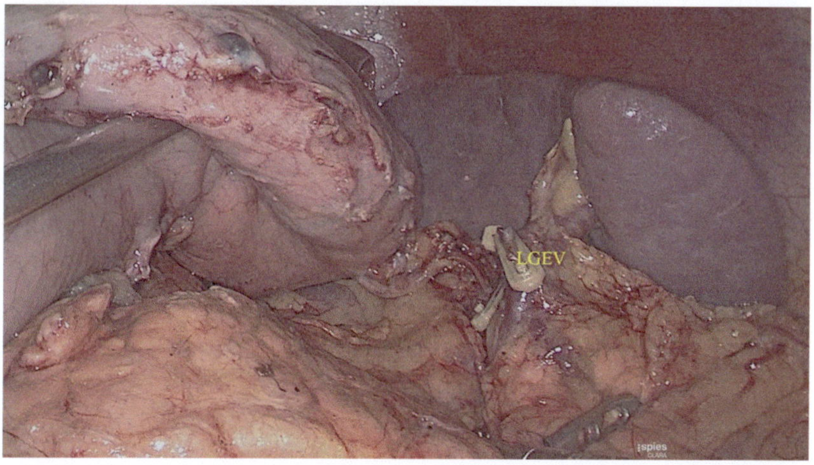

Fig. 4.20 The greater curvature of the stomach is bared

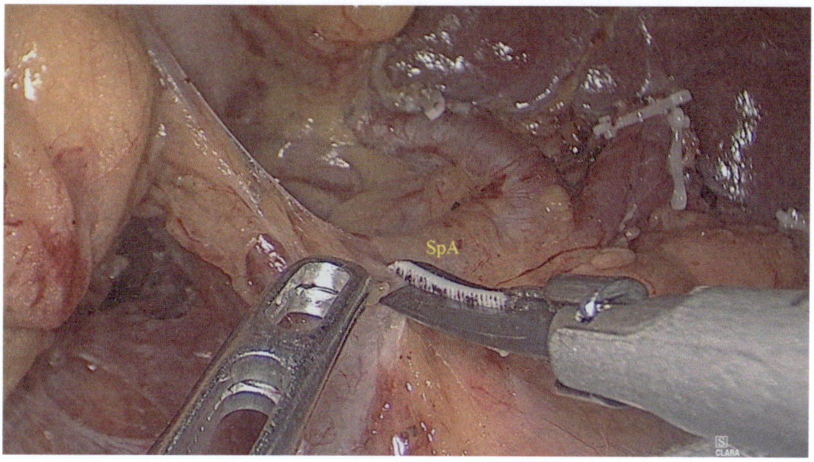

Fig. 4.21 Dissection of LNs at the distal end of the SpA

PGV: Posterior gastric vessel; SpA: Splenic artery.

During the dissection, PGVs from the SpA are often encountered. The assistant clamps the PGVs and pulls them upwards. The surgeon's ultrasound scalpel dissects the fatty lymphatic tissue around the PGVs close to the trunk of the SpA (Fig. 4.22). Then, the PGVs are cut off at their root with vascular clamps (Fig. 4.23). This completes the dissection of No. 11d LNs.

SGV: Short gastric vessel.

SGV: Short gastric vessel; SpA: Splenic artery.

SGV: Short gastric vessel.

SpA: Splenic artery; SpV: Splenic vein.

SGV: Short gastric vessel.

In the third step, the LNs in the superior pole region of the spleen are dissected: the assistant gently lifts the fatty lymphatic tissue on the surface of the branches of the splenic vessels in the GSL. The surgeon uses the non-functional surface of the ultrasound scalpel along the anatomic space on the surface of the splenic lobar artery and vein to completely vascularize vessels in the splenic superior lobar area using meticulous sharp or blunt pushing, peeling, and dissection (Figs. 4.24

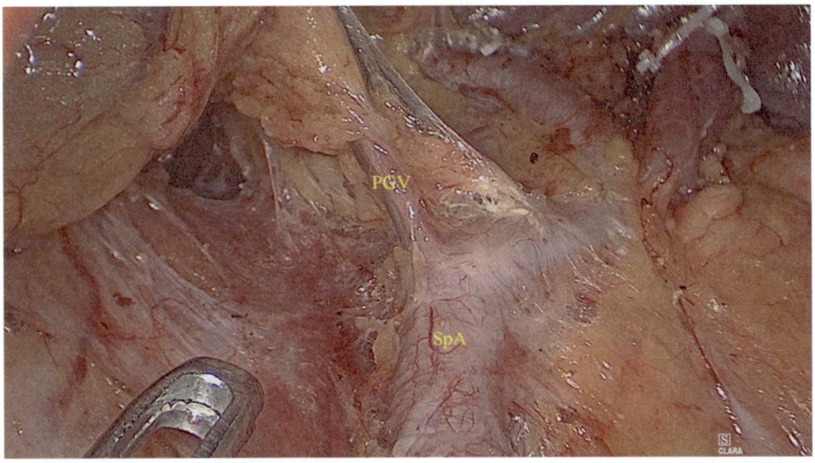

Fig. 4.22 The PGV is exposed and bare

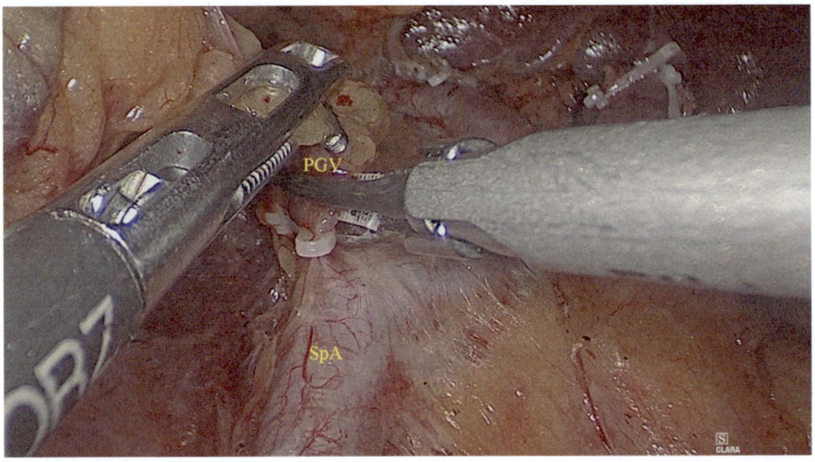

Fig. 4.23 The PGV is severed at its root

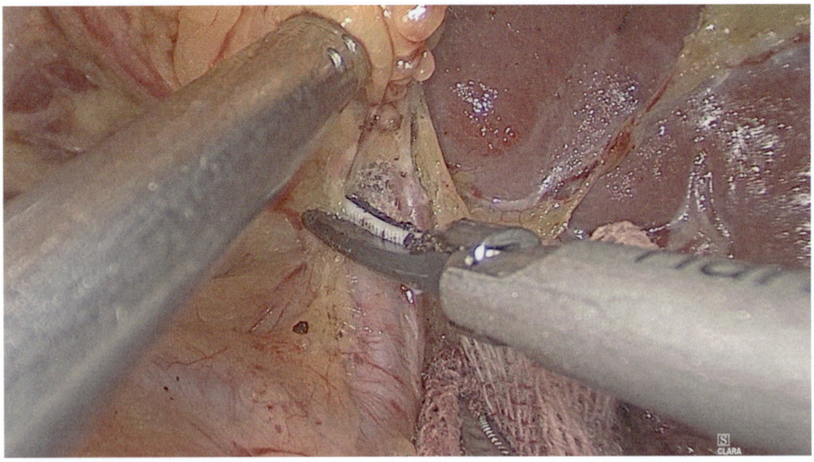

Fig. 4.24 The region of the superior lobar of the spleen is peeled sharply along the lobar vessels

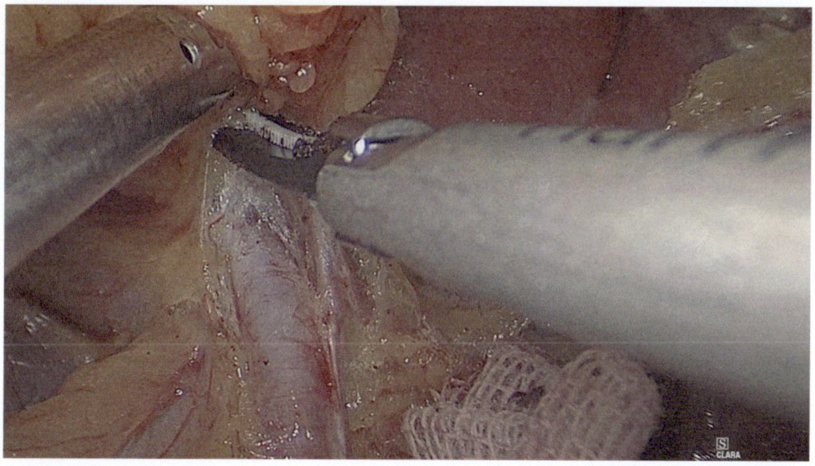

Fig. 4.25 The region of the superior lobar of the spleen is peeled bluntly along the lobar vessels

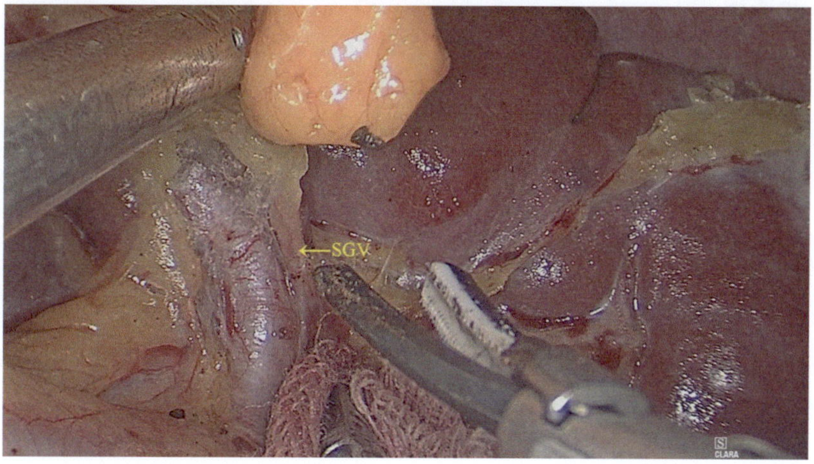

Fig. 4.26 Exposure of the second branch of the SGVs

and 4.25). During the dissection, one to three branches of the SGVs from the SLA often appear in the GSL (Figs. 4.26, 4.27, 4.28, and 4.29). The assistant should hold the SGVs and pull them upwards, while the surgeon's ultrasonic scalpel meticulously dissects the surrounding fatty lymphatic tissue, proceeding towards the roots of the vessels (Fig. 4.30).

SGV: Short gastric vessel.

SGV: Short gastric vessel.

The last SGV at the superior pole region of the spleen is usually short, making the fundus close to the splenic hilar (Fig. 4.31), and bleeding occurs easily if it is pulled incorrectly. At this time, the assistant should draw the gastric fundus towards the upper right side to fully expose the vessel, while the surgeon carefully dissects the surrounding fat lymphatic tissue and clamps and disconnects the blood vessels at their roots (Fig. 4.32).

SGV: Short gastric vessel; LGEV: Left gastroepiploic vessel; PGV: Posterior gastric vessel; LGA: Left gastric artery; SpA: Splenic artery.

SGV: Short gastric vessel; LGEV: Left gastroepiploic vessel; PGV: Posterior gastric vessel; SpA: Splenic artery.

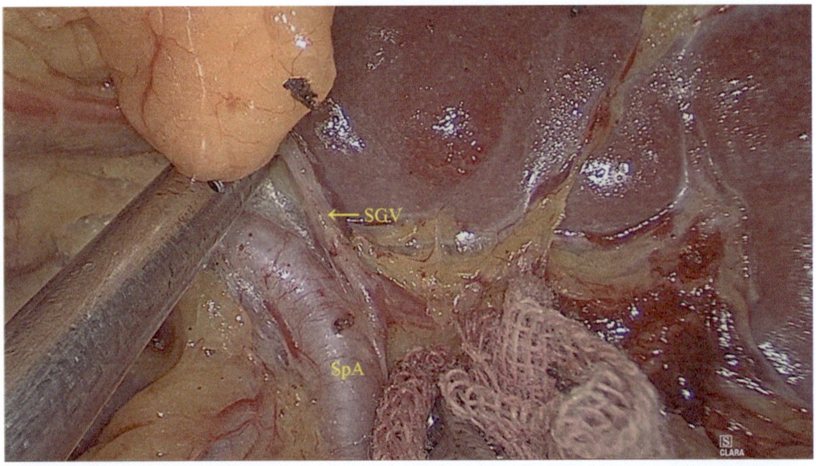

Fig. 4.27 The second branch of the SGVs is vascularized

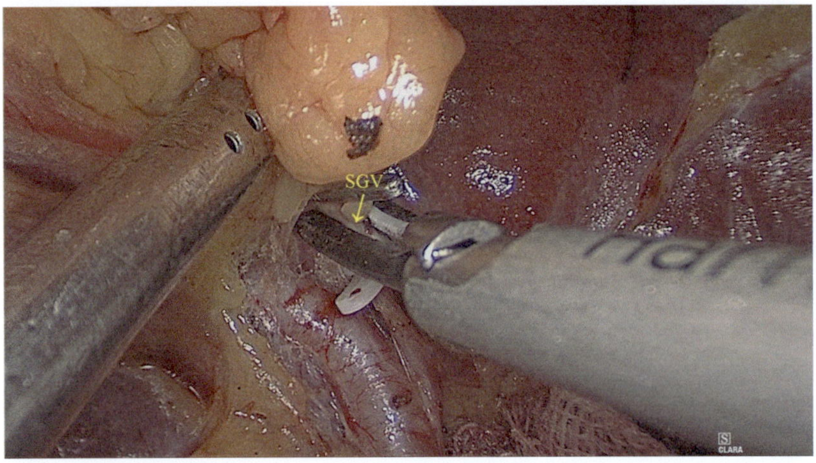

Fig. 4.28 The second branch of the SGVs is severed

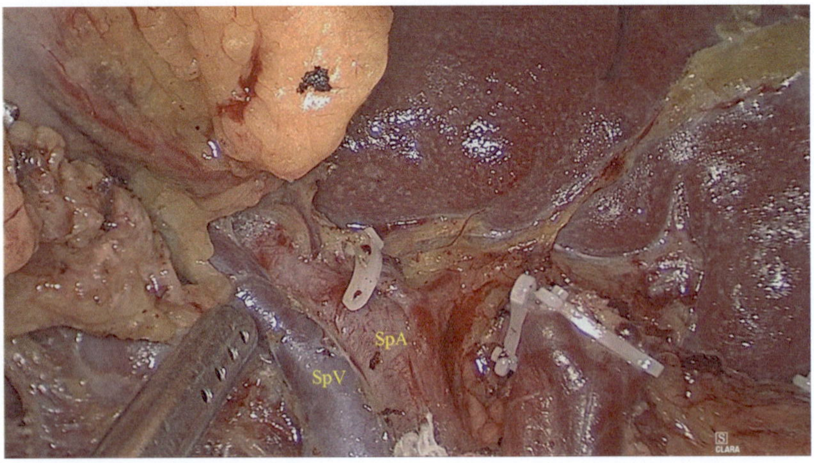

Fig. 4.29 The separation and exposure of the third branch of the SGVs

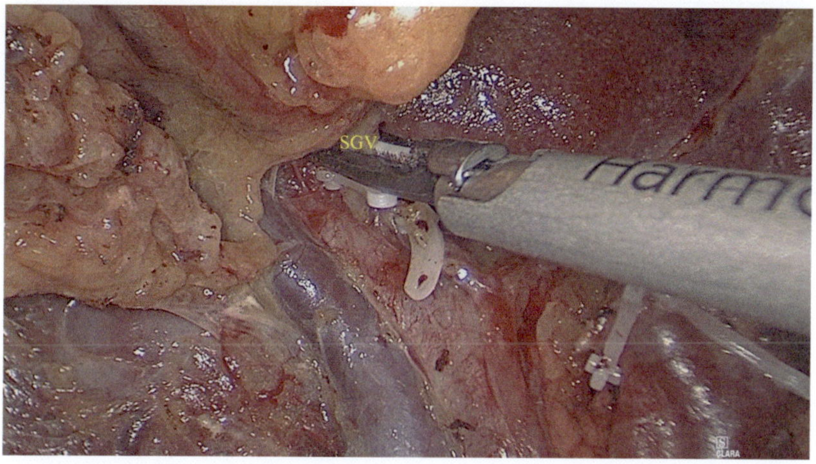

Fig. 4.30 The third branch of the SGVs is severed at its root

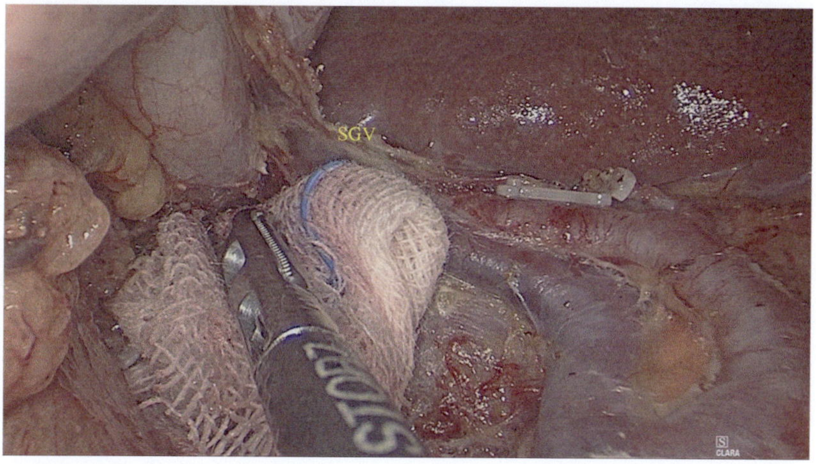

Fig. 4.31 The last SGV in the superior splenic pole region of the spleen is separated and exposed

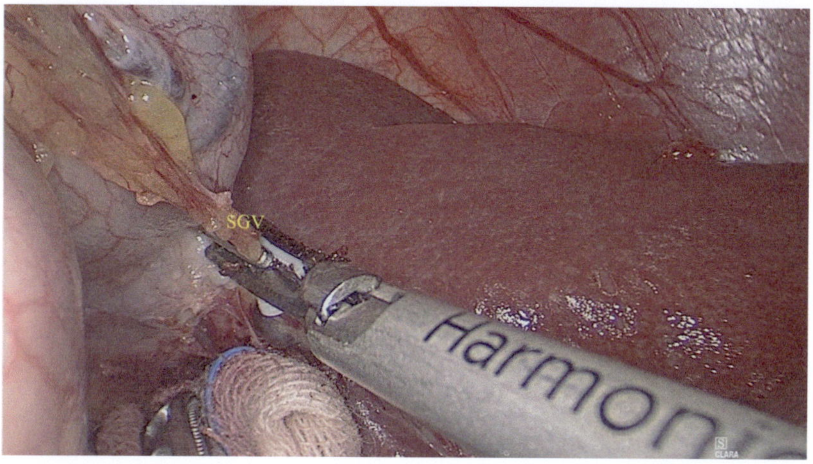

Fig. 4.32 The last SGV is cut off at its root in the superior pole region of the spleen

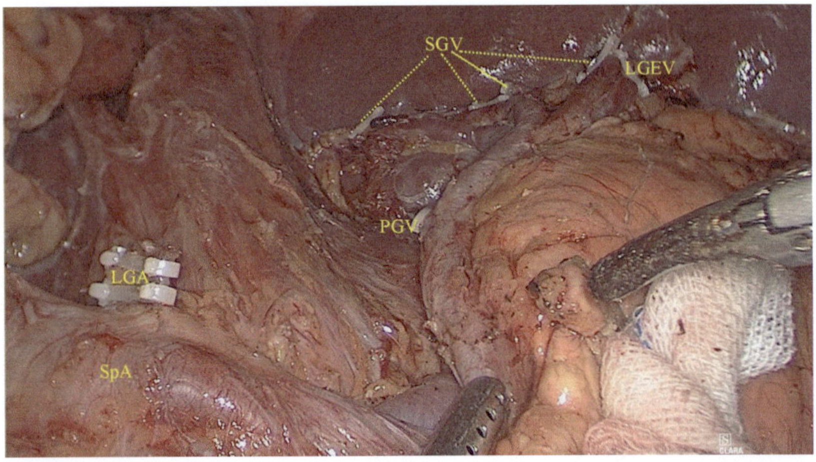

Fig. 4.33 Dissection of the SpA trunk region is completed

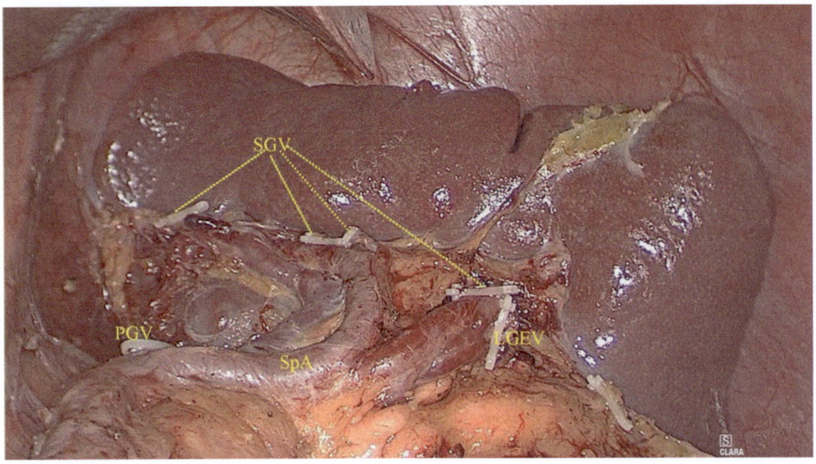

Fig. 4.34 Dissection of LNs in the splenic hilar area is completed

4.2 Operative Announcements of Laparoscopic Splenic Hilar Area LN Dissection for Gastric Cancer

4.2.1 Anatomy Associated with LN Dissection in the Splenic Hilar Area

4.2.1.1 Fascia and Intrafascial Space in the Splenic Hilar Area

Gastrosplenic and Splenorenal Ligaments

The spleen is connected with the stomach above the pancreas by the GSL (Figs. 4.35 and 4.36), while the spleen is connected with the kidney at the lateral abdominal wall by the SRL (Fig. 4.37).

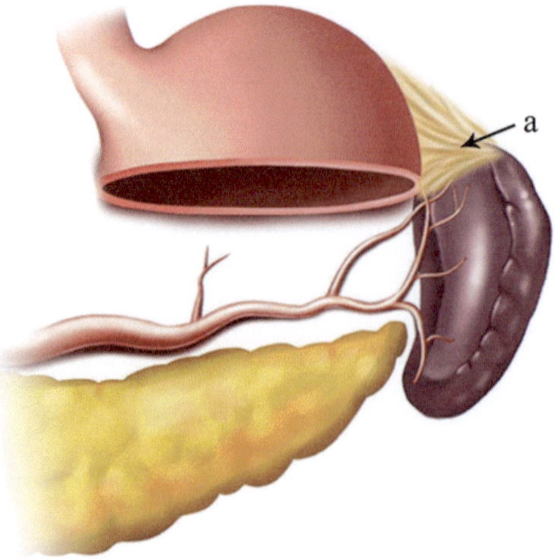

Fig. 4.35 The GSL (**a**) (Reproduced with permission from [1])

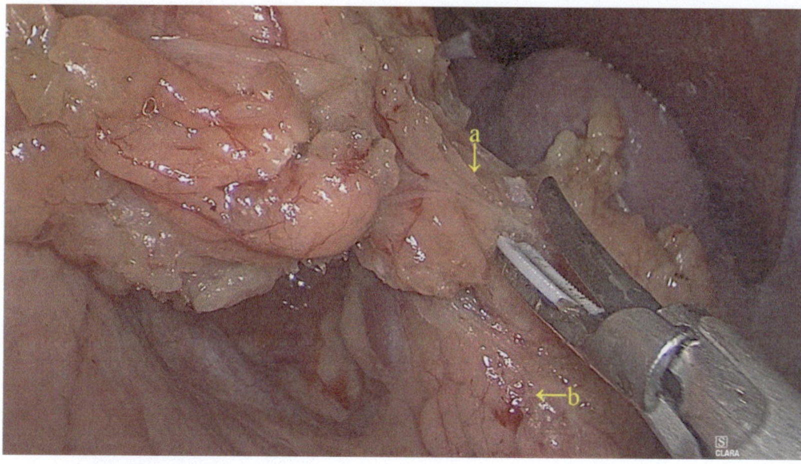

Fig. 4.36 The GSL (**a**) and the pancreastic tail (**b**)

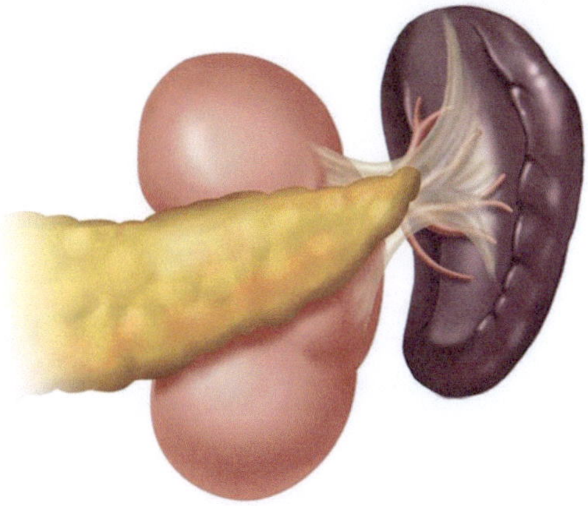

Fig. 4.37 Schematic of the SRL (Reproduced with permission from [1])

The front of the GSL is continuous with the APF at the pancreatic tail. By opening the AFP at the tail of the pancreas, the space in the GSL can be entered along the space above the pancreas. Ligaments around the splenic hilar can be dissected to expose the terminal branches of the SpA and the origin of the LGEA (Figs. 4.38, 4.39, and 4.40).

Toldt's Space (TS) and Gerota's Fascia

LGEV: Left gastroepiploic vessel; SpA: Splenic artery; PGA: Posterior gastric artery; SGV: Short gastric vessel.

TS is a complete boundary between the retropancreatic fascia and Gerota's fascia, which is widely distributed. The posterior area of the space is the prerenal fascia covering the left adrenal gland, left kidney, and renal vessels, and the posterior part of the pancreatic body and tail. The anterior inferior part communicates with the transverse colonic intrafascial space (Fig. 4.41).

4.2.1.2 Arterial Anatomy Associated with LN Dissection in the Splenic Hilar Area

SpA

SpV: Splenic vein; SGV: Short gastric vessel.

SGV: Short gastric vessel; LGEA: Left gastroepiploic artery; LPVS: lower pole vessels of the spleen

The SpA derives from the CA, which traverses left along the upper margin of the pancreas and emits the great pancreatic artery, caudal pancreatic artery, and several small arteries distributed in the parenchyma of the pancreas. It also emits the posterior gastric artery, short gastric artery, and the LGEA towards the posterior wall and the great curvature of the stomach (Figs. 4.42, 4.43, and 4.44).

Relationship Between the Course of the SpA and the Pancreas

The course of the SpA is closely related to the pancreas. According to the data of 319 patients undergoing laparoscopic spleen-preserving splenic hilar LN dissection in our institution, there are four common types of SpA:

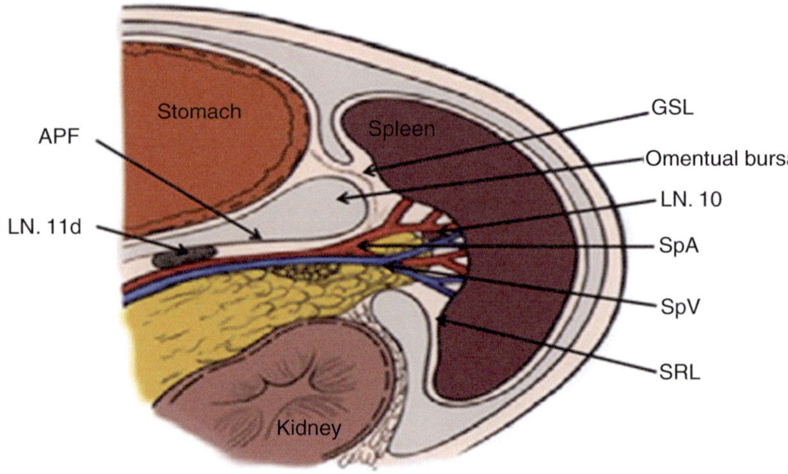

Fig. 4.38 The GSL and the SRL are mutually linked (Reproduced with permission from [1])

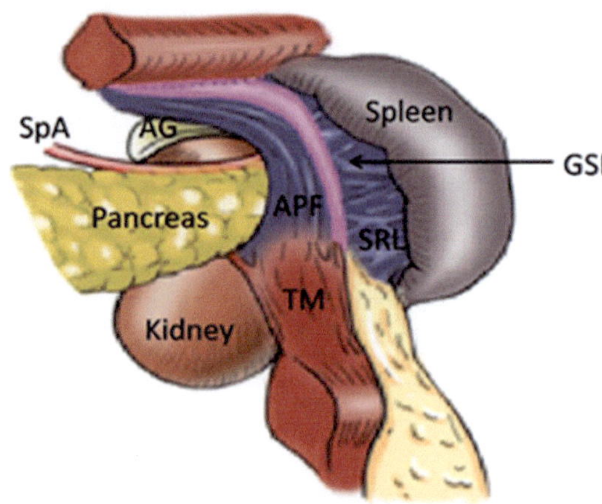

Fig. 4.39 The GSL and the SRL are mutually linked (Reproduced with permission from [1])

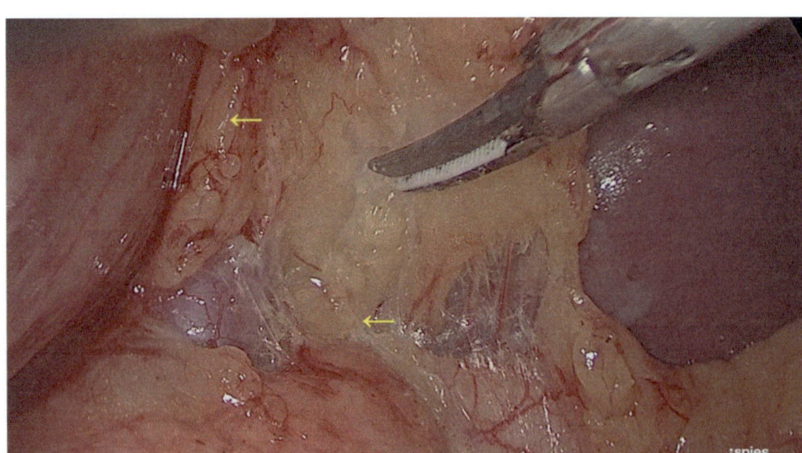

Fig. 4.40 The GSL and the SRL are mutually linked

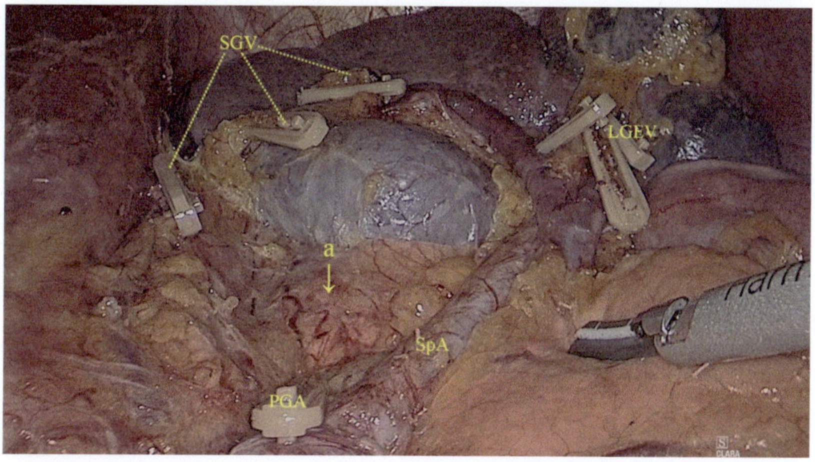

Fig. 4.41 Gerota's fascia (**a**)

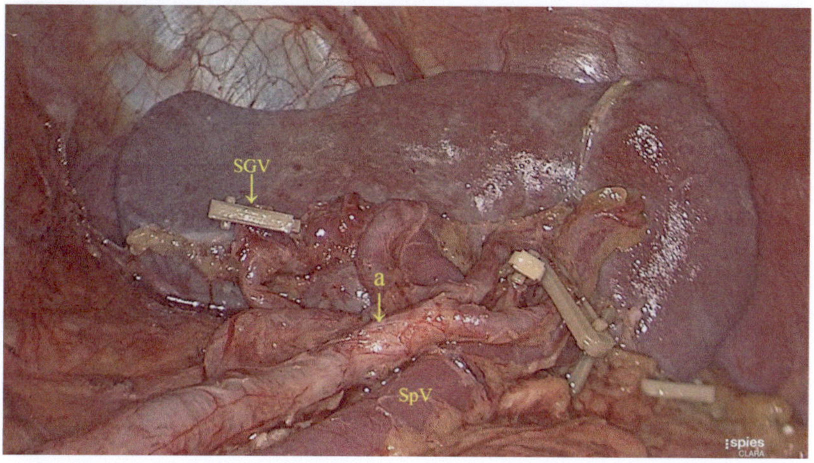

Fig. 4.42 SpA (**a**)

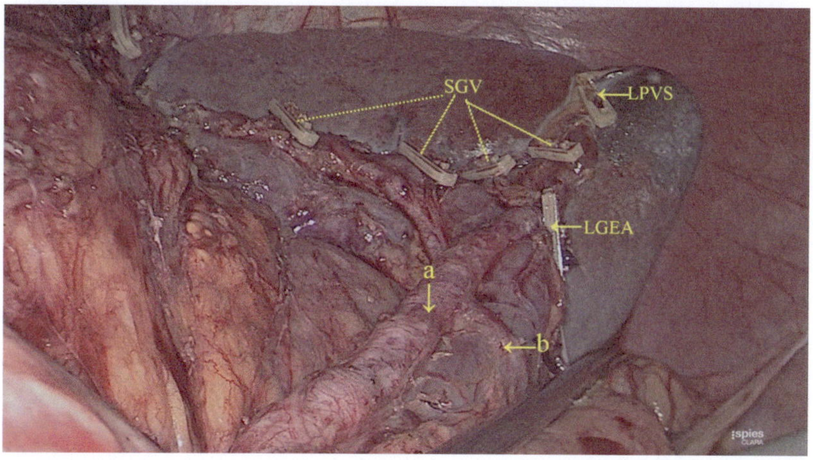

Fig. 4.43 Caudal pancreatic artery (**b**) from the SpA (**a**)

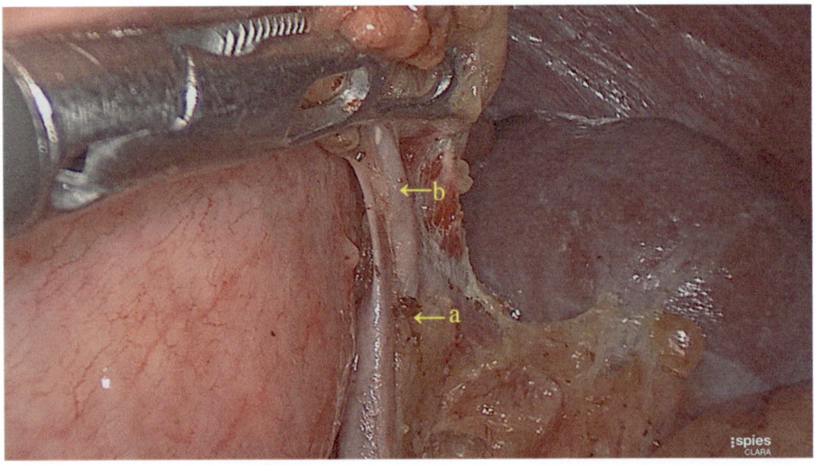

Fig. 4.44 The SpA (**a**) gives rise to the LGEA (**b**) before reaching the spleen

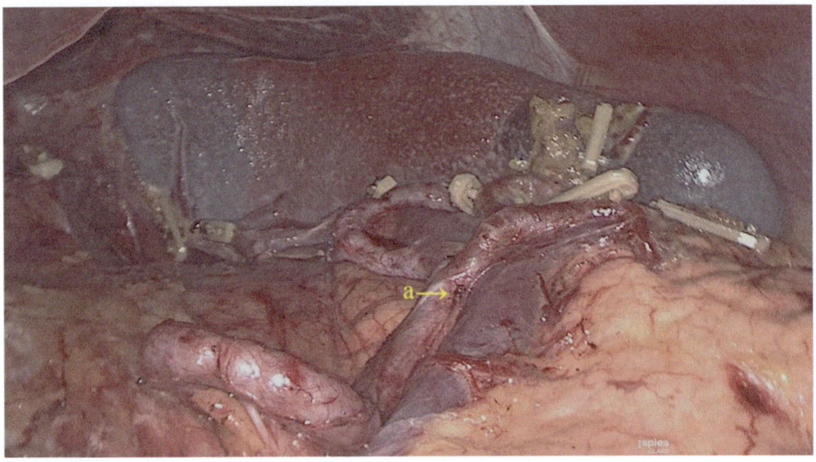

Fig. 4.45 Type I SpA (**a**)

Type I: the SpA derived from the CA to the splenic hilar along the suprapancreatic course in 87 cases (27.2%) (Fig. 4.45).

Type II: the middle half of the SPA took either a retro- or intrapancreatic course in 213 cases (66.8%) (Fig. 4.46);

Type III: the distal half of the SPA followed either a retro- or intrapancreatic course in 13 cases (4.1%) (Fig. 4.47);

Type IV: the distal three-fourths of the SpA were entirely embedded in the substance of the pancreas or followed a retropancreatic course in six cases (1.9%) (Fig. 4.48).

Branches of the SpA

SLA

The SLA is the terminal branch of the SpA at the splenic hilar. According to the data of 319 patients in our department, it is anatomically divided into four types:

Rare one-branched type: the SpA passed tortuously through the splenic hilar without dividing into terminal branches in 22 cases (6.9%) (Fig. 4.49);

Two-branched type: the superior lobe and inferior lobe of splenic artery were dissected by the SpA at the splenic hilar in 252 cases (79.0%) (Fig. 4.50).

Three-branched type: the superior lobar arteries, middle lobar arteries, and inferior lobar arteries of the spleen were disposed by the SpA in the splenic hilar in 43 cases (13.5%) (Fig. 4.51);

Rare multiple branched type: the SpA dissected from the splenic door producing 4-7 branches into the spleen in 2 cases (0.6%) (Fig. 4.52).

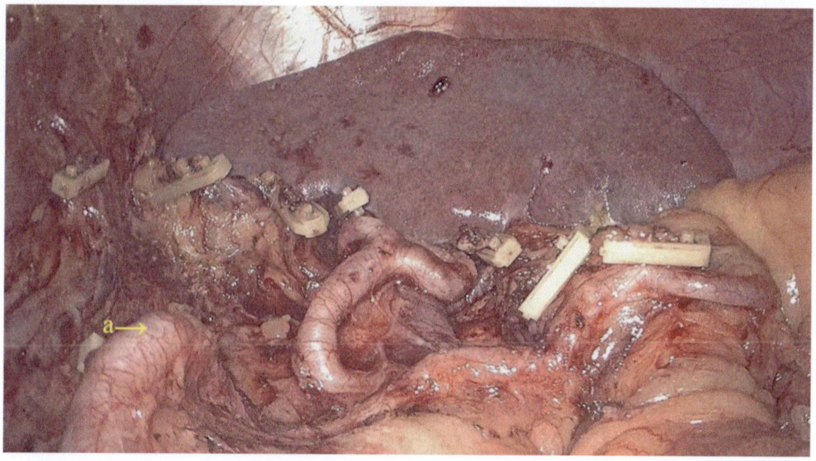

Fig. 4.46 Type II SpA (**a**)

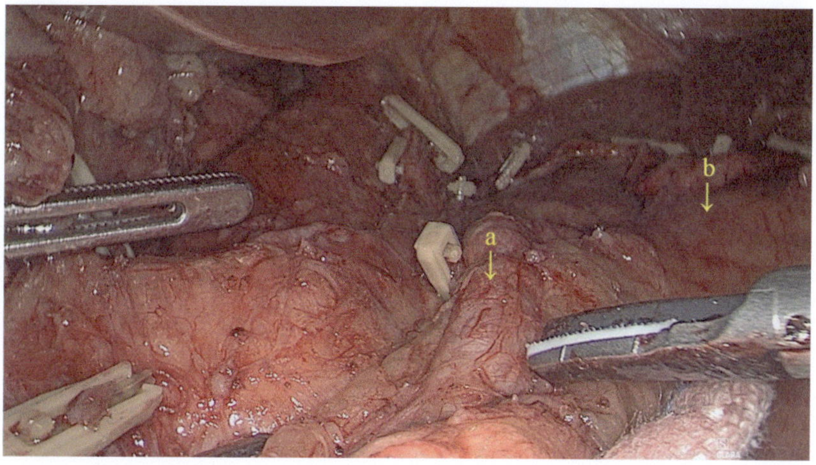

Fig. 4.47 Type III SpA (**a**), pancreatic tail (**b**)

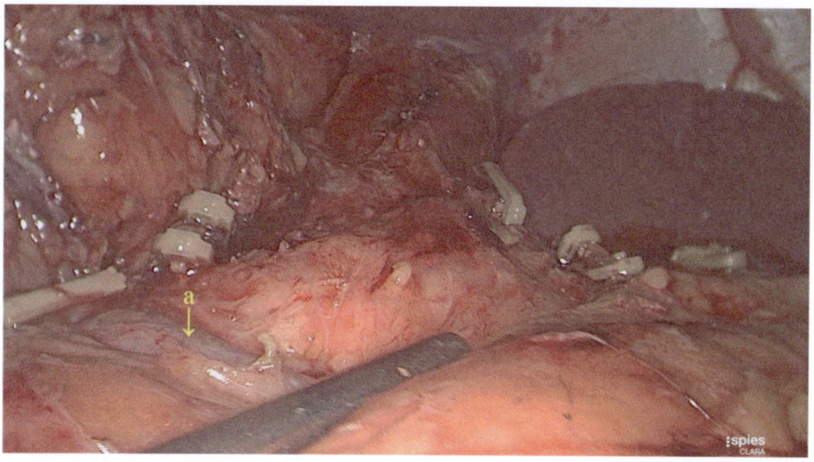

Fig. 4.48 Type IV SpA (**a**)

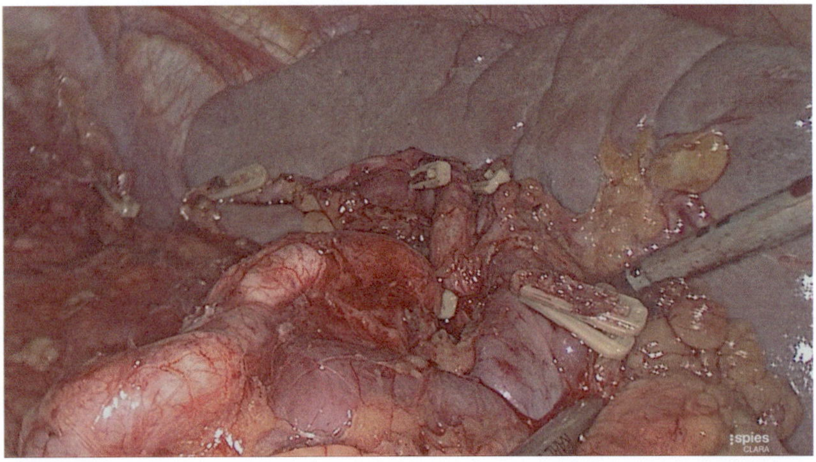

Fig. 4.49 One-branched type

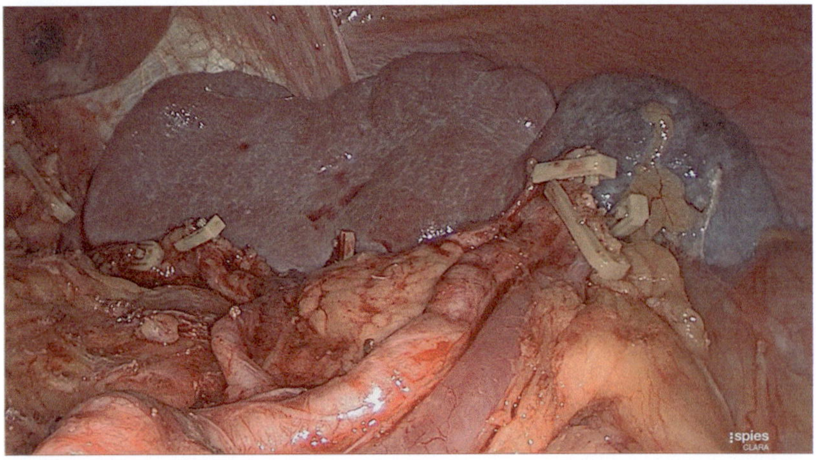

Fig. 4.50 Two-branched type

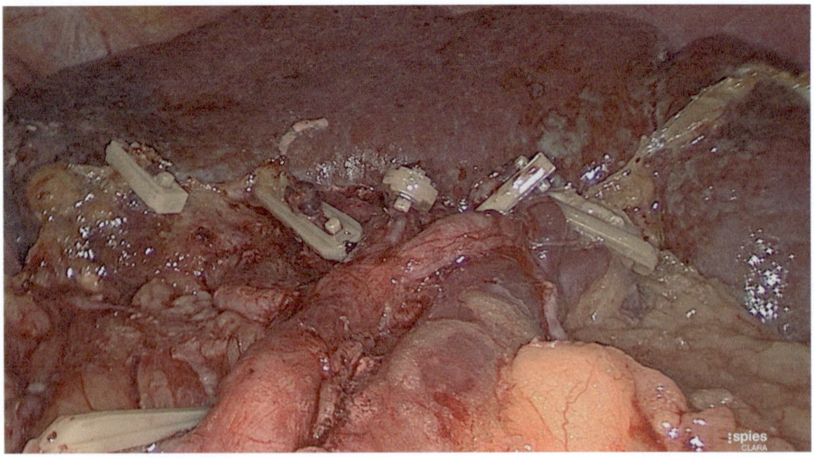

Fig. 4.51 Three-branched type

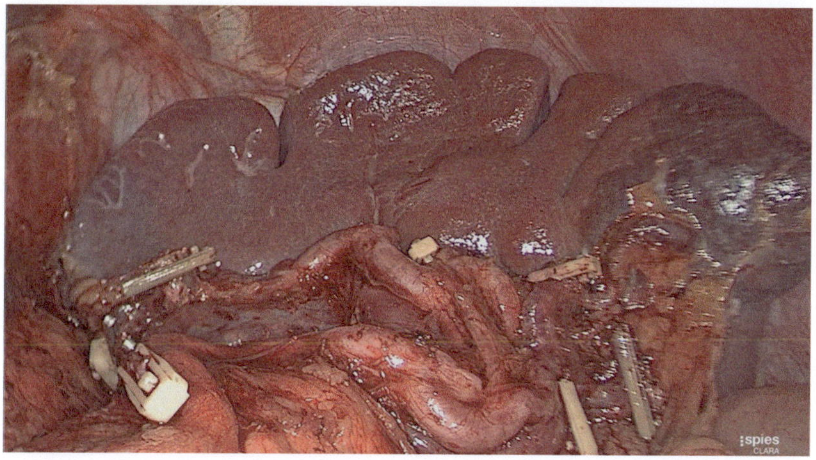

Fig. 4.52 Multiple branched type

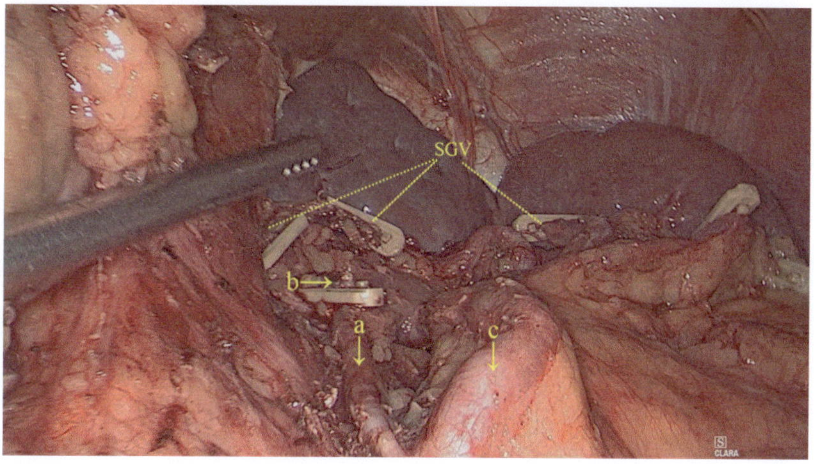

Fig. 4.53 Splenic upper-pole artery (SUPA) (**a**), PGA (**b**), and SpA (**c**)

Splenic Pole Artery (SPoA).

SGV: Short gastric vessel.

SpV: Splenic vein; LGEA: Left gastroepiploic artery.

The SPoA is an artery that enters the superior and/or inferior poles of the spleen without passing through the splenic hilar. Most of the SUPA originates from the trunk of the SpA, with some from the SLA. Most of the SLPA originates from the LGEA or ISLA, with some from the trunk of the SpA. Of 319 patients in our department, 53 cases (16.6%) had SUPA, and only 16 cases (5.0%) had SLPA (Figs. 4.53 and 4.54).

LGEA.

The LGEA is a branch of the SpA, ISLA, or SLPA. The LGEA branches derives from the LGEA and runs between the two anterior layers of the greater omentum in the GSL, and from left to right along the great curvature of the stomach. The LGEA then sends out several branches to the anterior and posterior walls and omentum of the stomach, forming an arch to the great curvature of the stomach with the RGEA (Figs. 4.55, 4.56, and 4.57).

Short Gastric Artery (SGA).

The SGA originates from the trunk of the SpA or its branches. There are four SGASs in total, and occasionally some branches originate from the LGEA (Figs. 4.58 and 4.59).

SGAs are located in the layers of the GSL and are distributed outside of the fundus of the stomach. Because shorter SGAs are closer to the spleen, more attention should be paid to total gastrectomies in such cases (Fig. 4.60).

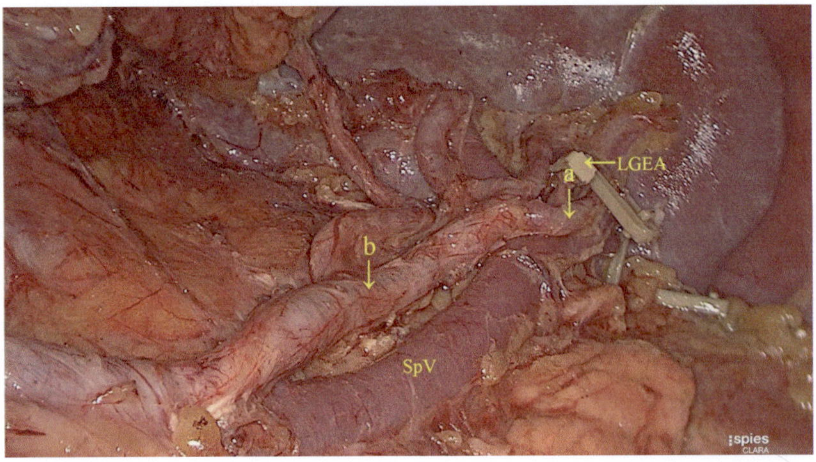

Fig. 4.54 The SLPA (**a**) from the SpA (**b**)

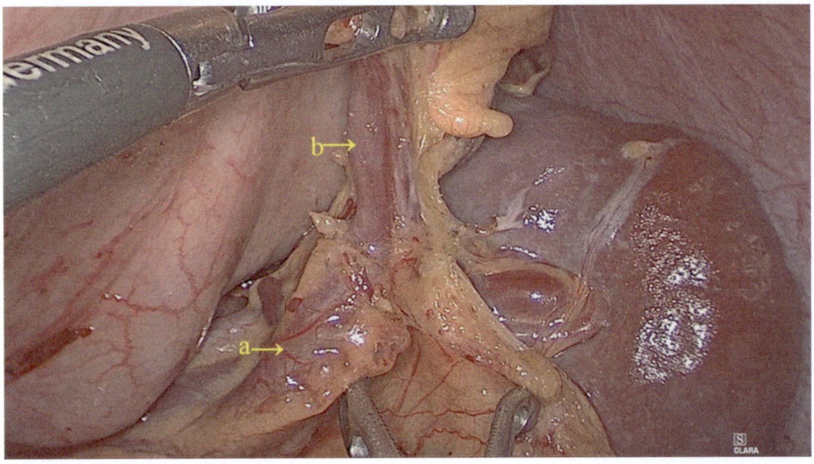

Fig. 4.55 The SLPA (**a**) from the LGEA (**b**)

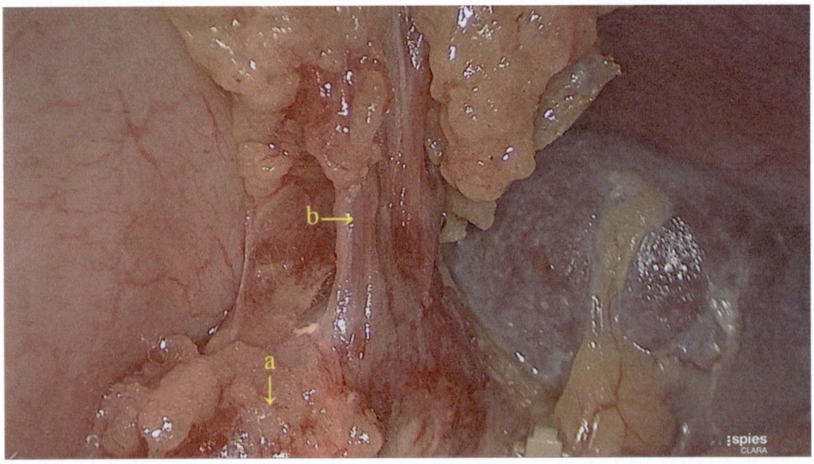

Fig. 4.56 The SLPA (**b**) from the SpA (**a**)

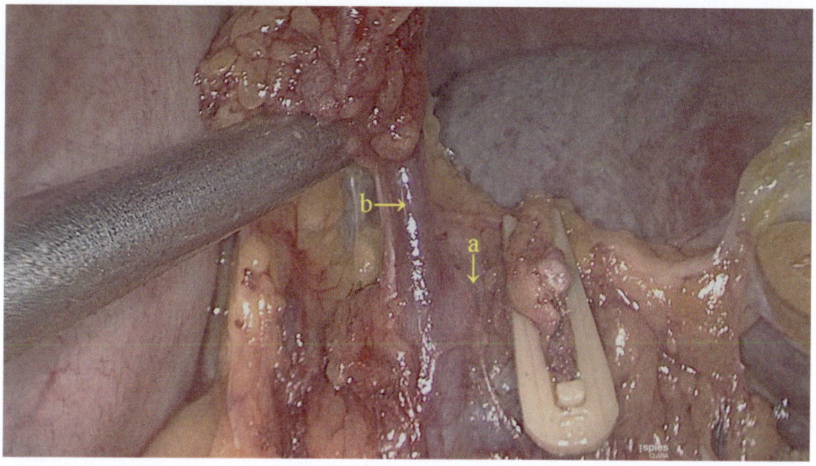

Fig. 4.57 The ISLA (**a**) from the LGEA (**b**)

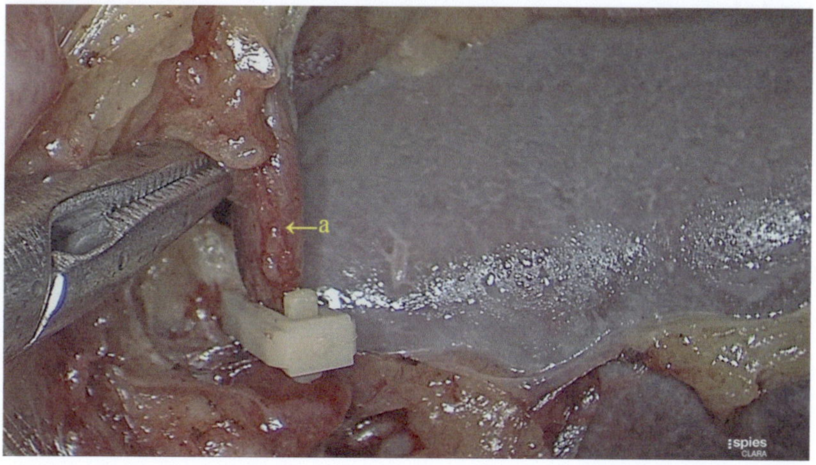

Fig. 4.58 The SGAs (**a**) originates from the trunk or branches of the SpA

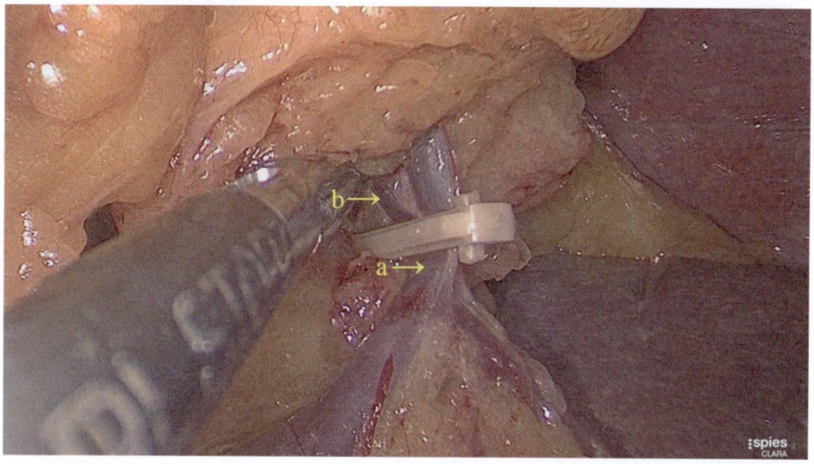

Fig. 4.59 The LGEA (**a**) from SGVs (**b**)

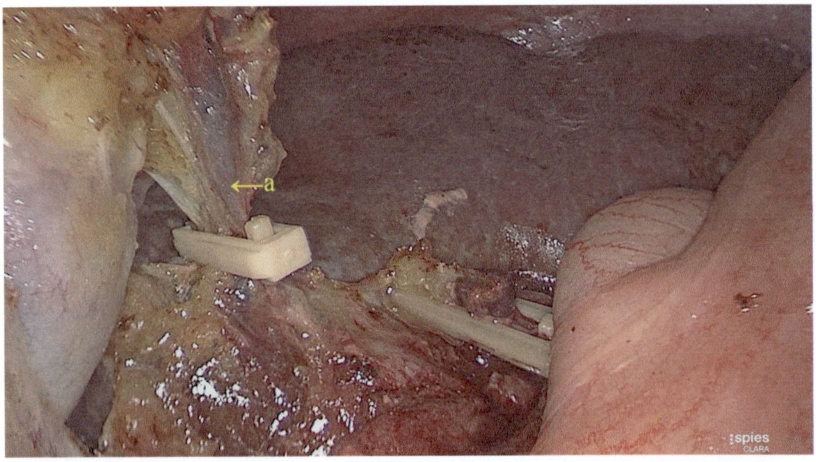

Fig. 4.60 The SGVs (**a**) at the superior pole region of the spleen are short, and the fundus of the stomach is close to the superior pole region of the spleen

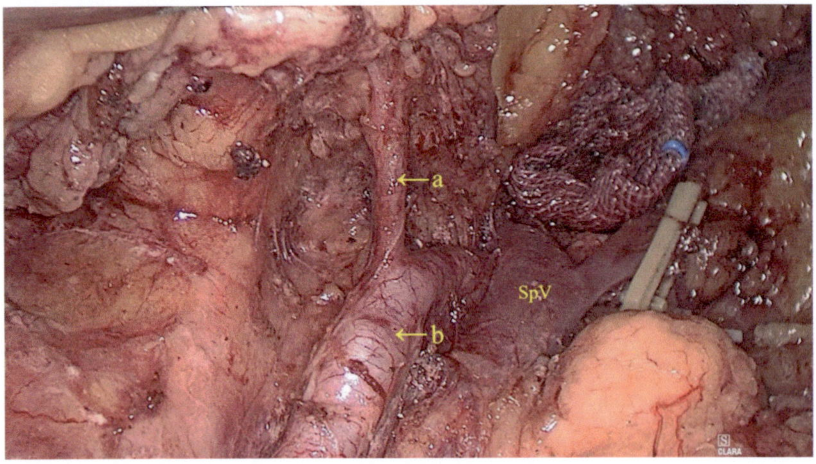

Fig. 4.61 The PGA (**a**) originates from the trunk of the SpA (**b**)

PGA

SpV: Splenic vein.

At the posterior wall of the stomach, the PGA originates from the SpAT and its branches. It mostly derives from the trunk of the SpA (Fig. 4.61), with some from the SUPA (Fig. 4.62). The probability of PGA occurrence was around 60.0%–80.0%, and was associated with an ascending vein of the same name after the omentum bursa.

Classification of the Terminal Branches of the SpA

According to the distance from furcation of the artery and the splenic hilar region, the terminal branches of the SpA are divided into the distributed type and concentrated type. The concentrated type often sends out branches within 2 cm of the splenic hilum. The trunk of the SpA is relatively long, and the SLA is relatively short and concentrated (Figs. 4.63 and 4.64).

The distance between the terminal branches of the SpA and the splenic hilum of the distributed type is generally more than 2 cm. The branches of the SLA are longer and smaller in diameter, and are often accompanied by the SPoA (Figs. 4.65 and 4.66). Data of 319 patients in our department showed that 205 cases (64.3%) were the concentrated type, and 114 cases (35.7%) were the distributed type.

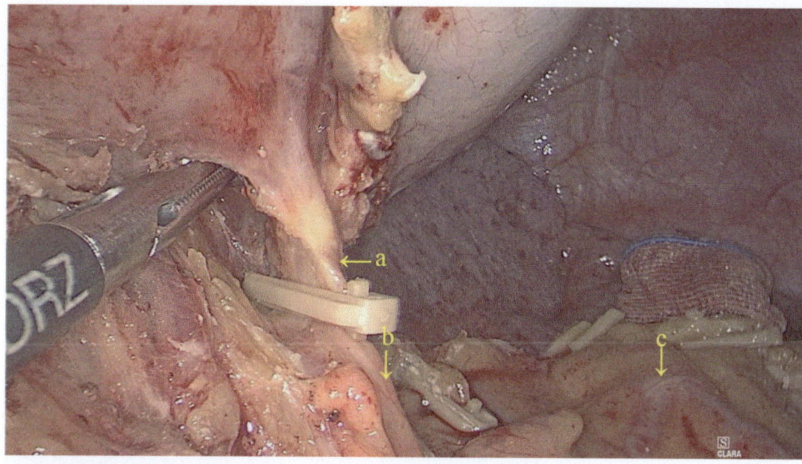

Fig. 4.62 The PGA (**a**) originates from the SUPA (**b**), or SpA (**c**)

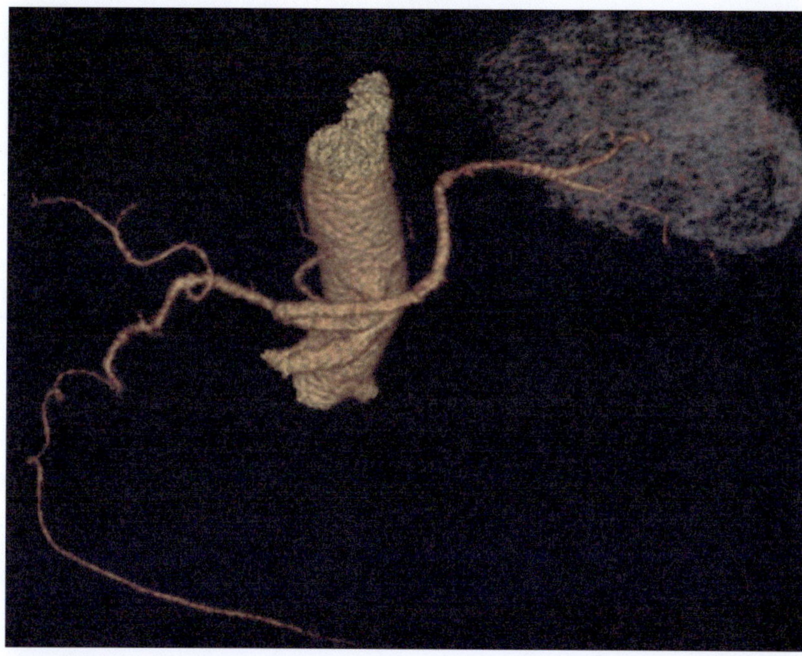

Fig. 4.63 Concentrated type of SpA terminal branches (3D computed tomography [CT])

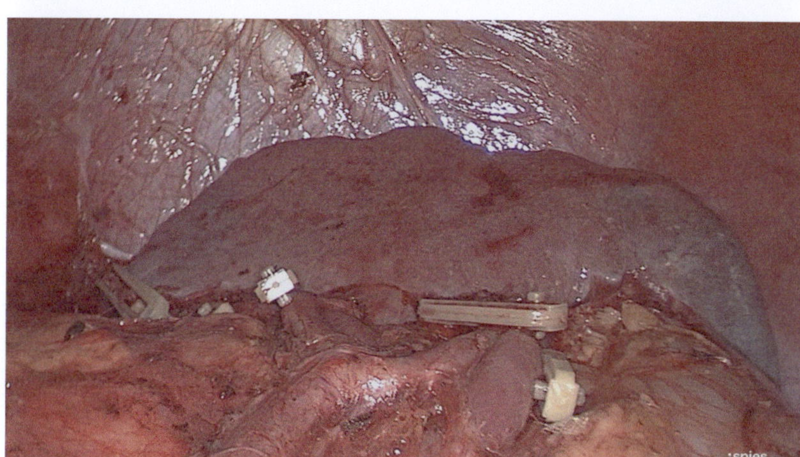

Fig. 4.64 Concentrated type of SpA terminal branches

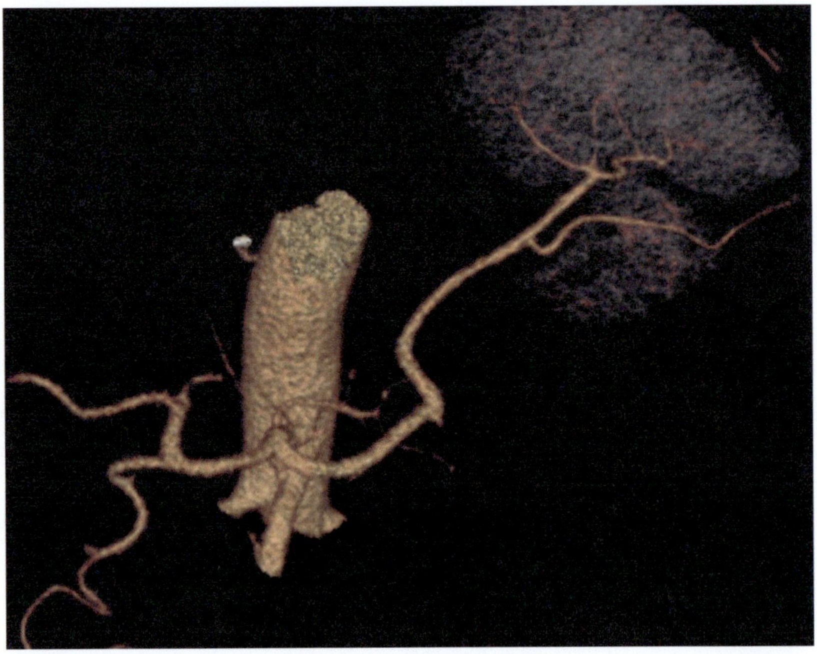

Fig. 4.65 Distributed type of SpA terminal branches (3D CT)

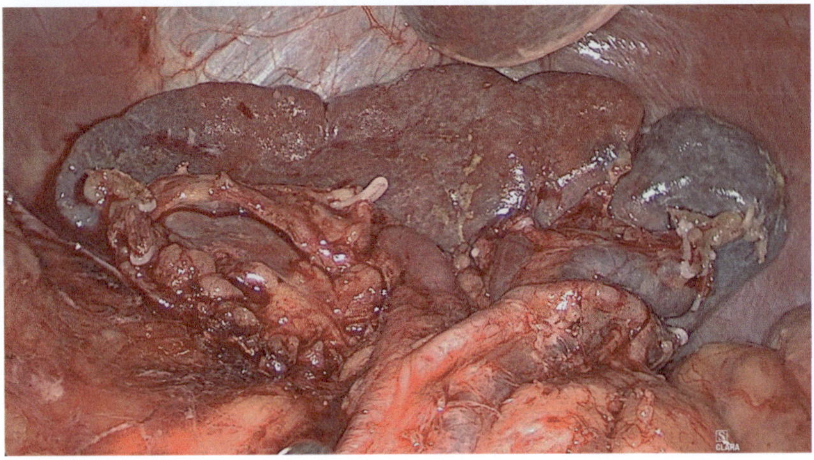

Fig. 4.66 Distributed type of SpA terminal branches

4.2.1.3 Veins Associated with LN Dissection in the Splenic Hilar Area

LGEV

The LGEV is accompanied by an artery of the same name and flows into the SpV (Figs. 4.67 and 4.68).

SpV

LGEV: Left gastroepiploic vein; LGEA: Left gastroepiploic artery.

The SpV is composed of splenic lobar veins at the splenic hilar, and also receives blood from the splenic polar vein (SPoV), branches of the pancreatic vein, short gastric vein, the LGEV, and the inferior mesenteric vein during the journey. It is

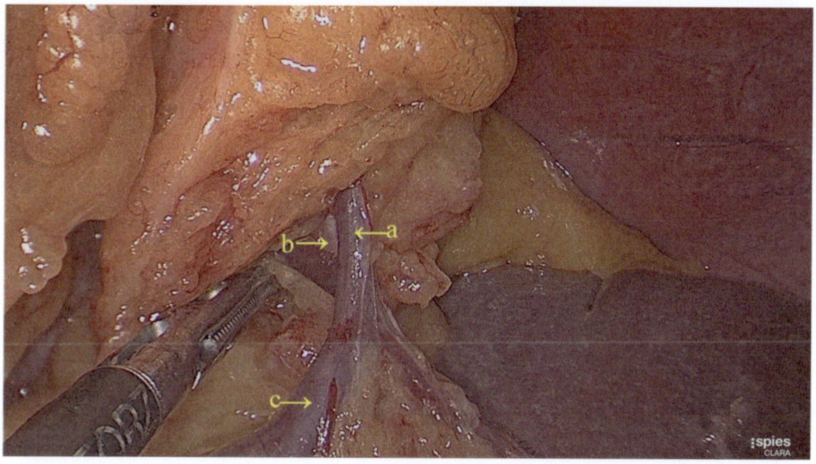

Fig. 4.67 The LGEV (**a**) is accompanied by an artery of the same name (**b**) and flows into the SpV (**c**)

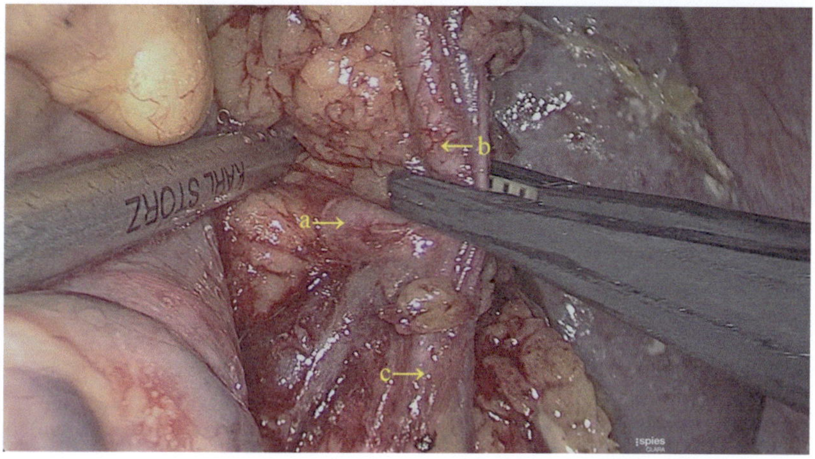

Fig. 4.68 The junction of the SGV (**a**) from the LGEV (**b**) with the SpA (**c**)

often accompanied by the splenic artery, but is not as circuitous (Fig. 4.69).

4.2.1.4 LN Anatomy Associated with LN Dissection in the Splenic Hilar Area

No. 4 LNs (LNs Around the Greater Curvature of the Stomach)

No. 4 LNs were named as three substations according to their accompanying arteries.

No. 4d LNs.

Definition of No. 4d LNs.

No. 4d LNs are located between the two layers of the mesogastrium and are attached to the greater curvature of the stomach along the RGEA. The boundary between No. 4d LNs and No. 6 LNs is the first branch of the RGEA entering the gastric wall. The right side of the branch (including the branch) is No. 6 LNs and the left is No. 4d LNs (Fig. 4.70).

No. 4d LN metastasis (Fig. 4.71).

No. 4sa LNs.

Definition of No. 4sa LNs.

LGEA: Left gastroepiploic artery.

No. 4sb LNs are located between the two layers of the mesogastrium and are attached to the greater curvature of the stomach in the GSL along the LGEA. The dividing line between No. 4sb LNs and No. 10 LNs is the first branch of the LGEA entering the gastric wall. LNs located at the distal end of the branch (including the branch)

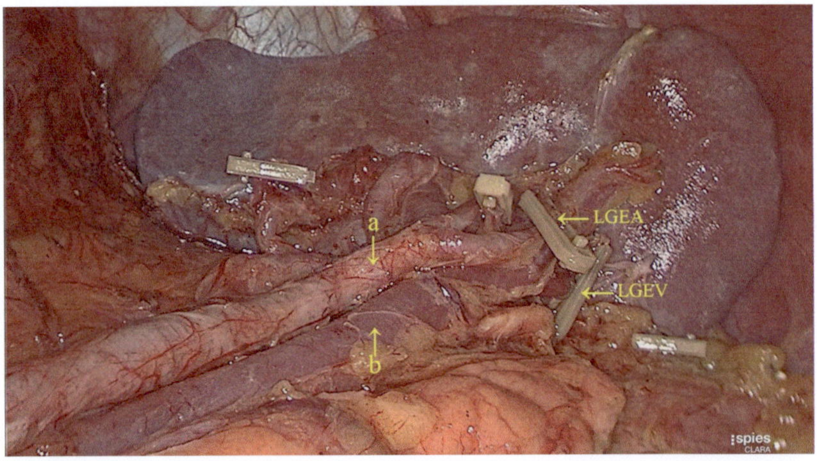

Fig. 4.69 The SpV (**a**) accompanies the SpA (**b**)

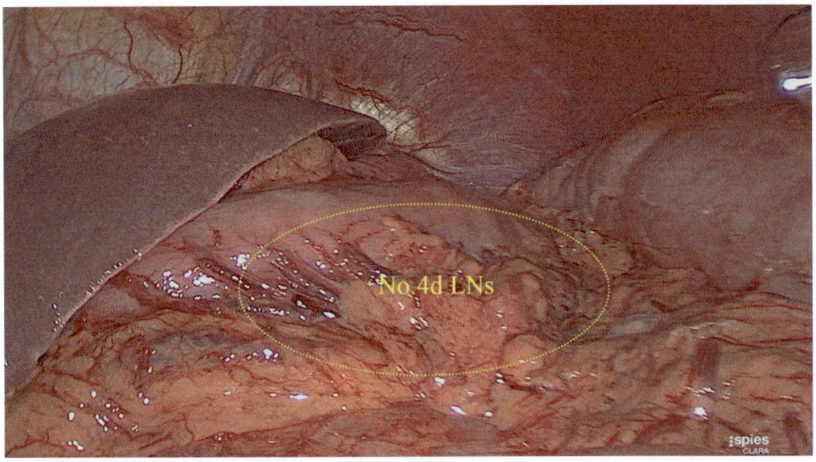

Fig. 4.70 The scope of No. 4d LNs

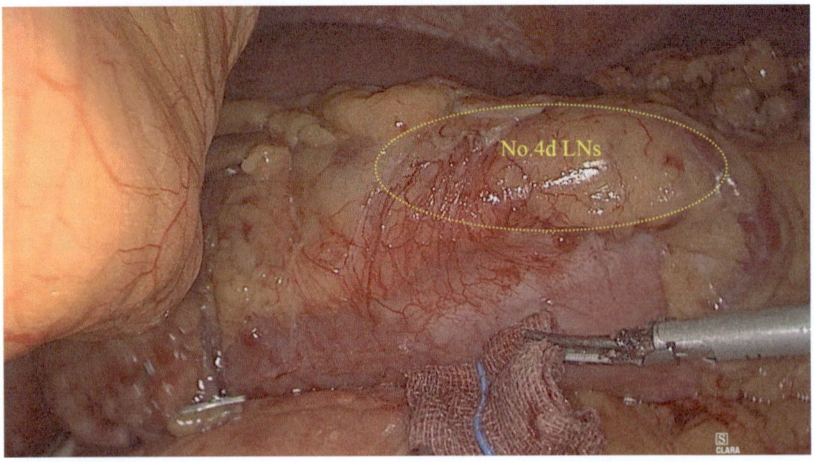

Fig. 4.71 No. 4d LN metastasis

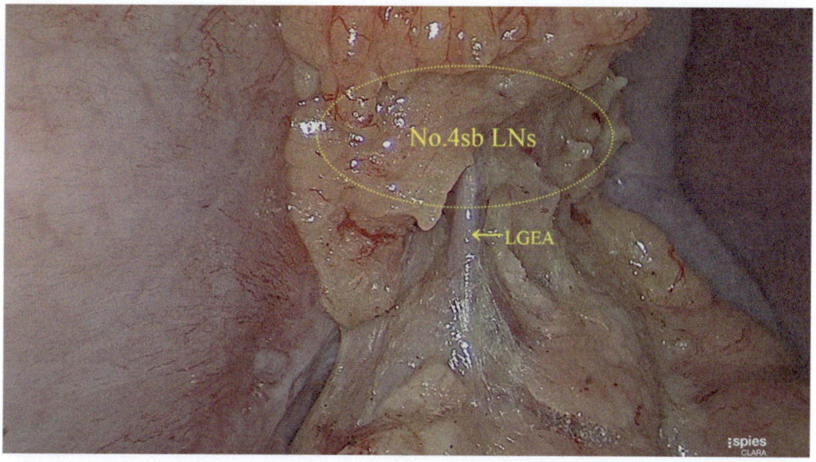

Fig. 4.72 The scope of No. 4sb LNs

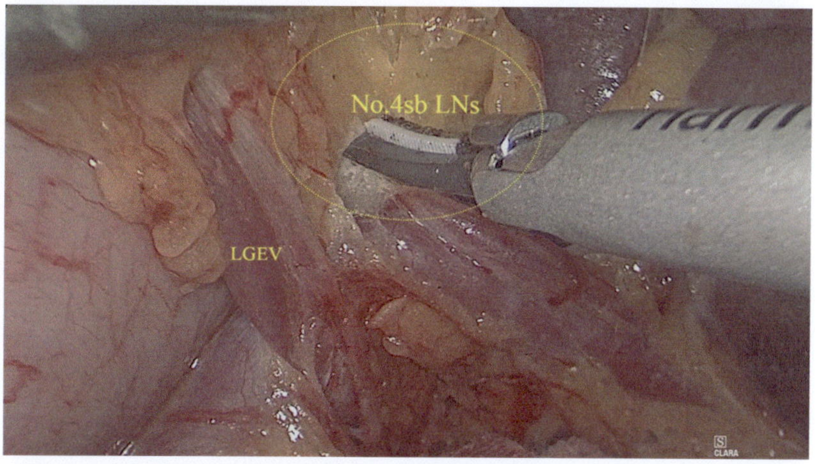

Fig. 4.73 No. 4b LN metastasis

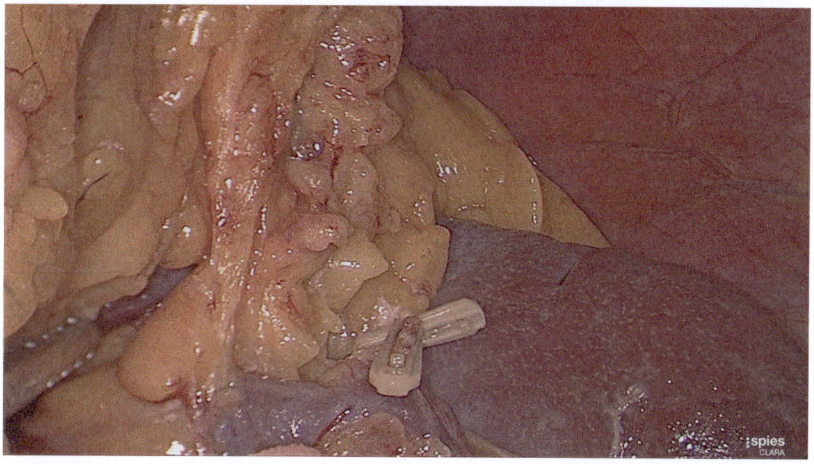

Fig. 4.74 No. 4b LN metastasis (appearance after dissection)

belong to No. 4sb LNs, and the proximal end of the branch vessel and LNs in the splenic hilum belong to No. 10 LNs (Fig. 4.72).

No. 4b LN metastasis (Figs. 4.73 and 4.74).

LGEV: Left gastroepiploic vessel.

No. 4sa LNs.

Definition of No. 4sa LNs.

SpA: Splenic artery; LGEA: Left gastroepiploic artery; SGV: Short gastric vessel.

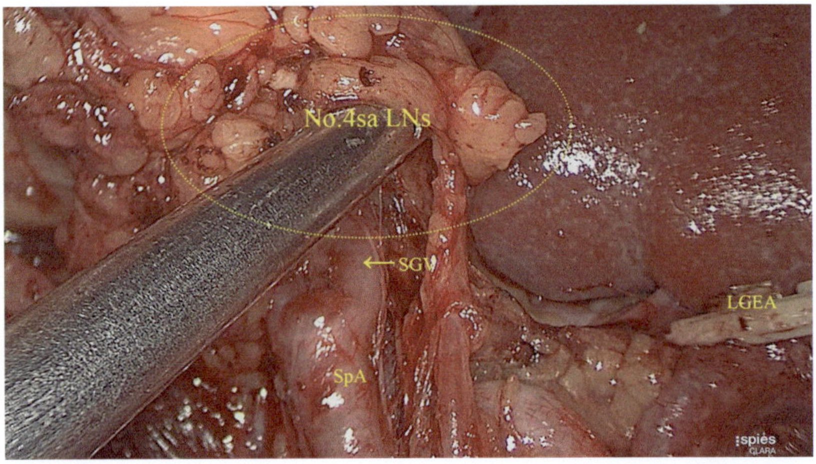

Fig. 4.75 The scope of No. 4sa LNs

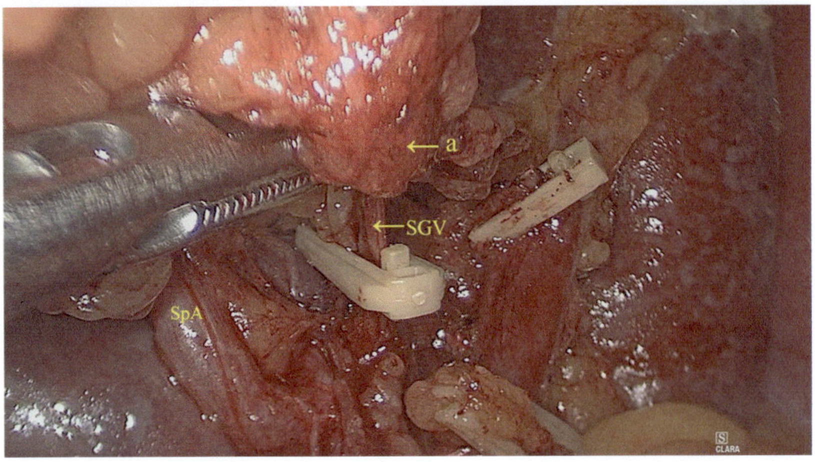

Fig. 4.76 No. 4sa LNs (**a**)

No. 4sa LNs are located on the gastric wall between the two layers of the mesogastrium and are attached to the greater curvature of the stomach along the SGAs (Fig. 4.75).

No. 4sa LN metastasis (Fig. 4.76).

SGV: Short gastric vessel; SpA: Splenic artery.

An ICG display of No. 4 LNs is seen in Figs. 4.77 and 4.78.

No. 10 LNs (LNs Located at the Splenic Hilar)

Definition of No. 10 LNs.

SGV: Short gastric vessel; SpA: Splenic artery; SpV: Splenic vein.

No. 10 LNs are located at the splenic hilum and are distributed along the vessels from the pancreas tail to enter the spleen. The boundary between No. 10 LNs with No. 11 LNs is the end of the pancreas tail (Fig. 4.79).

No. 10 LN metastasis (Figs. 4.80 and 4.81).

An ICG display of No. 10 LNs is seen in Figs. 4.82 and 4.83.

No. 11 LNs (LNs Along the SpA Trunk)

Definition of No. 11 LNs.

No. 11 LNs are distributed along the trunk of the SpA, including LNs behind the pancreas. Based on lymphatic flow and clinical needs, No. 11 LNs are divided into two subtypes with the midpoint of the SpA as the boundary. The side near the CA is classified as No. 11p LNs, and the side near the splenic hilum is classified as No. 11d LNs (Fig. 4.84).

No. 11 LN metastasis (Fig. 4.85).

LGEV: Left gastroepiploic vessel.

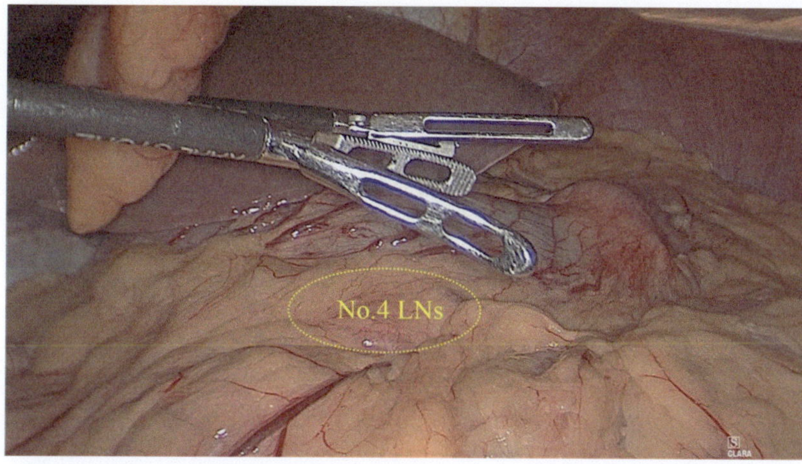

Fig. 4.77 Intraoperative view of No. 4 LNs

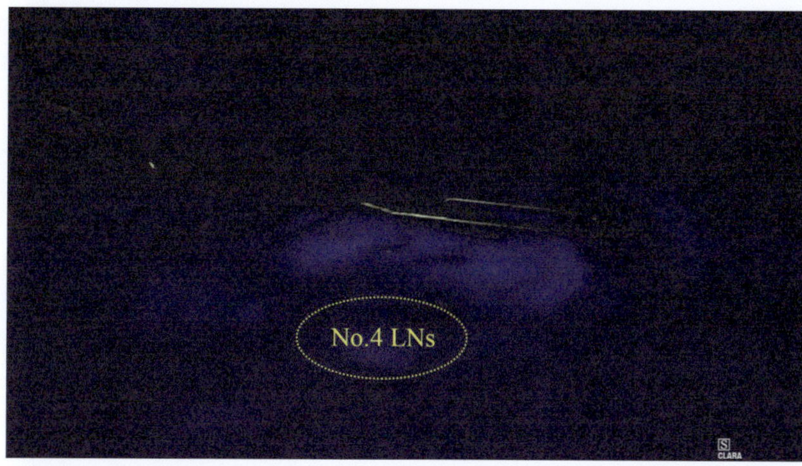

Fig. 4.78 ICG display of No. 4 LNs

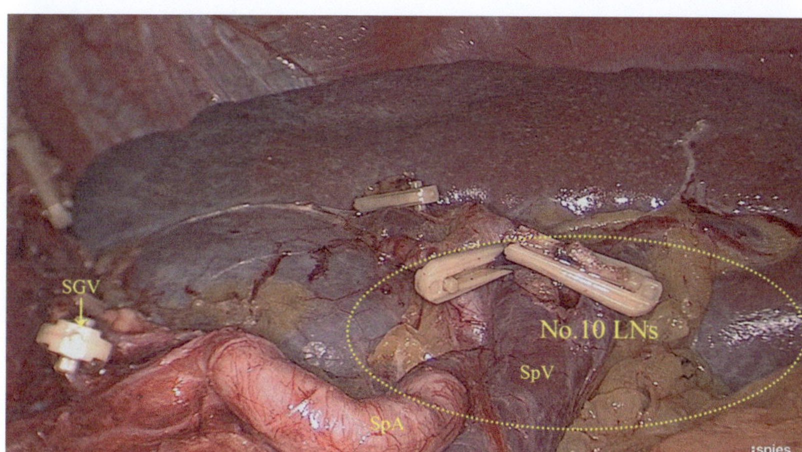

Fig. 4.79 The scope of No. 10 LNs

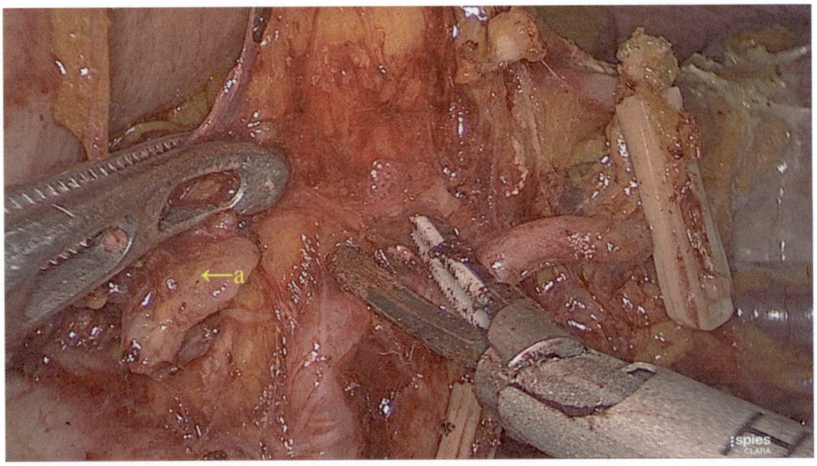

Fig. 4.80 No. 10 LNs metastasis (**a**)

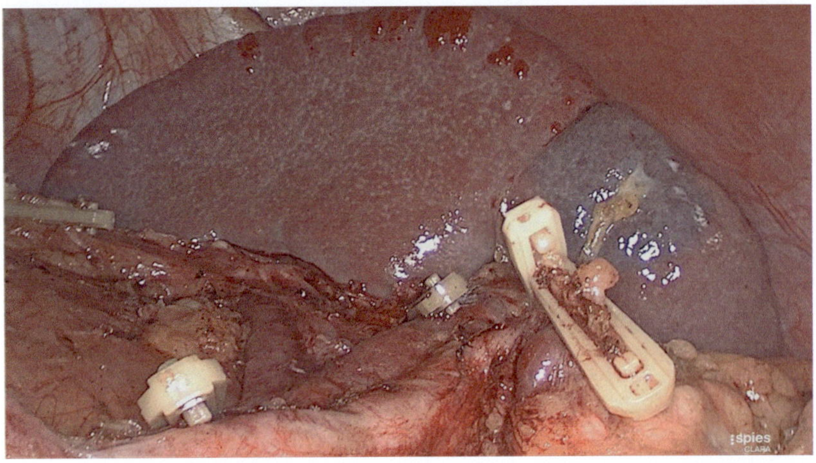

Fig. 4.81 No. 10 LNs metastasis (appearance after dissection)

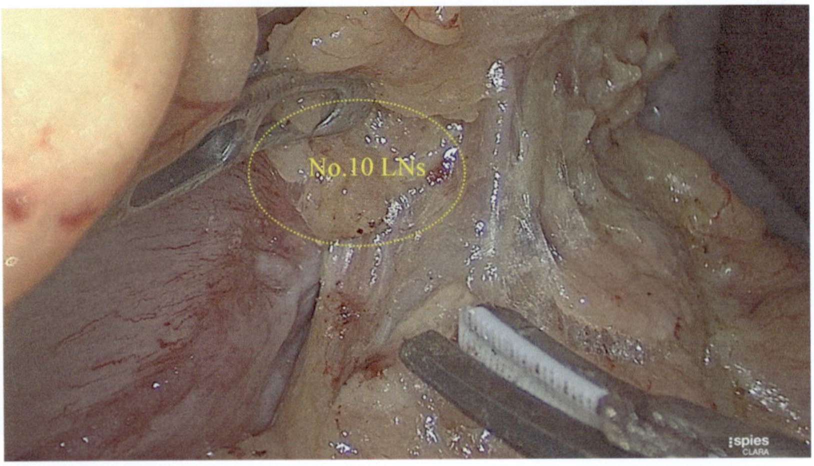

Fig. 4.82 Intraoperative view of No. 10 LNs

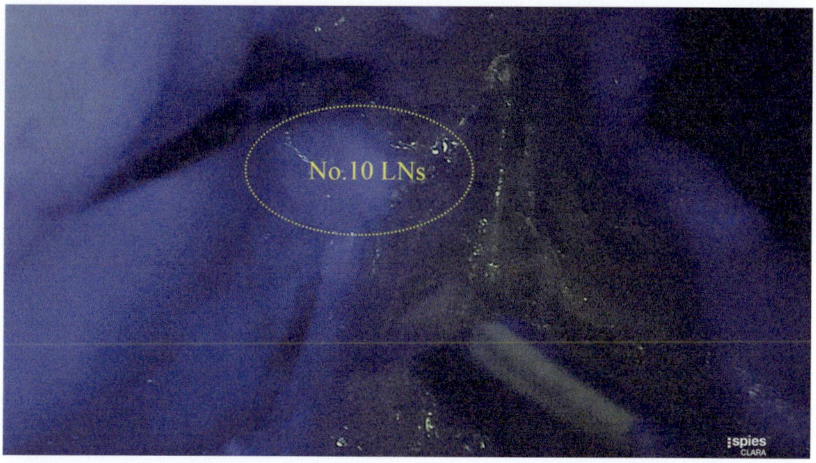

Fig. 4.83 ICG display of No. 10 LN metastasis

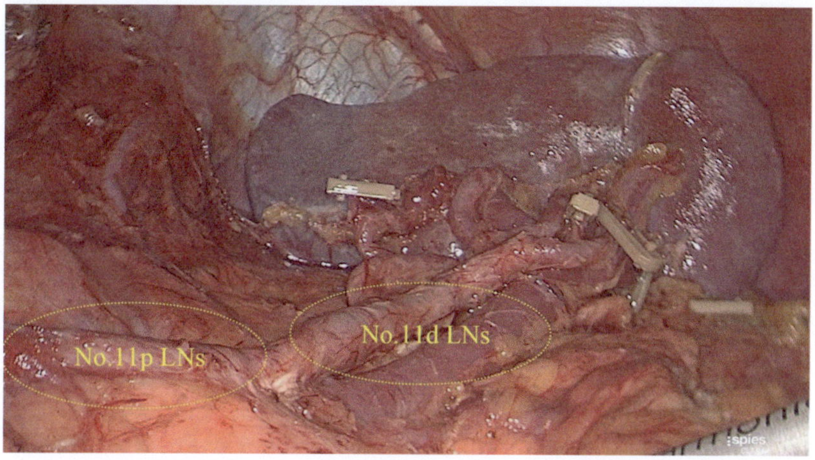

Fig. 4.84 Scope of No. 11 LNs

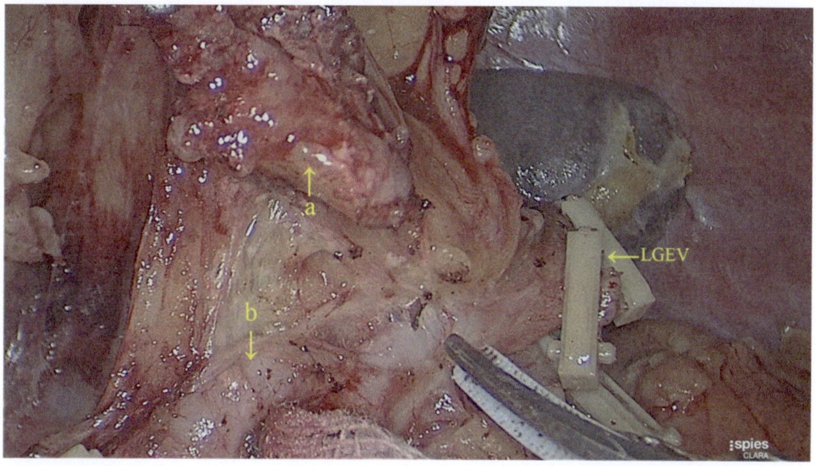

Fig. 4.85 No. 11 LN metastasis (**a**), SpA (**b**)

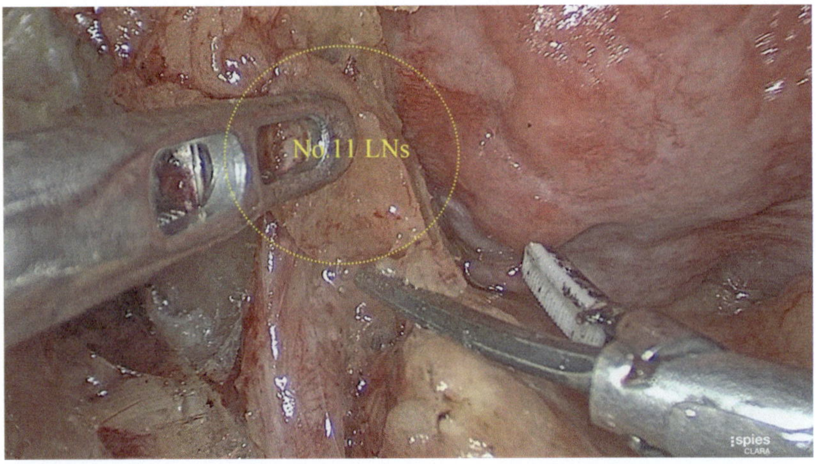

Fig. 4.86 Intraoperative view of No. 11 LNs

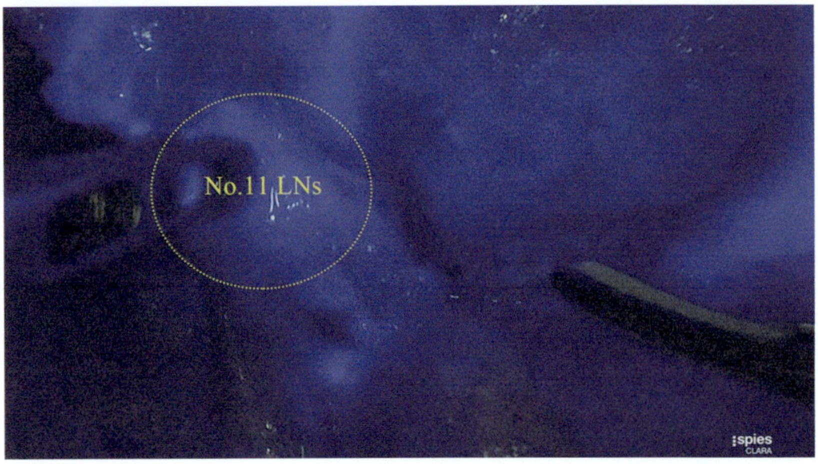

Fig. 4.87 ICG display of No. 11 LN metastasis

An ICG display of No. 11 LNs is seen in Figs. 4.86 and 4.87.

4.2.2 Intraoperative Announcements of Laparoscopic Splenic Hilar Area LN Dissection for Gastric Cancer

Before dissection of LNs in this area, the gastric body should be pushed down to the lower right, then the omentum should be overturned and pushed over the anterior wall of the stomach so that the body of the stomach and the omentum do not block the visual field during surgery. Some patients have adhesion between omentum tissue and the spleen (Fig. 4.88). In these cases, the assistant should pay attention to the strength and angle of the traction tissue to avoid splenic tears and bleeding from improper exertion (Fig. 4.89). Therefore, GSL adhesion should be released before LN dissection (Fig. 4.90).

LPVS: Lower pole vessels of the spleen.

After opening the pancreatic anterior fascia in the direction of the fascia anterior extension to the tail of the pancreas, the SRL space along the posterior space of the pancreatic anterior fascia can be gradually enlarged. LLVSs or LPVSs can then be exposed by stripping through this space (Fig. 4.91).

SUPA:splenic upper-pole artery; SpA: Splenic artery; SpV: Splenic vein.

Splenic ischemia is mostly caused by cutting off the wrong branches of the splenic blood supply during surgery. In particular, during dissection

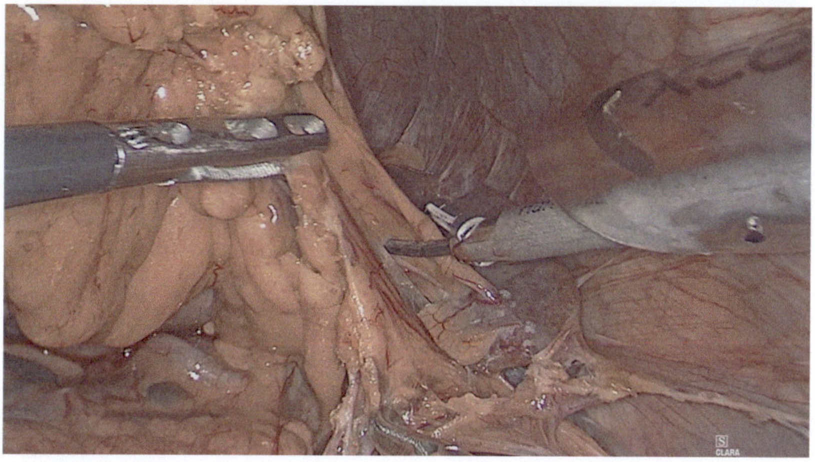

Fig. 4.88 Adhesions between the spleen and the omentum

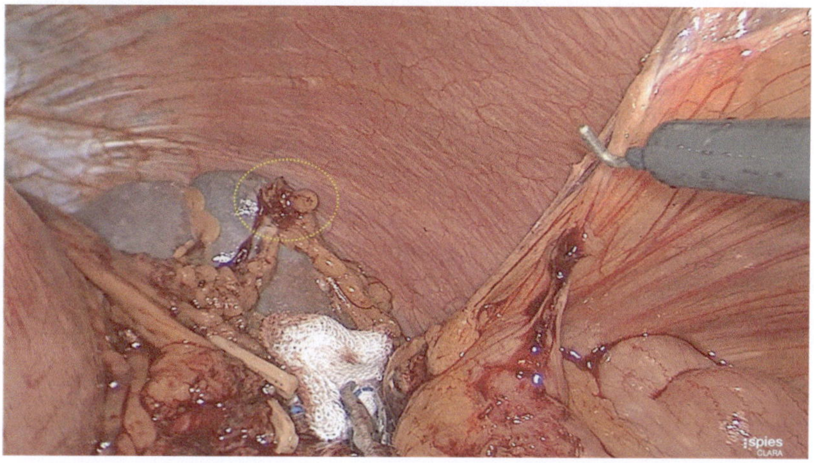

Fig. 4.89 The excessive force of pulling spleen adhesions leads to bleeding of the splenic capsule

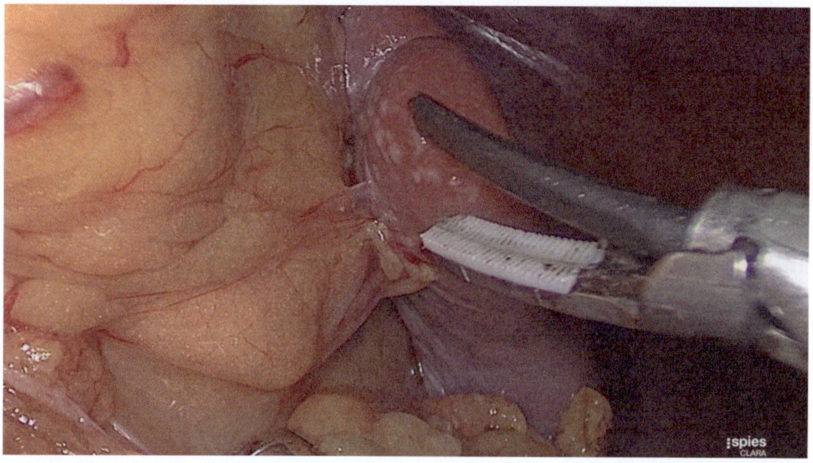

Fig. 4.90 Spleen adhesions should be released before further surgery

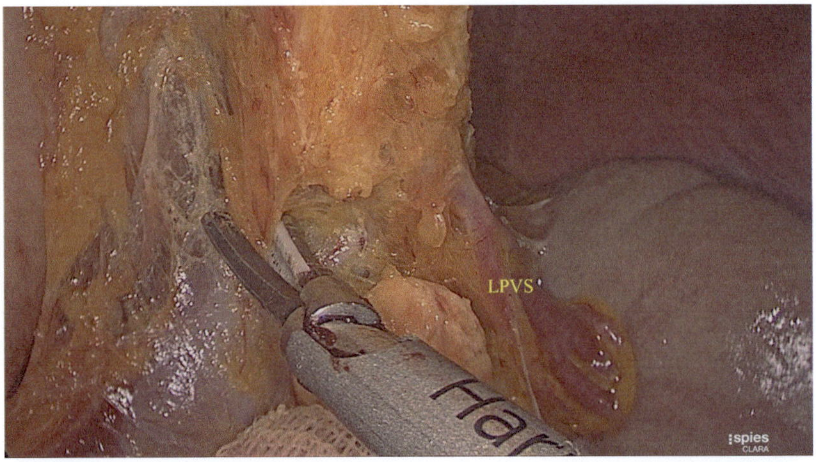

Fig. 4.91 The LPVSs can be exposed by dissection through the SRL space

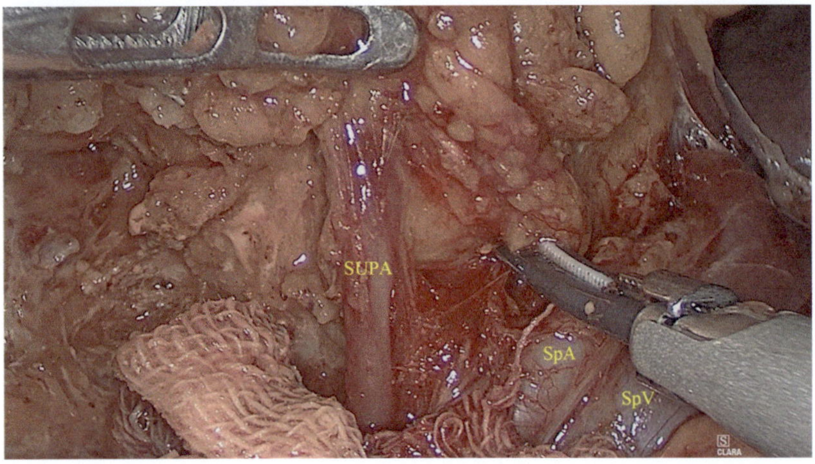

Fig. 4.92 The splenic upper-pole vessel branching from the SpAT is usually lifted and may be mistaken as the posterior gastric vessel

of the distal part of the SpAT, splenic upper-pole vessel branching from the SpAT is usually lifted and may be mistaken as the posterior gastric vessel (Fig. 4.92). Attention should therefore be paid to the branches of blood vessels in this area, which should be preserved when it is not possible to discriminate between them.

SGV: Short gastric vessel; SpA: Splenic artery; PGA: Posterior gastric artery; Panc: Pancreas.

SpA: Splenic artery; LGEV: Left gastroepiploic vein; LGEA: Left gastroepiploic artery; PGA: Posterior gastric artery.

The relationship between the spleen and the pancreatic tail is very close. About 50% of patients had a distance of only 1 cm between the spleen and the pancreatic tail, while 30% had direct contact with the splenic hilar region. Among these latter patients, 49.5% had the pancreatic tail was close to the middle of the splenic hilar region in 49.5%, and the tail of the pancreas was close to the lower pole in 42.5%. Additionally, 8.3% of patients had the tail of the pancreas close to the upper pole of the spleen (Figs. 4.93, 4.94 and 4.95).

LGEV: Left gastroepiploic vein; LGEA: Left gastroepiploic artery; SpA: Splenic artery; SpV: Splenic vein; SGV: Short gastric vessel.

Care should be taken not to injure the pancreatic tail when dissecting LNs on the dorsal side of the splenic vessels. We suggest that LNs behind the splenic portal vessels should only be cleaned when the pancreatic tail is located in the lower pole of the spleen and is at an appropriate distance from the splenic hilar region. LN dissection in the splenic hilus should be carried out on the

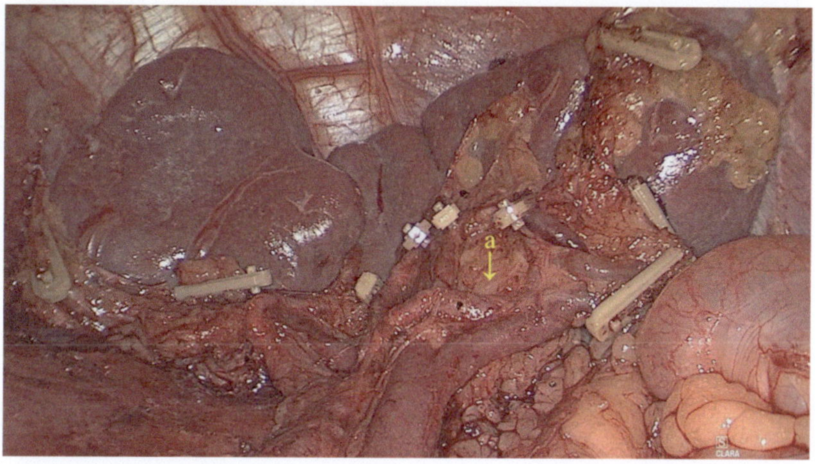

Fig. 4.93 The pancreatic tail (**a**) is in close proximity to the middle of the splenic hilar region

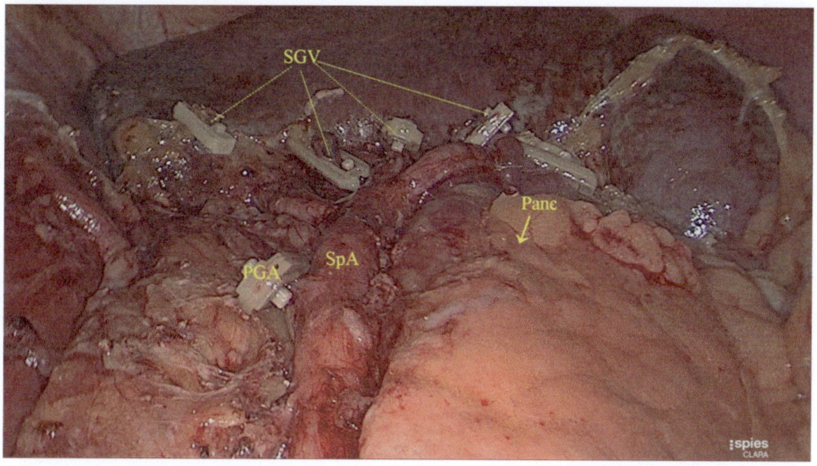

Fig. 4.94 The pancreatic tail is close to the lower pole of the spleen

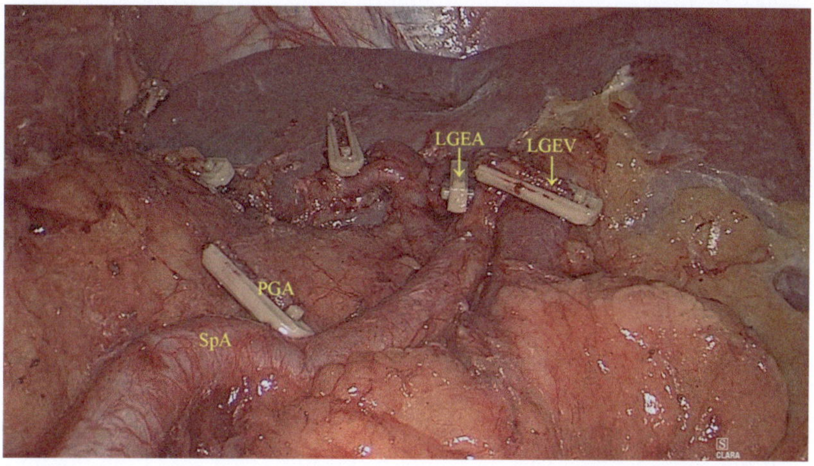

Fig. 4.95 The pancreatic tail is close to the upper pole of the spleen

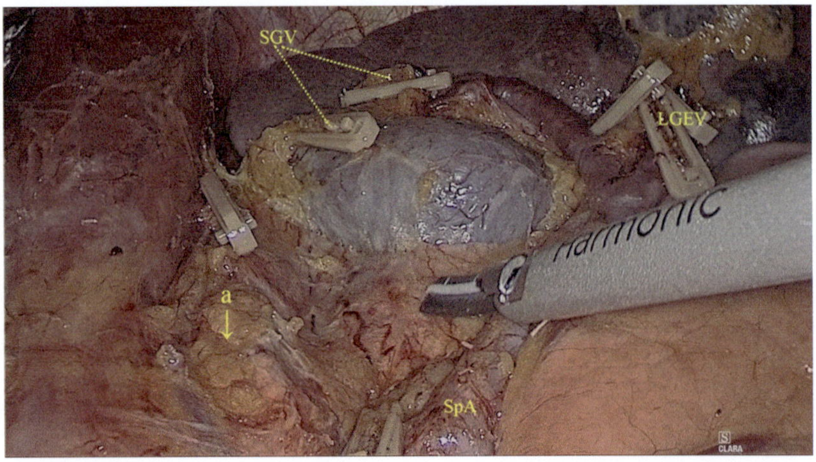

Fig. 4.96 The adrenal gland (**a**) should be distinguished from the lymphatic adipose tissue to prevent damaging it

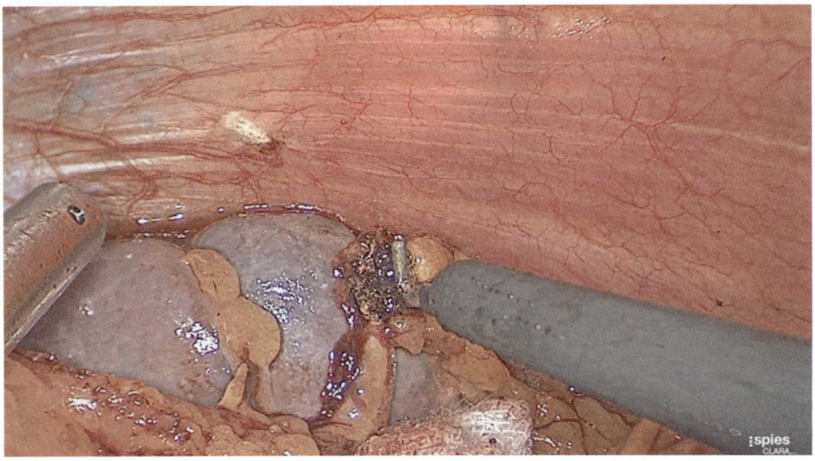

Fig. 4.97 The surgeon should use the hook parallel to the surface of the bleeding site

surface of Toldt's fascia, and the operating plane should not be too deep to prevent injury to Gerota's fascia (Fig. 4.96).

The treatment of splenic hemorrhage is difficult because superficial lacerations can cause more bleeding, resulting in an unclear field of vision. However, if the hemorrhage is too massive to control, the surgeon should use a bipolar coagulation hook (90–100 W) with a spray-coagulating model and with the hook parallel to the surface of the bleeding site, so that the spleen parenchyma scabs over to stop the bleeding (Fig. 4.97).

LGEV: Left gastroepiploic vessel.

SpA: Splenic artery; SpV: Splenic vein.

If the corresponding vessels cannot be identified, it is not advisable to break them blindly. Instead, the surgeon should fully expose the RPS on the superior margin of the pancreatic tail and further expose the vessel towards the distal terminal to determine its route. In general, the LGEV should be removed from the root after exposure to the splenic vessel to avoid splenic ischemia caused by incorrect transection of the splenic lobe vessel (Figs. 4.98 and 4.99).

LGEV: Left gastroepiploic vessel.

In the course of distal subtotal gastrectomy, one or two SGVs should continue to be disconnected after amputation of the LGEV (Fig. 4.100). When naked, the surgeon can use an ultrasonic scalpel to open an operating hole in the vascularized area from the middle of the great curvature of the stomach. This facilitates the complete

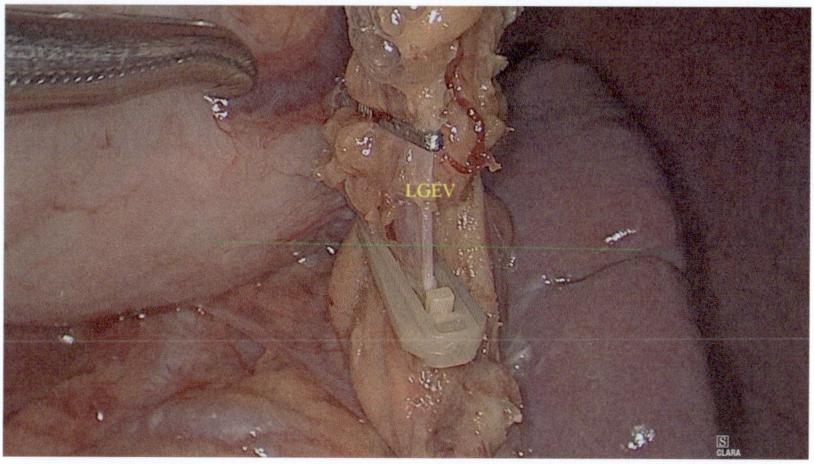

Fig. 4.98 Exposing the root of the LGEV and severing the LGEV above the green dotted line level

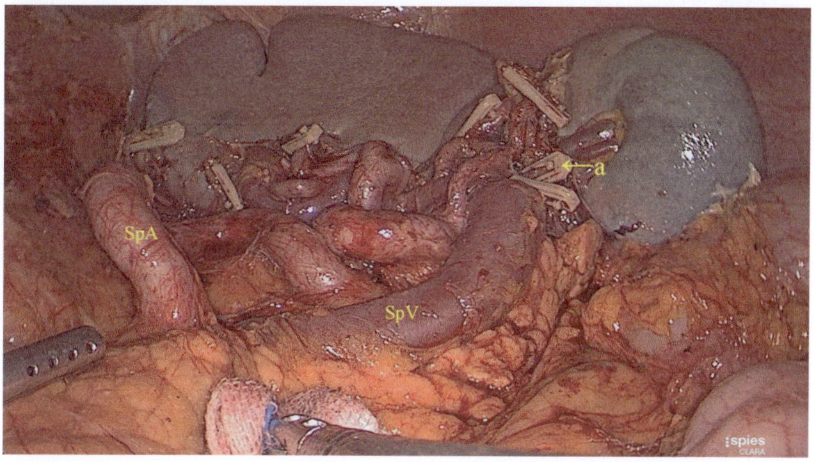

Fig. 4.99 The LPVSs (**a**) are severed, causing splenic ischemia

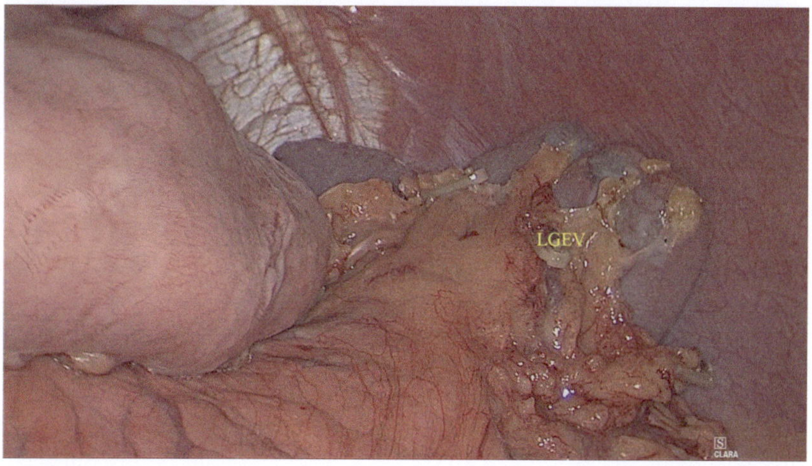

Fig. 4.100 One or two SGVs continue to disconnect towards the great curvature of the stomach after severing the LGEV

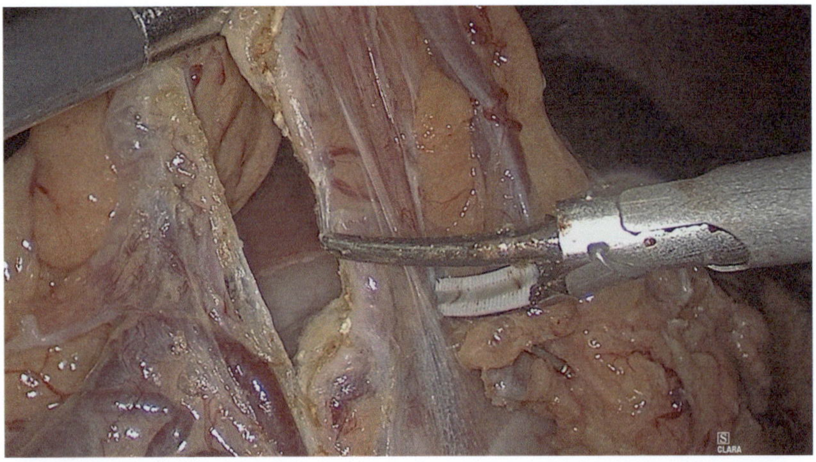

Fig. 4.101 The surgeon opens an operating hole in the vascularized area of the great curvature of the stomach with an ultrasound scalpel

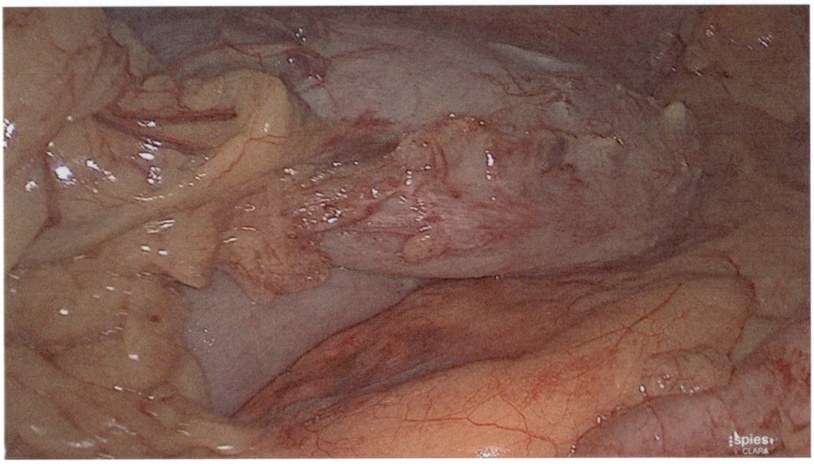

Fig. 4.102 The greater curvature of the stomach after exposing

clamping of the vessels when the great curvature of the stomach is naked (Figs. 4.101 and 4.102).

LGA: Left gastric artery; SpA: Splenic artery; SpV: Splenic vein; SGV: Short gastric vessel.

Although the initial position of the splenic artery is relatively fixed (arising from the CA in 98% of cases), the SpA runs within the parenchyma of the pancreas in some patients. During dissection, the surgeon should therefore pay attention to the boundary between the lymphatic tissues around the SpA and pancreatic parenchyma. Pancreatic tissue should not be dissected because LN resection will cause complications such as intraoperative hemorrhage and postoperative pancreatic fistulae (Fig. 4.103).

SpA: Splenic artery; SpV: Splenic vein.

During dissection, special attention should be paid to distinguish the space between the circuitous vessels and the LNs. Moreover, the trunk of the tortuous splenic artery, resembling a swollen LN, should not be dissected to avoid hemorrhage or splenic ischemia (Fig. 4.104).

SpV: Splenic vein.

SpV: Splenic vein.

Continuity of the dissected lymphatic fatty tissue should be maintained to facilitate pulling by the assistant and exposure of the anatomic space (Figs. 4.105 and 4.106).

SGV: Short gastric vessel.

SGVs of the stomach (usually 4–7 branches) should be disconnected during splenic hilar LN dissection. The GSL should be separated layer by

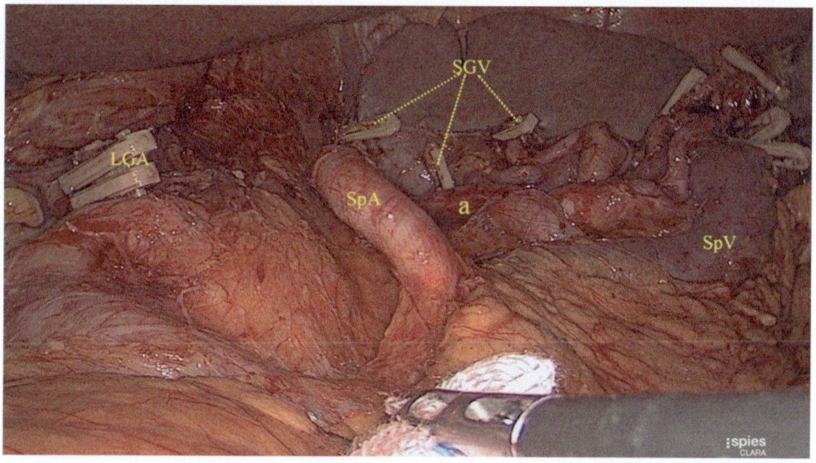

Fig. 4.103 The pancreas should be protected during dissection because a portion of the SpA (**a**) runs within the pancreatic parenchyma

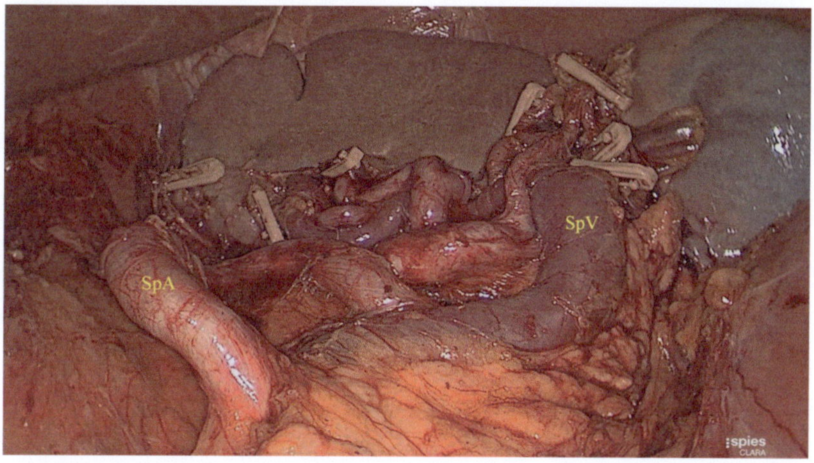

Fig. 4.104 A severely tortuous splenic artery

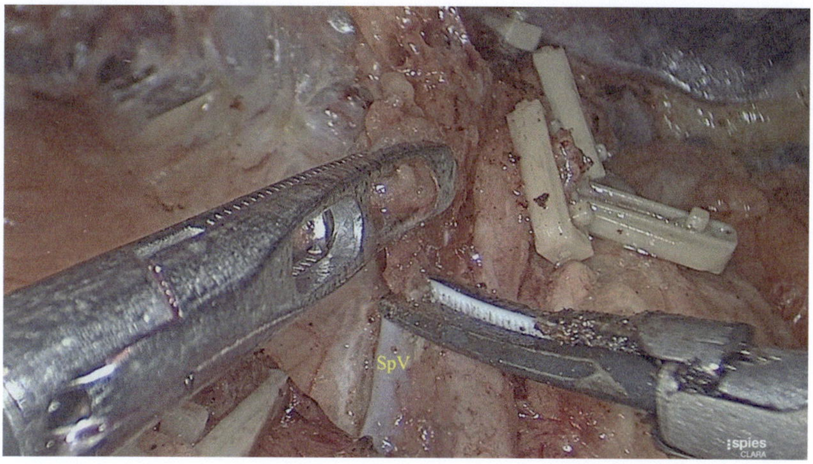

Fig. 4.105 Sharp separation of lymphatic fatty tissues on the surface of the vein with an ultrasonic scalpel

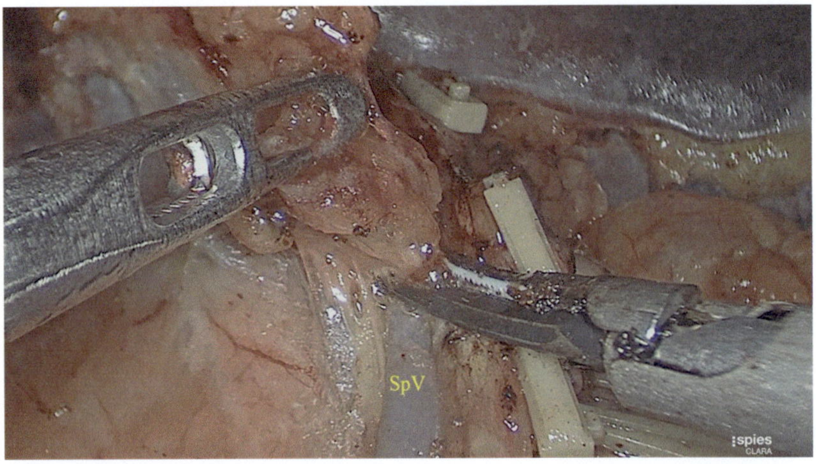

Fig. 4.106 Maintaining continuity of lymphatic tissues on the surface of blood vessels

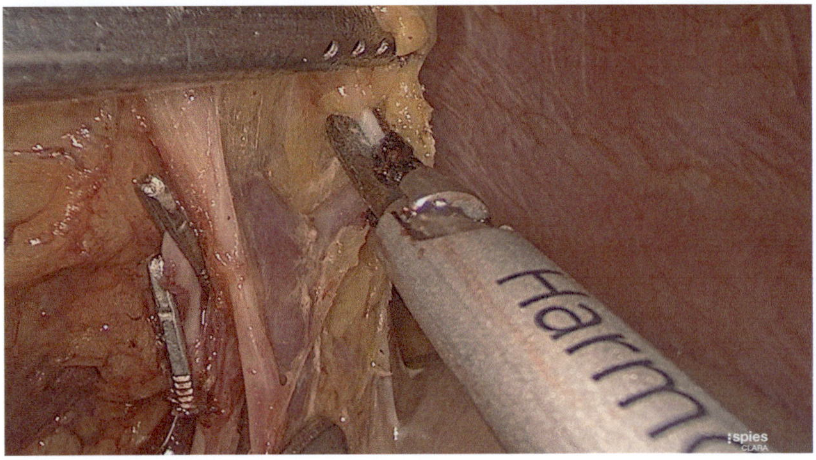

Fig. 4.107 Separating the GSL by dividing the fascia of the splenic side

layer when the SGVs are exposed. The fascia of the splenic side should be cut first, and an inboard fascial incision should then be made (Figs. 4.107 and 4.108). Ultrasound scalpels should not be used to hold large numbers of tissues to prevent bleeding caused by incomplete blood vessel closure. The farther away from their root, the more the SGV branches increase, and the greater the need for blood vessels to be cut off and an increased risk of injury (Figs. 4.109 and 4.110).

SGV: Short gastric vessel.

When LNs are dissected to the upper pole of the spleen, attention should be paid to the existence and characteristics of the SGVs in the stomach. The gastric fundus should not be pulled hard, and the vessel should be cut off after it is denuded to avoid bleeding caused by the incomplete closure of blood vessels by the ultrasonic scalpel (Figs. 4.111 and 4.112).

SGV: Short gastric vessel.

The upper pole of the spleen in some patients is supplied by the SGVs of the stomach, and partial ischemia of the spleen may occur after the SGVs are disconnected (Fig. 4.113).

PGA: Posterior gastric artery.

ULVSs often only have arteries and travel straight to the superior splenic lobe without passing through the splenic hilar. In such cases, the assistant lifts the body of the stomach, and the surgeon compresses the pancreas using their hand while maintaining tension of the PGA for easy identification and dissociation. When the

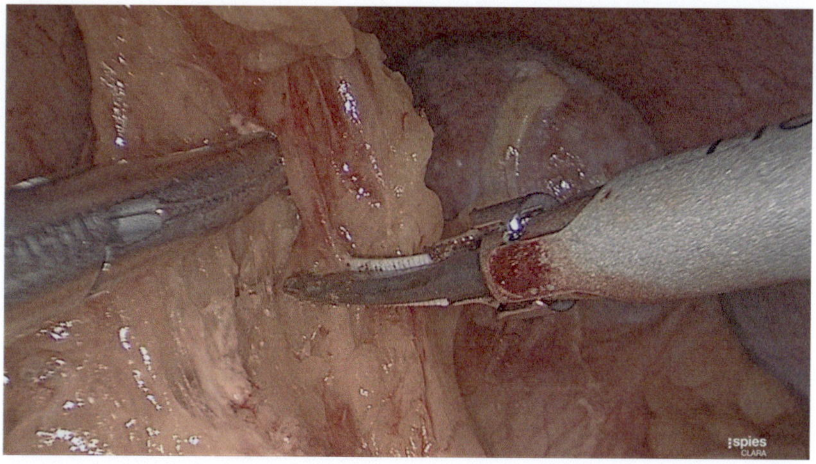

Fig. 4.108 Separating the GSL by dividing the inboard fascia

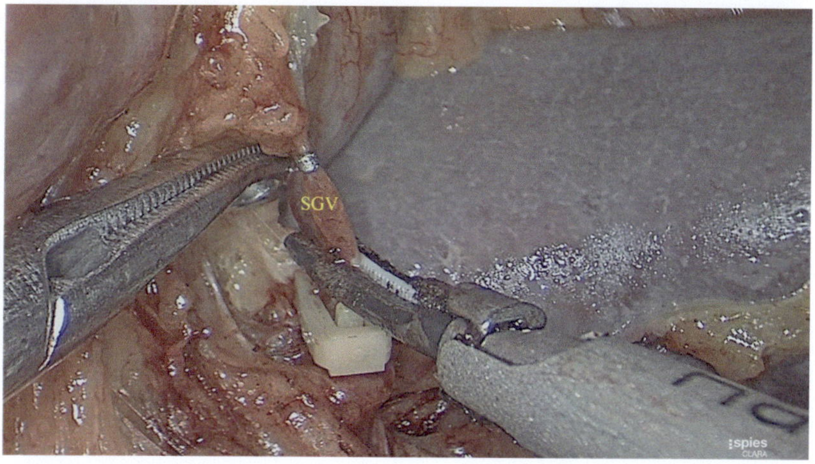

Fig. 4.109 LNs should be dissected close to the splenic hilar vessels, and SGVs should be cut off at their root

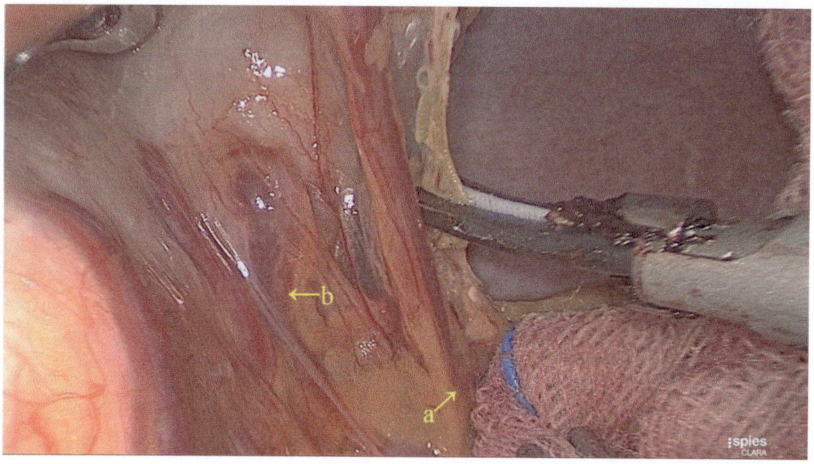

Fig. 4.110 SGVs (**a**) are removed from the root, and their branches (**b**) may need additional attention

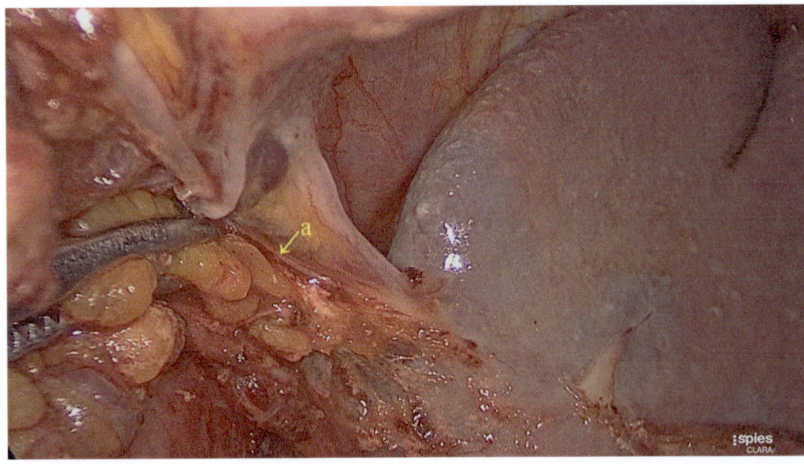

Fig. 4.111 The last SGV (**a**) is short, and the stomach fundus is close to the spleen

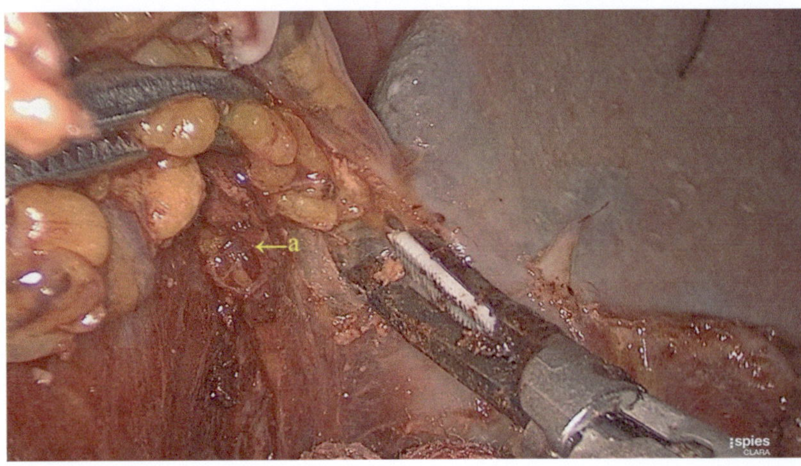

Fig. 4.112 The SGV (**a**) flows directly into the upper pole of the spleen

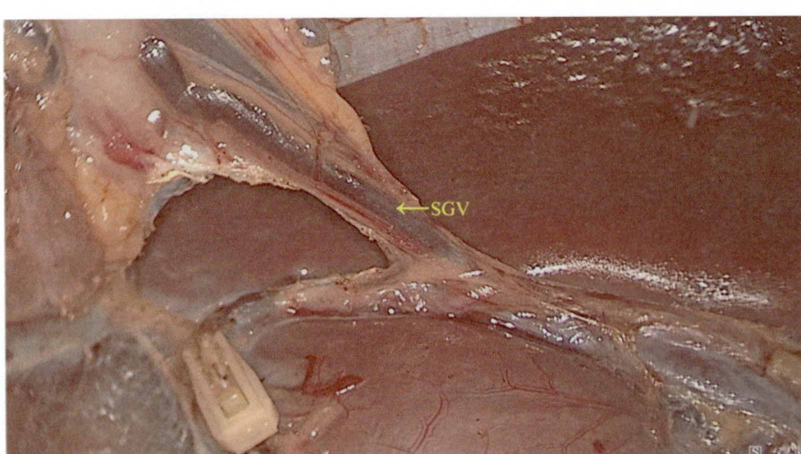

Fig. 4.113 The SGVs supply the upper pole of the spleen

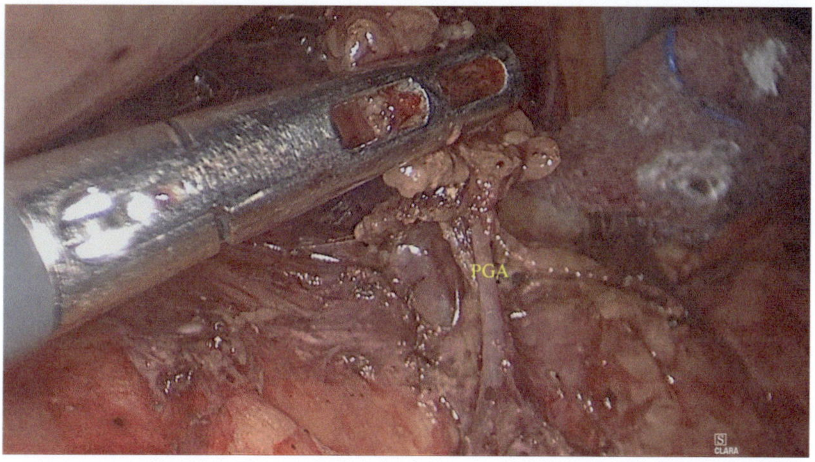

Fig. 4.114 The PGA is vascularized and severed at its root

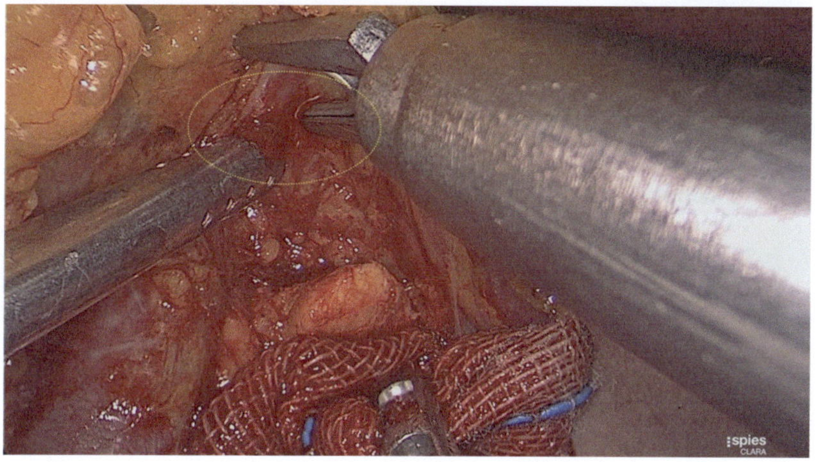

Fig. 4.115 The surgeon uses atraumatic forceps to gently clip the bleeding point, and the titanium clips are ligated to stop bleeding

root of the PGA is vascularized, priority should be given to cutting it to facilitate exposure of the splenic hilar region (Fig. 4.114).

Controlling bleeding is one of the difficulties in splenic hilar LN dissection. If the amount of bleeding is large and the assistant cannot expose the bleeding point, the surgeon should quickly press on it with a large gauze to provide temporary control. The assistant should then suction the blood and re-adjust the position to expose the bleeding site. The surgeon should stop bleeding by using titanium clips to ligate both the upper and lower parts of the bleeding site (Figs. 4.115 and 4.116).

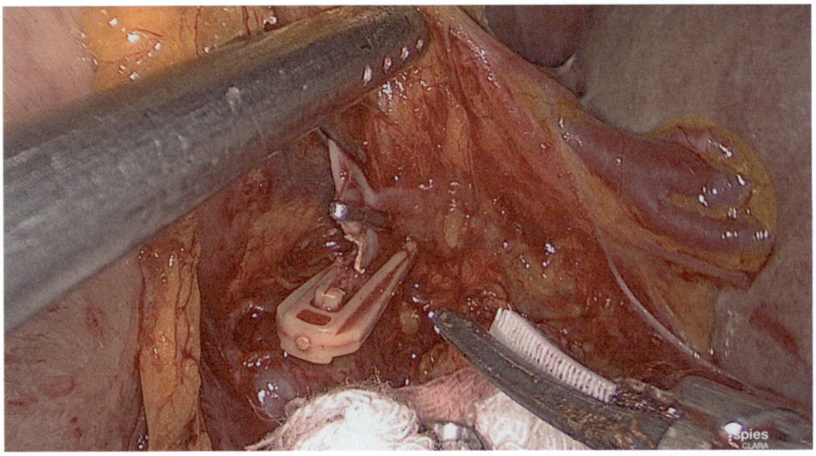

Fig. 4.116 Once hemostasis is successfully stopped

Clarification

All images of the chapter come from FuJian Medical University gastric surgery database and video database.

References

1. Huang C-M, Zheng C-H, editors. Laparoscopic gastrectomy for gastric cancer: Springer; 2015.
2. Huang CM, Chen QY, Lin JX, et al. Huang's three-step maneuver for laparoscopic spleen-preserving No. 10 lymph node dissection for advanced proximal gastric cancer. Chin J Cancer Res. 2014;26(2):208–10.
3. Wang JB, Huang CM, Zheng CH, et al. Laparoscopic spleen-preserving No. 10 lymph node dissection for advanced proximal gastric cancer in left approach: a new operation procedure. World J Surg Oncol. 2012;10:241–7.
4. Huang CM, Chen QY, Lin JX, et al. Laparoscopic spleen-preserving No. 10 lymph node dissection for advanced proximal gastric cancer using a left approach. Ann Surg Oncol. 2014;21(6):2051.
5. Huang CM, Chen QY, Lin JX, et al. Laparoscopic spleen-preserving splenic hilar lymphadenectomy performed by following the perigastric fascias and the intrafascial space for advanced upper-third gastric cancer. PLoS One. 2014;9(3):e90345.
6. Huang CM, Lin JX. Laparoscopic spleen-preserving splenic hilar lymph node dissection for proximal gastric cancer. Chin J Gastrointest Surg. 2012;15(8):784–6.

Laparoscopic Cardial Area LN Dissection for Gastric Cancer

5

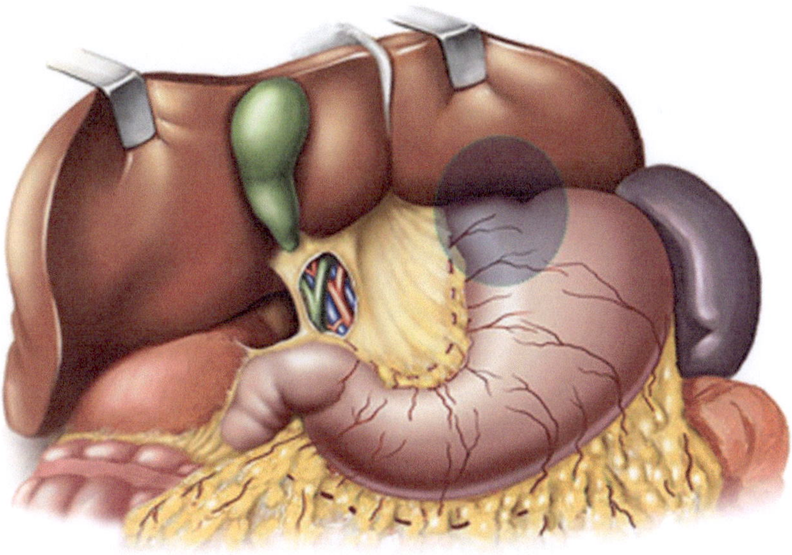

Fig. 5.1 Cardial area (Reproduced with permission from [1])

5.1 Operative Steps for LN Dissection in the Cardial Area

5.1.1 Baring the Gastric Lesser Curvature and Dissection of No.1 and No. 3 LNs

5.1.1.1 Operative Approach

No. 1 and No. 3 LNs are excised by the posterior gastric approach, taking the avascular area of the posterior wall of the gastric lesser curvature as the surgical entry point (Fig. 5.2). The gastric anterior wall and the HGL are used to ward off the liver making it easier to expose the posterior wall of the gastric lesser curvature. The cutting direction of the ultrasonic scalpel is parallel to the gastric lesser curvature to aid division of the HGL along the gastric lesser curvature. The surgeon should use the ultrasonic scalpel to completely clamp and divide the vessels of the gastric lesser curvature to avoid vascular bleeding.

C.-M. Huang et al., *Atlas of Laparoscopic Gastrectomy for Gastric Cancer*,
https://doi.org/10.1007/978-981-13-2862-6_5

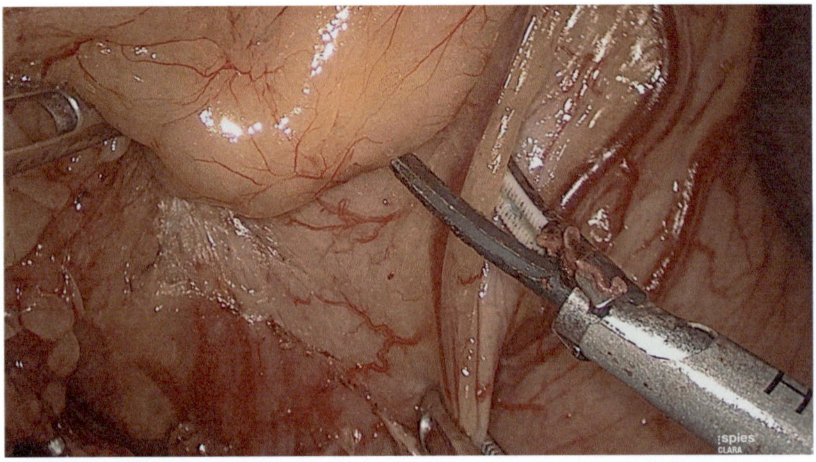

Fig. 5.2 Excising No. 1 and No. 3 LNs using the posterior gastric approach

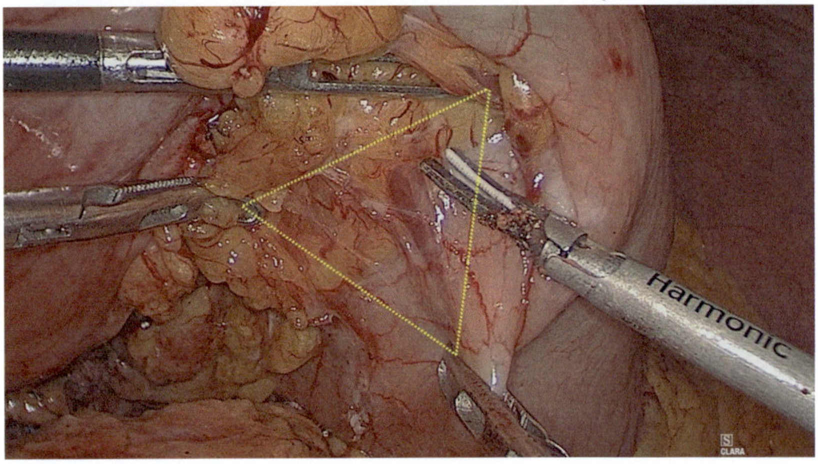

Fig. 5.3 Triangle traction maintains tension on the posterior wall of the gastric body

5.1.1.2 Exposure Methods

The assistant turns the greater curvature of the gastric body over to the head side. Using the left-hand grasper, they then clamp the GPF at the lesser curvature, and use the right-hand grasper to clamp the lesser omentum at the posterior wall of the upper gastric lesser curvature to unfold it on both sides. The surgeon then pulls down the back wall of the gastric body to form a triangulation by clamping the posterior wall of the gastric body. This maintains tension on the HGL at the upper gastric lesser curvature and the posterior wall of the gastric body (Fig. 5.3), improving the surgical space.

5.1.1.3 Operative Procedures

The ultrasonic scalpel opens the posterior lobe of the HGL in the avascular area at the posterior wall of the gastric lesser curvature (Fig. 5.4). Then the posterior lobe of the HGL and vessels of the posterior gastric wall against the gastric wall are separated and divided (Fig. 5.5). Next, the gastric wall towards the anterior lobe of the HGL is separated (Fig. 5.6), and this is continued to transect the anterior lobe of the HGL and the anterior gastric wall (Fig. 5.7). The dissection proceeds upwards until it reaches the cardia (Fig. 5.8), and this is separated down near the gastric angle (Fig. 5.9). Finally, the gastric lesser

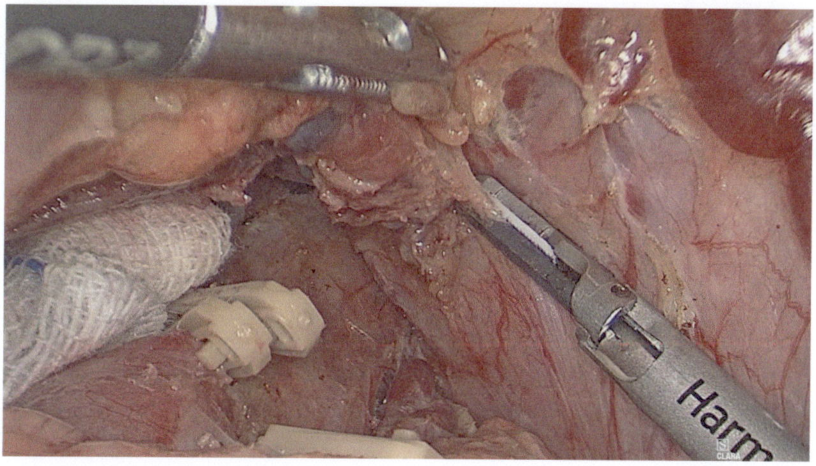

Fig. 5.4 The posterior lobe of the HGL is opened in the avascular area at the posterior wall of the gastric lesser curvature

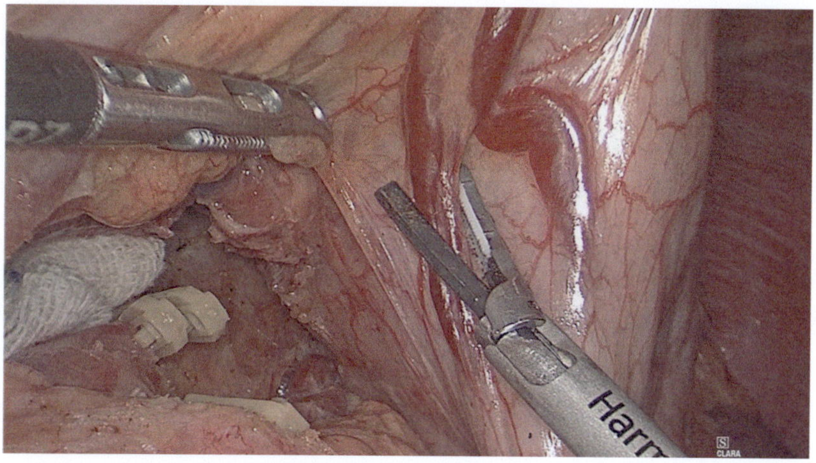

Fig. 5.5 The posterior lobe of the HGL and the vessels of the gastric posterior wall are divided to denude the posterior wall of the gastric lesser curvature

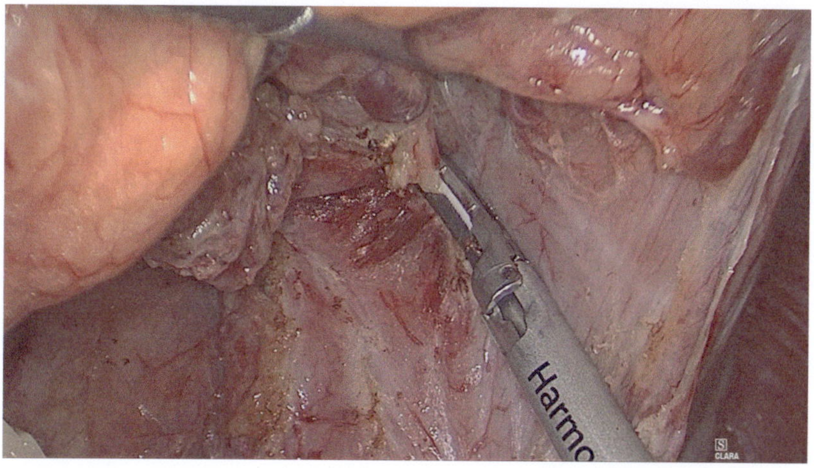

Fig. 5.6 The anterior lobe of the HGL is opened in the avascular area at the posterior wall of the gastric lesser curvature

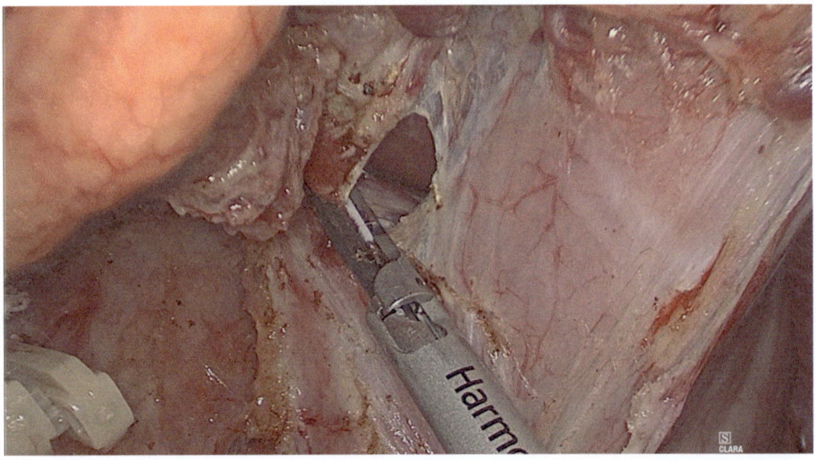

Fig. 5.7 The anterior lobe of the HGL and the vessels of the gastric anterior wall are divided to denude the anterior wall of the gastric lesser curvature

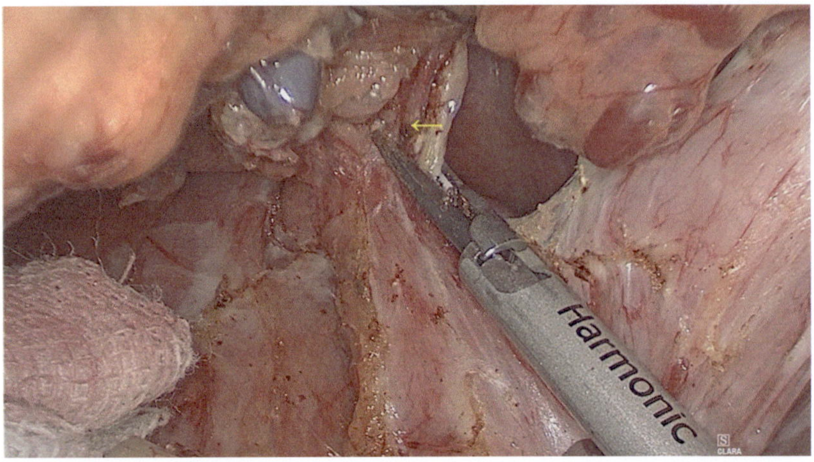

Fig. 5.8 The dissection proceeds upwards along the gastric lesser curvature until the cardia is reached

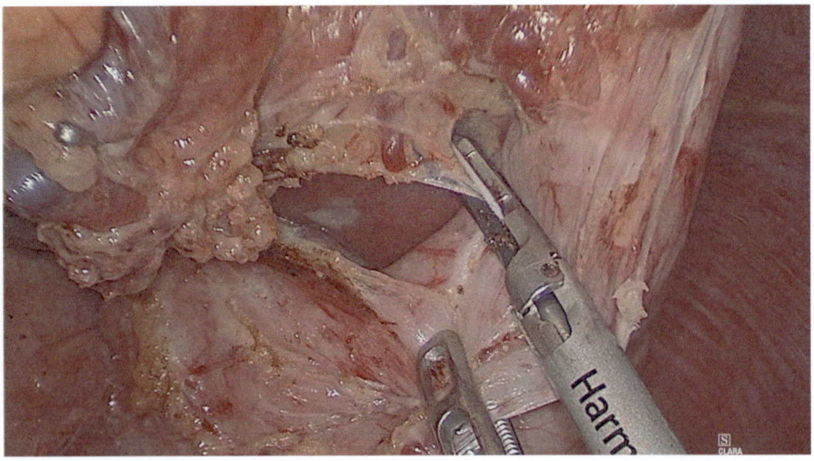

Fig. 5.9 The dissection proceeds downwards along the gastric lesser curvature until the gastric angle is reached

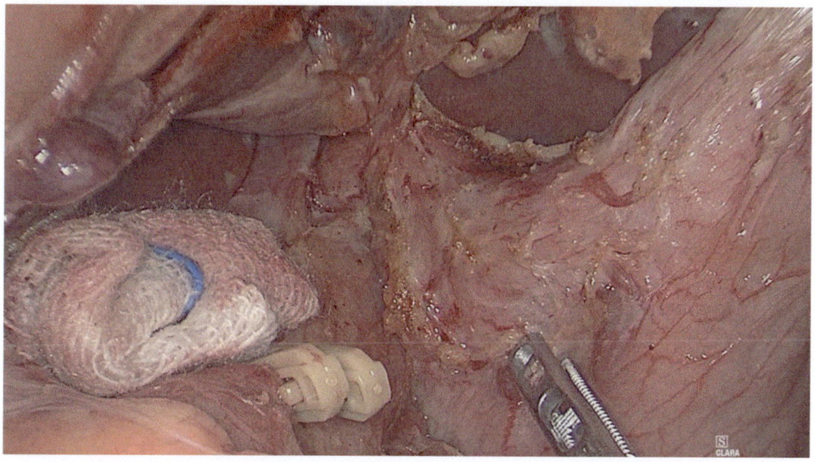

Fig. 5.10 The gastric lesser curvature is fully bared, and dissection of No. 3 LNs is accomplished

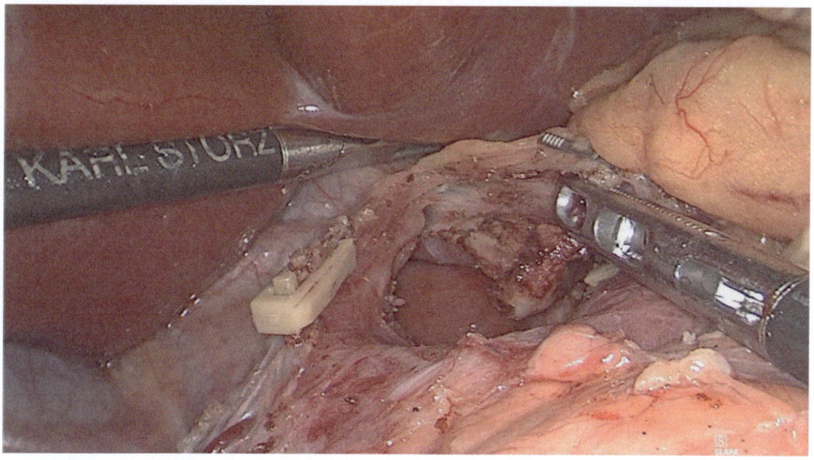

Fig. 5.11 The assistant lifts up the left lobe of the liver to expose the HDL from the front

curvature is thoroughly exposed to complete the dissection of No. 3 LNs (Fig. 5.10).

The assistant turns the gastric wall back to the normal position and holds the grasper, lifting up the left lateral external lobe of the liver along the lower hepatic margin until the left phrenic angle. The surgeon's left hand presses the gastric corner to tighten the HGL and exposes the anterior segment of the HDL from the front (Fig. 5.11). Next, the ultrasonic scalpel is used to separate upwards to the first hepatic hilum through the window created on the right side of the anterior segment of the HDL. Subsequently, the HGL is transected from the lower edge of the liver to the cardia (Figs. 5.12 and 5.13). Finally, No. 1 and No. 3 LNs are removed (Fig. 5.14).

5.1.2 Baring the Left Side of the Esophagus and Dissection of No. 2 LNs

After excising No. 4sa and No. 10 LNs, the assistant moves the separated omentum and GSL to the right lower abdomen and pulls the gastric wall down to the right side to expose the left region of the cardia (Fig. 5.15).

T ultrasonic scalpel is used to separate the GPL from the upper pole of the spleen along the diaphragm to the esophageal hiatus. When separated to the left of the diaphragm, the assistant pulls the wall of the gastric fundus and cardia towards the upper right side to reveal the crus. Synchronously, the surgeon uses the ultra-

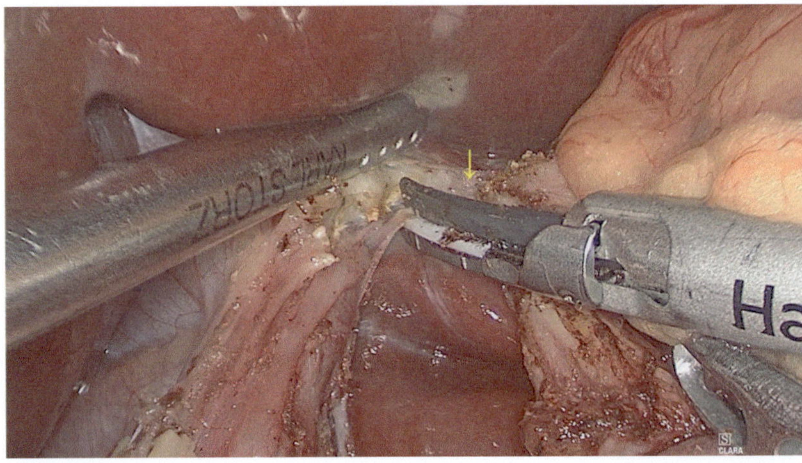

Fig. 5.12 The HGL is transected along the inferior edge of the liver

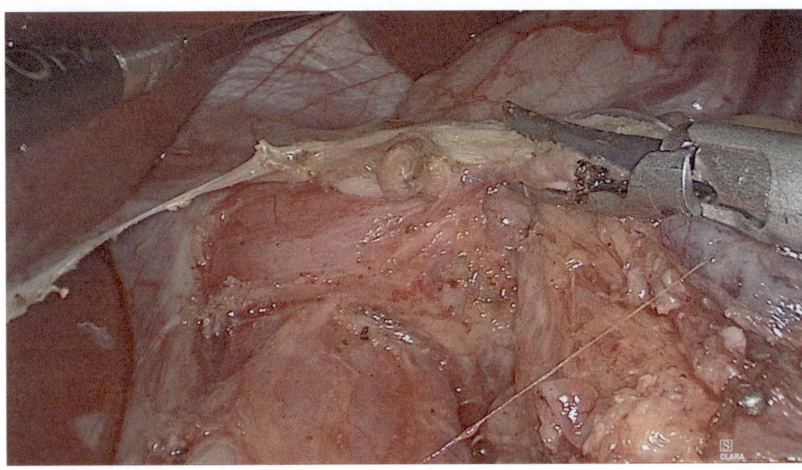

Fig. 5.13 The HGL is transected along the inferior edge of the liver until the cardia is reached

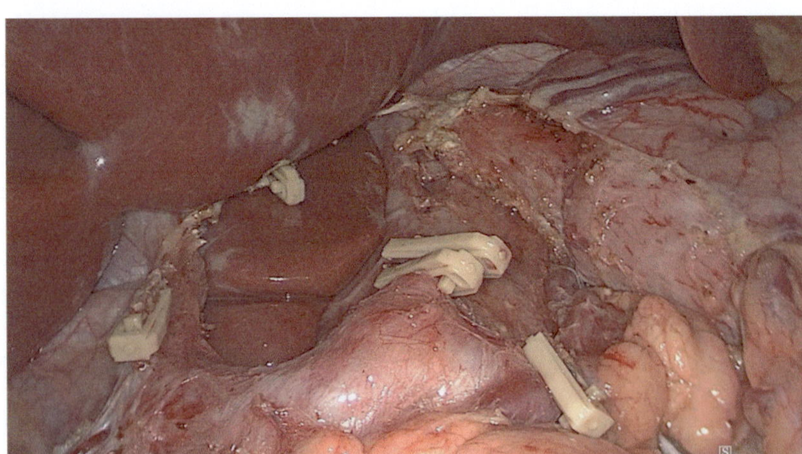

Fig. 5.14 No. 1 and No. 3 LNs are removed

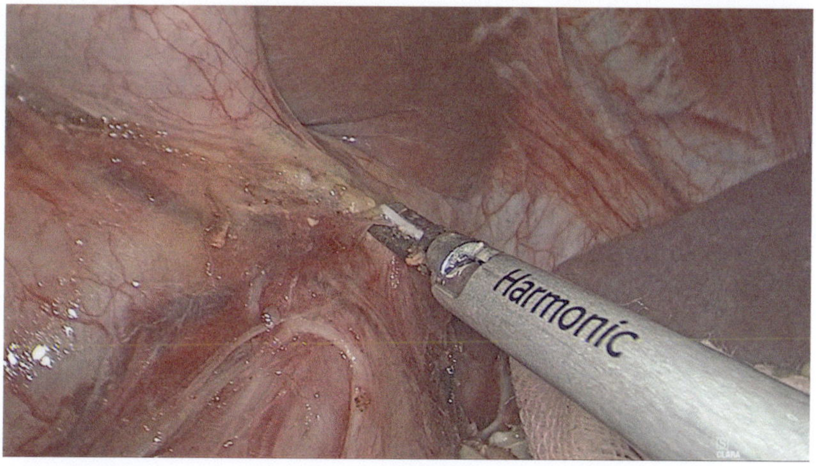

Fig. 5.15 The left aspect of the cardia is exposed

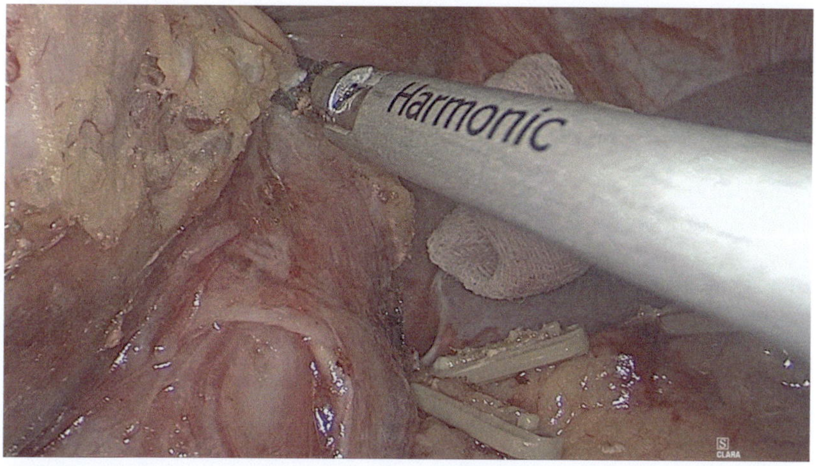

Fig. 5.16 The left side of the GPL is transected along the left diaphragmatic crus to dissect No. 2 LNs

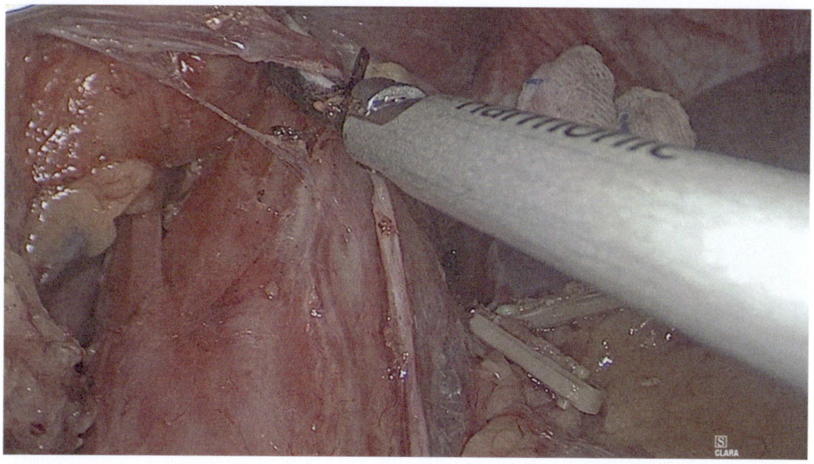

Fig. 5.17 Baring of the lower part of the left side of the esophagus

sonic scalpel to separate adipose lymphoid tissue on the left side of the esophagus and cardia against the left diaphragmatic crus (Fig. 5.16), thus baring the lower left side of the esophagus (Fig. 5.17).

At this point, it is important to note that the fundus branches of the LIPA supply the gastric fundus. The LIPA should be isolated and divided from the fundus at the root (Figs. 5.18 and 5.19) to complete the No. 2 LN dissection (Fig. 5.20).

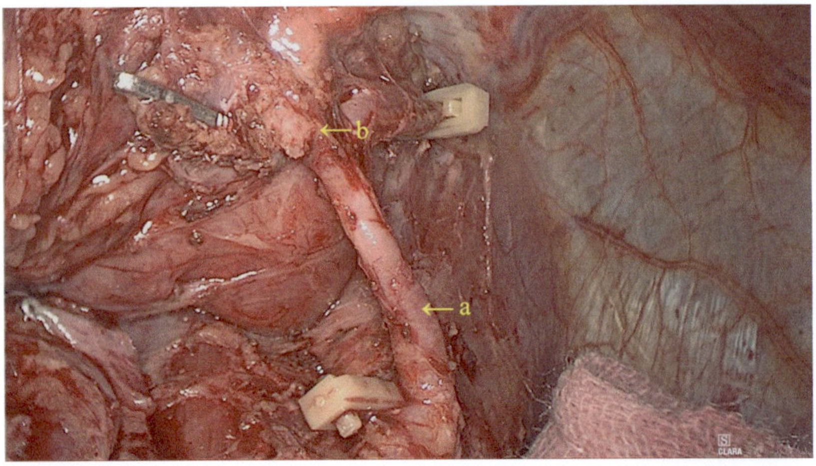

Fig. 5.18 The left inferior phrenic artery (LIPA) (**a**) and its fundic branch (**b**) are isolated

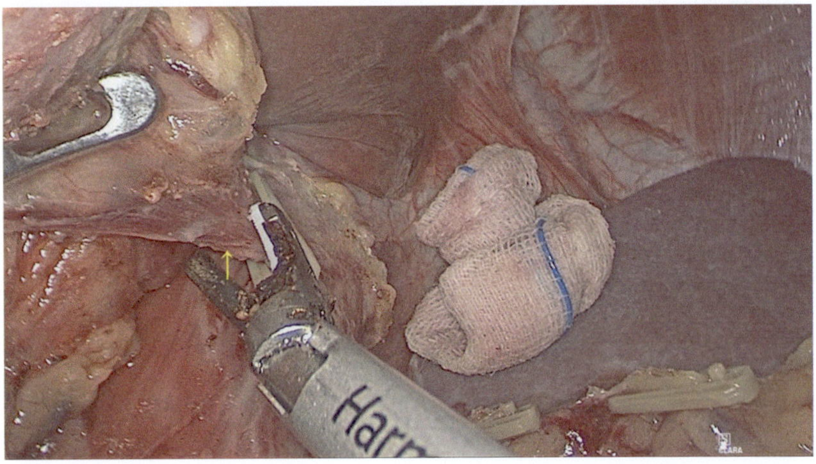

Fig. 5.19 Division of the fundic branch of the LIPA

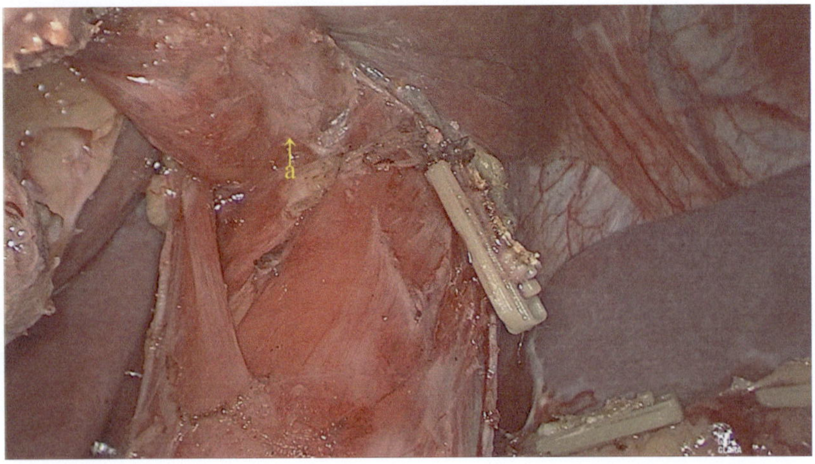

Fig. 5.20 Dissection of No. 2 LNs is accomplished; the left side of the esophagus (**a**)

5.2 Operative Announcements of Laparoscopic Cardial Area LN Dissection for Gastric Cancer

5.2.1 Anatomy Associated with LN Dissection in the Cardial Area

5.2.1.1 Fascia and Intrafascial Space in the Cardial Area

GPL

The GPL comprises the cranial part of the DM that extends upwards to the diaphragm which is continuous with the upper portion of the GSL and the SRL. It is a peritoneal fold between the gastric fundus (close to the cardia) and the left crus of the diaphragm. The fundic branch of the LIPA and the PGAs usually run into the gastric fundus through the GPL (Figs. 5.21 and 5.22).

Hepatogastric Ligament

The HGL derives from the primitive ventral mesogastrium, and arises from the right margin of phrenic and venous ligament fissures. It adheres to the lower left side of the abdominal esophagus and the gastric lesser curvature which is continuous with the hepatoduodenal ligament (Figs. 5.23 and 5.24).

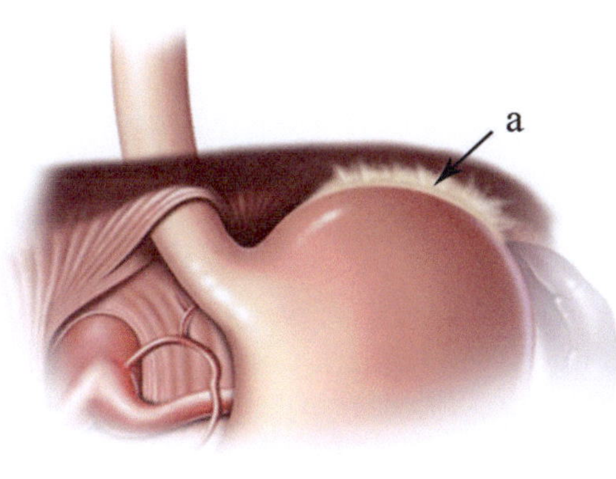

Fig. 5.21 The anterior aspect of the GSL (**a**) (Reproduced with permission from [1])

Arteries Associated with LN Dissection in the Cardial Area

Terminal Branch of the LGA

After emitting from the CA, the LGA travels towards the upper left side until it is just below the lesser curvature of the cardia, where it enters the HGL. It has two descending branches near the gastric wall, and runs downwards and to the right along the anterior and posterior sides of the gastric lesser curvature. Around 4–6 branches supply the anterior and posterior gastric walls, and anastomose with the right gastric artery to form a small curved artery arch (Figs. 5.25 and 5.26).

Fundic Branch of the LIPA

The gastric fundus branch of the LIPA arises from the abdominal aorta and passes upwards to divide into the left and right inferior phrenic arteries, which are terminal branches of the left inferior phrenic artery. The left inferior phrenic artery bypasses the posterior side of the cardiac area, and its fundic branch runs through the GPL to supply the gastric fundus (Fig. 5.27).

5.2.1.2 Veins Associated with LN Dissection in the Cardial Area

LGA: Left gastric artery.

The coronary vein comprises venous branches from the anterior and posterior walls of the gastric lesser curvature. They flow in the direction of the cardia within the lesser omentum, and then drain into the SpV or the PV. Partial vein from the esophageal veins and the submucosal venous plexus may form the short gastric veins or the posterior gastric vein (PGV) to end in the SV, and then communicate with the superior vena cava. This forms the portal-caval venous collateral circulation (Fig. 5.28).

5.2.1.3 LN Anatomy of the Cardial Area

No. 1 LNs (Right Paracardial LNs)

Definition of No. 1 LNs.

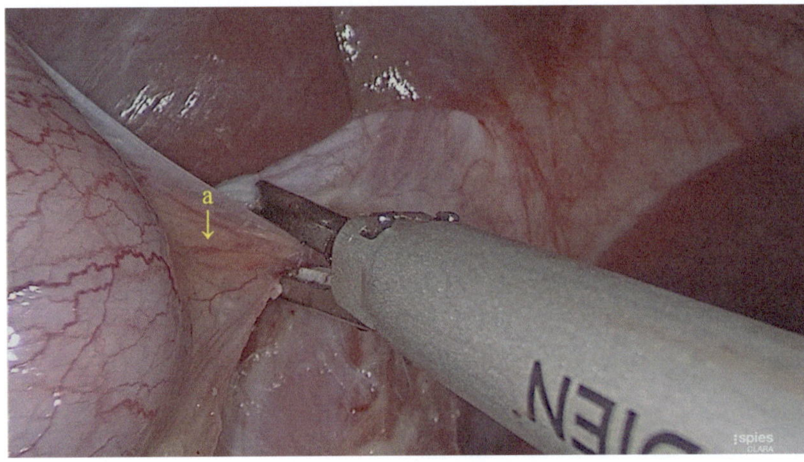

Fig. 5.22 GSL (**a**)

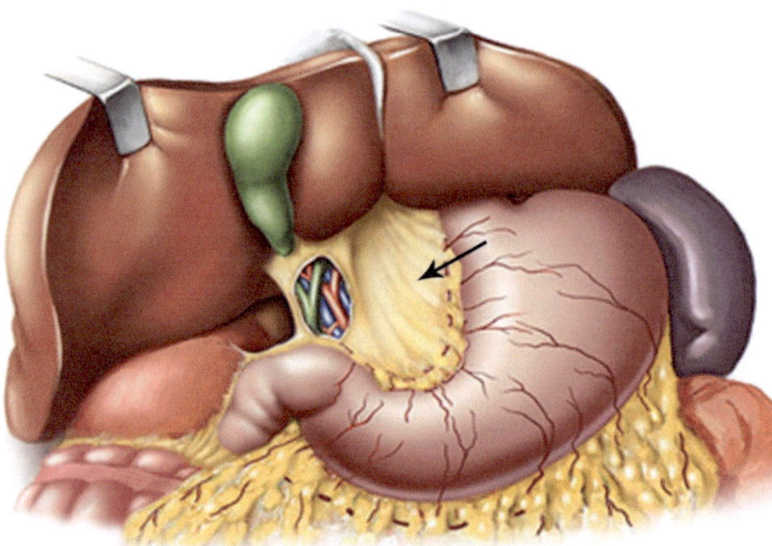

Fig. 5.23 Schematic of the HGL (arrowed) (Reproduced with permission from [1])

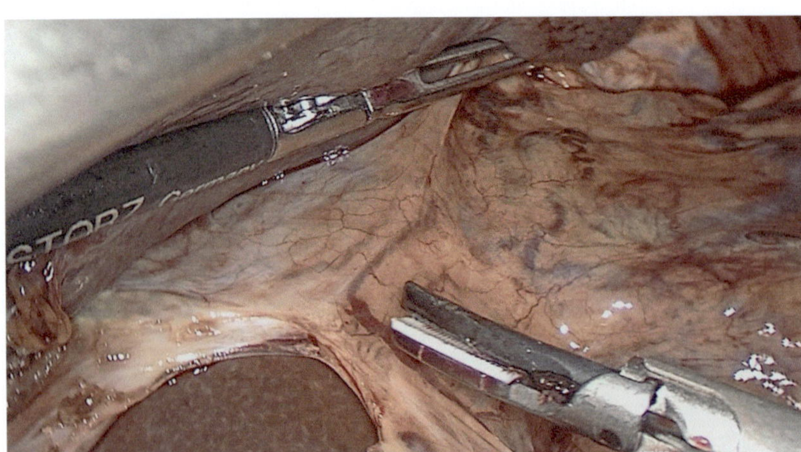

Fig. 5.24 HGL

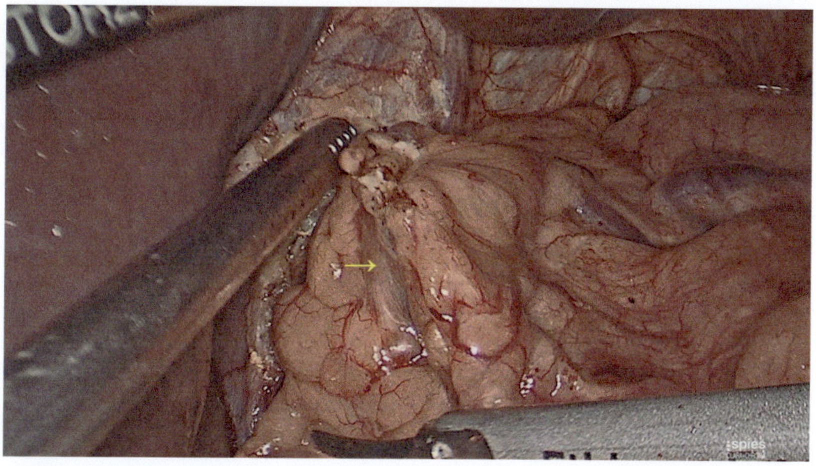

Fig. 5.25 The LGA has ascending branches (arrowed)

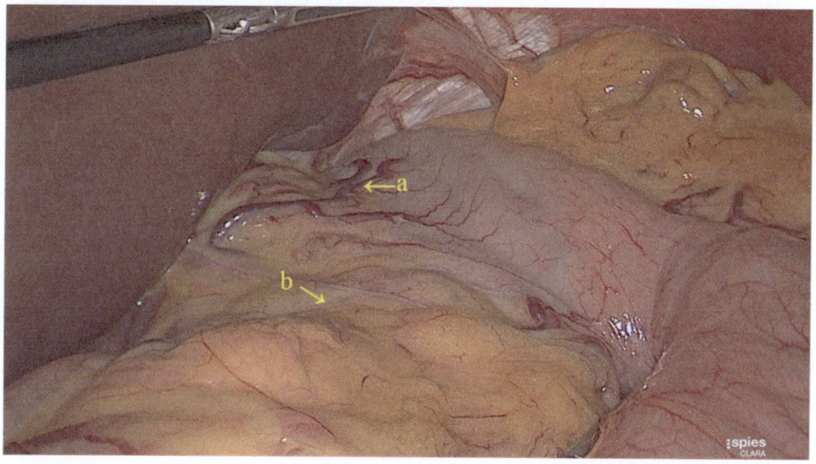

Fig. 5.26 The LGA has anterior (**a**) and posterior (**b**) gastric branches

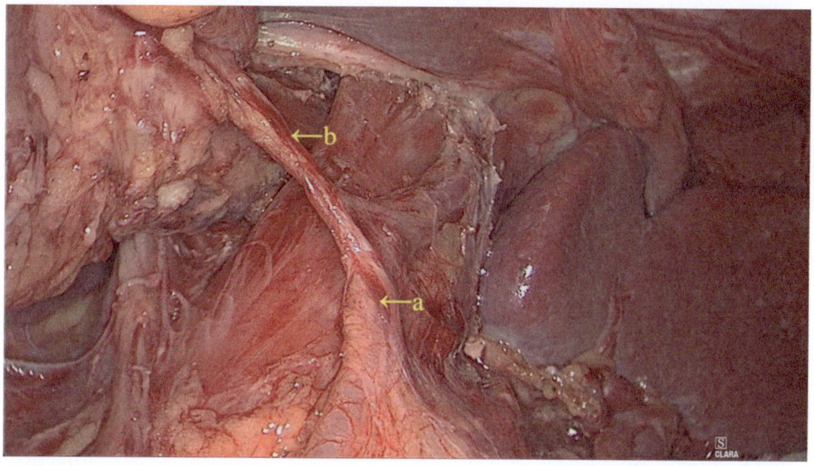

Fig. 5.27 The LIPA (**a**) gives off the fundic branch (**b**) to supply the fundus

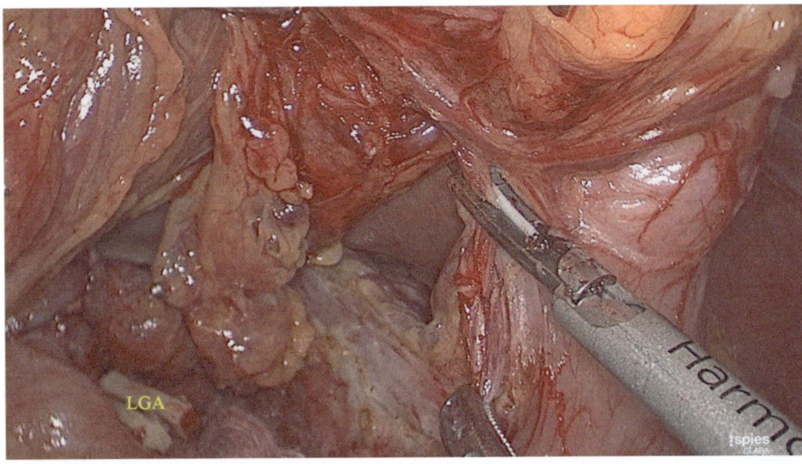

Fig. 5.28 The venous branches from the anterior and posterior walls of the gastric lesser curvature the join together to form the coronary vein

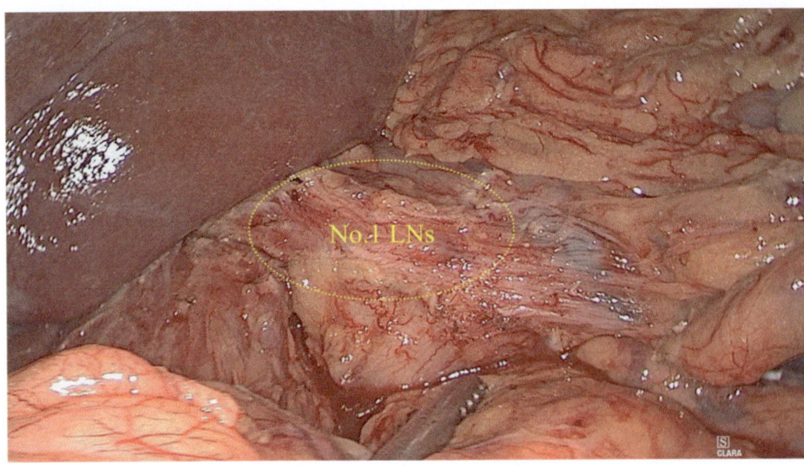

Fig. 5.29 The scope of No. 1 LNs

LNs above the first branch of the ascending LGA (cardia branch), those located at the right side of the cardia and the ascending branch of the left gastric artery or located in this branch of the blood vessel are all No. 1 LNs. Using the blood vessel (cardia branch) as a boundary, the LNs below are regarded as No. 3 LNs (Fig. 5.29).

No. 1 LNM can be seen in Fig. 5.30.

An ICG display of No. 1 LNs can be seen in Figs. 5.31 and 5.32.

No. 2 LNs (Left Paracardial LNs)

Definition of No. 2 LNs.

No. 2 LNs are distributed along the gastric fundus branch of the left inferior phrenic artery and are located at the anterior and posterior fundus on the left side of the cardia. No. 1 and No. 2 LNs are bordered by the esophageal axis (Fig. 5.33).

No. 2 LNM can be seen in Figs. 5.34 and 5.35.

An ICG display of No. 2 LNs can be seen in Figs. 5.36 and 5.37.

No. 3 LNs (LNs Along the Gastric Lesser Curvature)

Definition of No. 3 LNs.

GLC: Gastric lesser curvature.

No. 3 LNs are distributed along the left and right gastric arteries, and are included in the two layers of the lesser omentum along the gastric lesser curvature. The upper border is formed by the first branch of the ascending

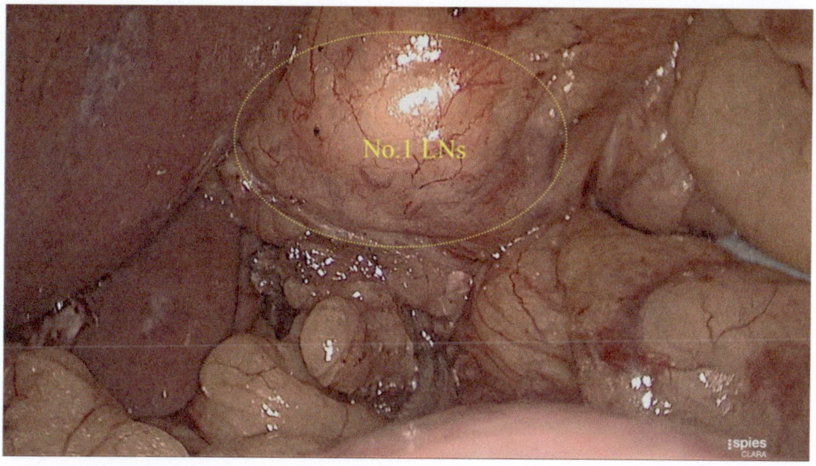

Fig. 5.30 Intraoperative view of No. 1 LNM

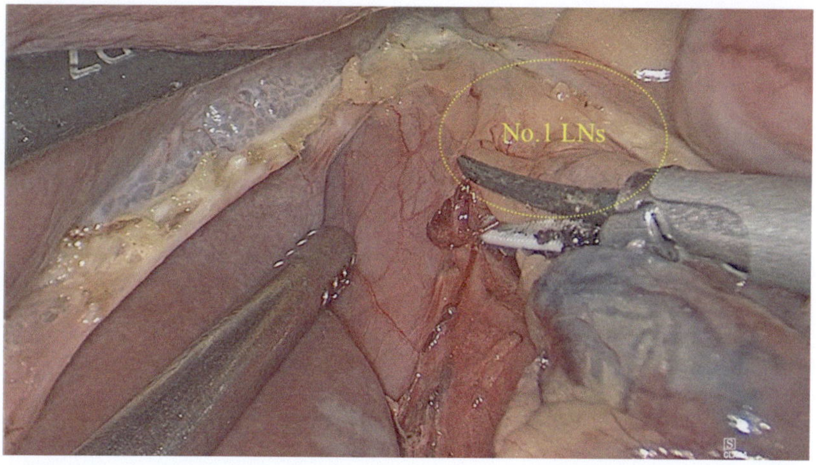

Fig. 5.31 View of No. 1 LNs with the naked eye

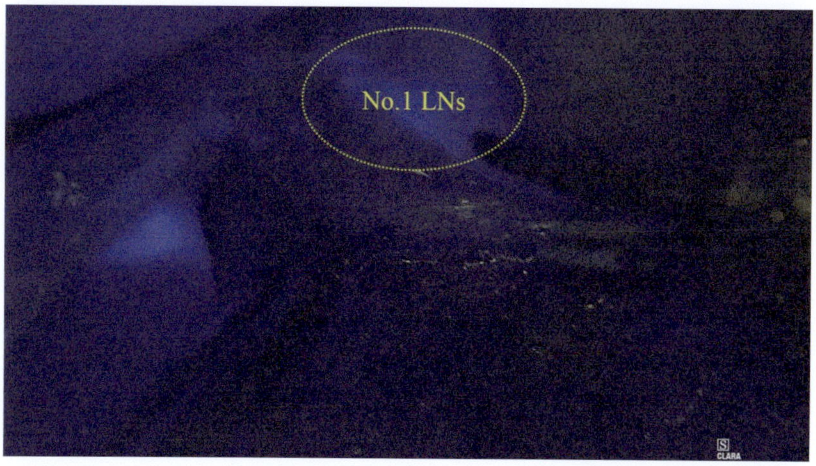

Fig. 5.32 ICG display of No. 1 LNs

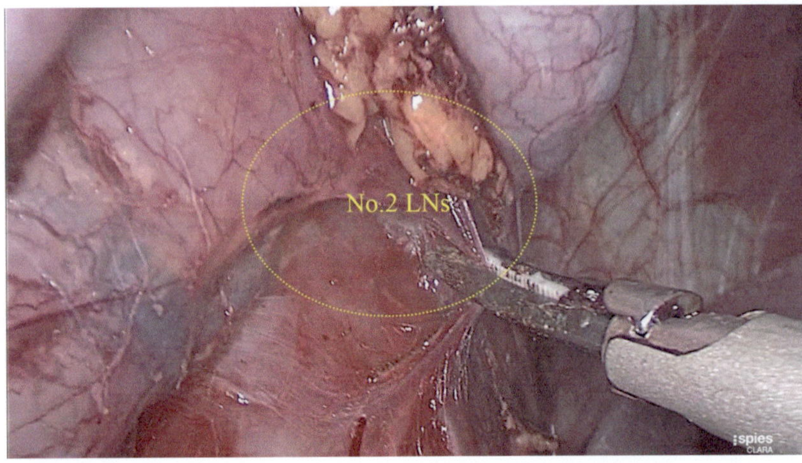

Fig. 5.33 The scope of No. 2 LNs

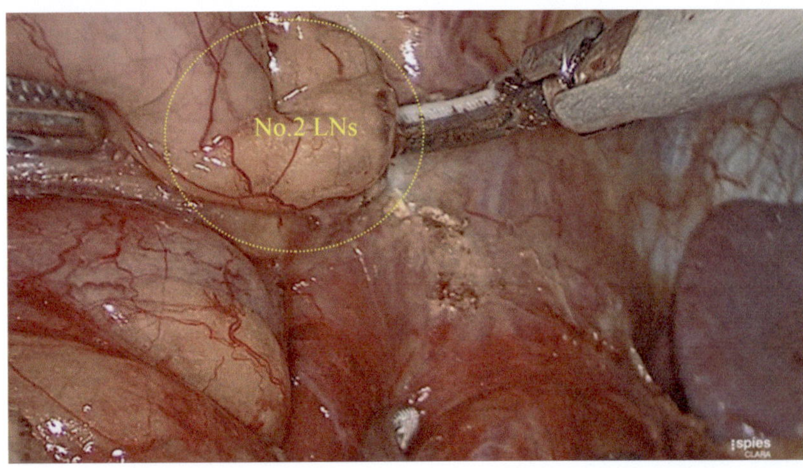

Fig. 5.34 Intraoperative view of No. 2 LNM

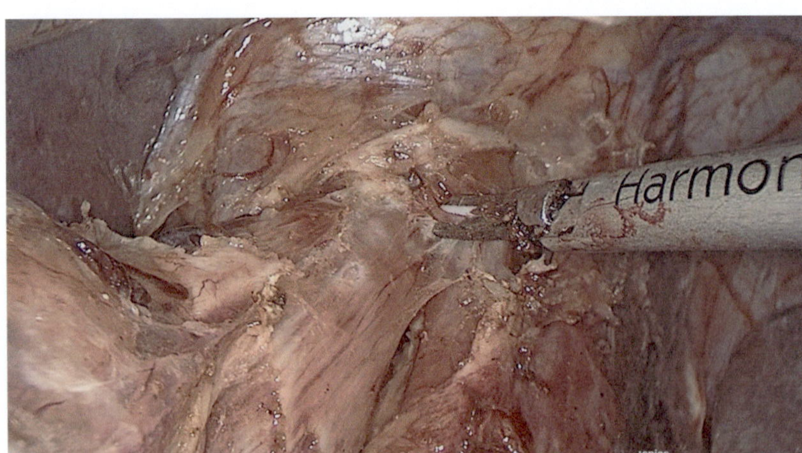

Fig. 5.35 No. 2 LNM (after dissection)

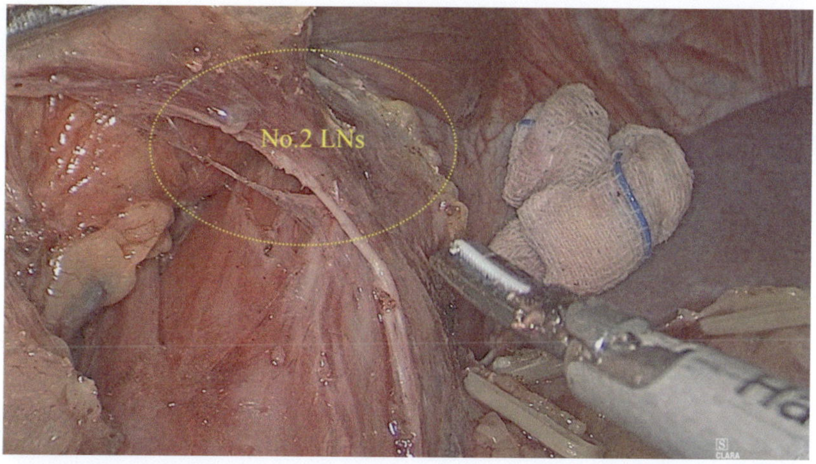

Fig. 5.36 View of No. 2 LNs with the naked eye

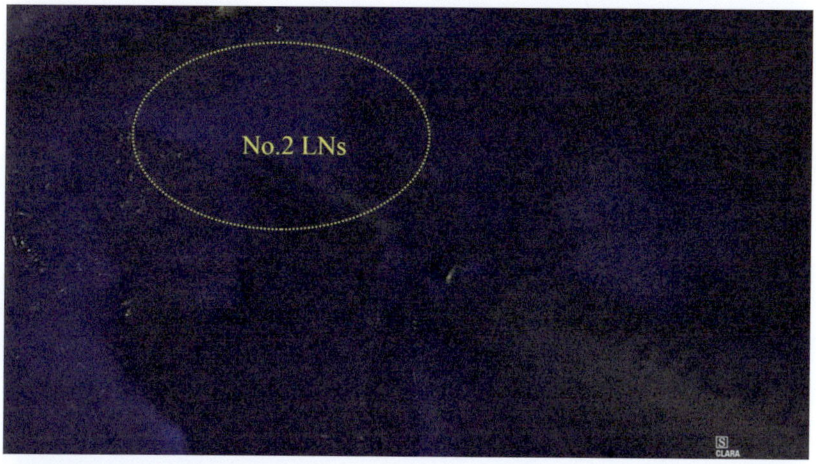

Fig. 5.37 ICG display of No. 2 LNs

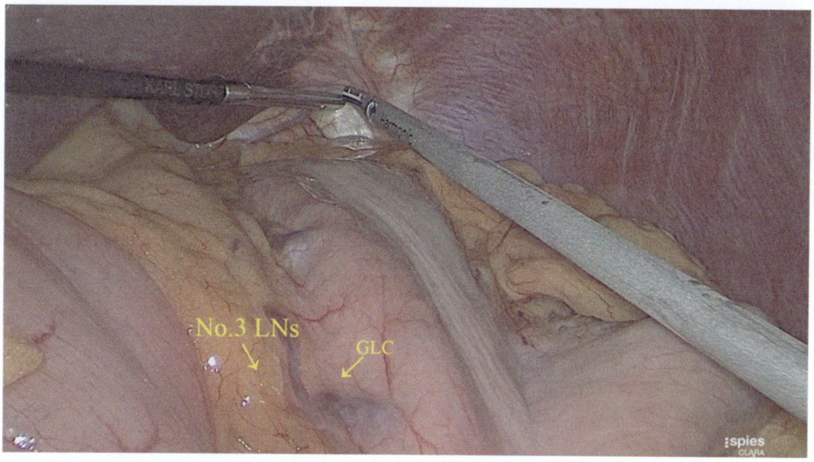

Fig. 5.38 The scope of No. 3 LNs

LGA which feeds the gastric walls (LNs on this branch of the blood vessel are not included). The lower border is the first left branch of the right gastric artery entering the gastric wall of the lesser gastric curvature (LNs located at the root of the vessel are classified as No. 5 LNs) (Fig. 5.38).

No. 3 LNM can be seen in Fig. 5.39.

An ICG display of No. 3 LNs can be seen in Figs. 5.40 and 5.41.

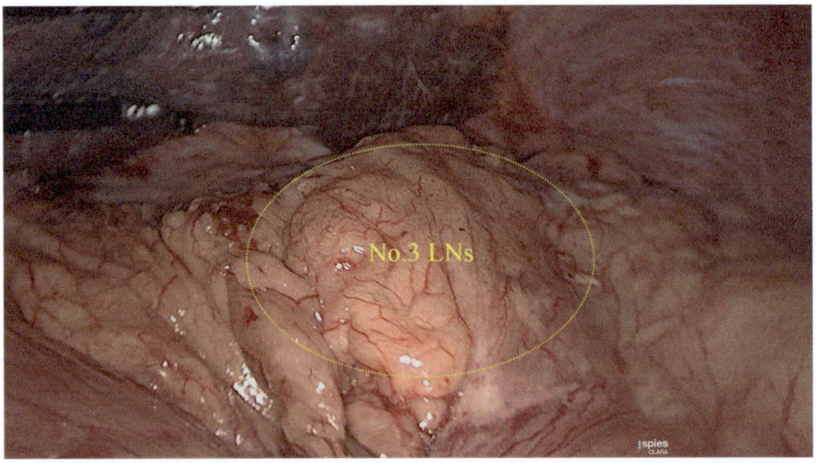

Fig. 5.39 Intraoperative view of No. 3 LNM

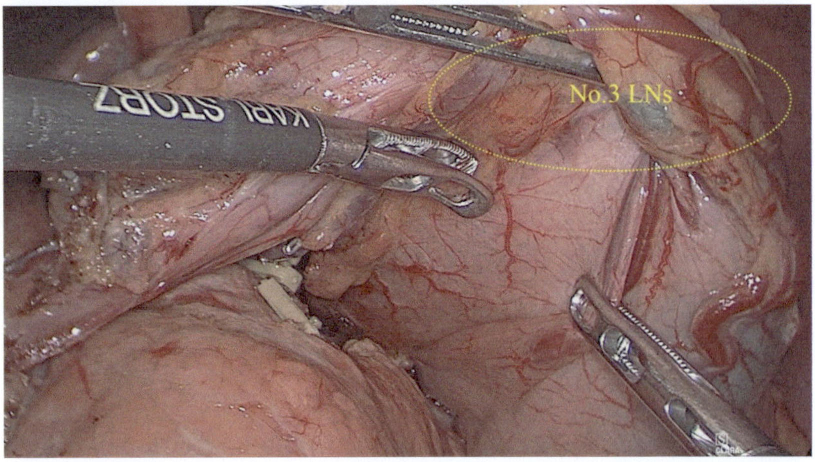

Fig. 5.40 View of No. 3 LNs with the naked eye

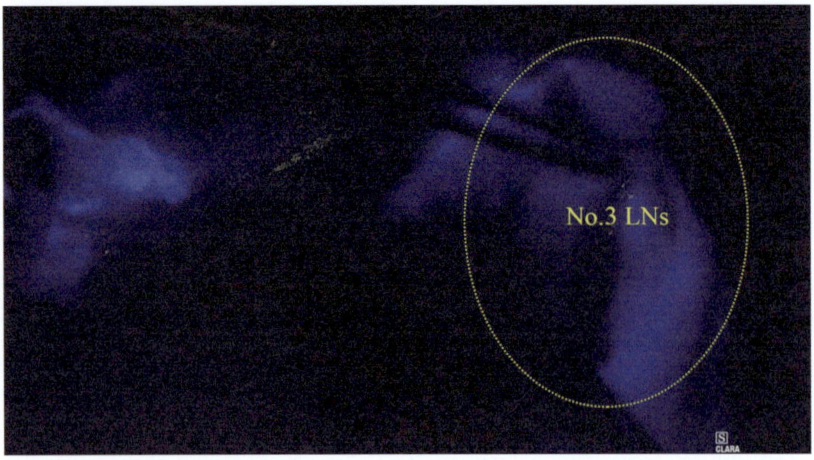

Fig. 5.41 An ICG display of No. 3 LNs

5.2.2 Intraoperative Considerations of LN Dissection in the Cardial Area

The surgeon's right hand holds the ultrasonic scalpel, baring the gastric curvature from the front wall to the posterior wall and from the lesser curvature side to the cardial side. The direction of surgery from the back to the front should coincide with that of the ultrasonic scalpel. This not only keeps the ultrasonic scalpel close to the lesser curvature for separation and maintains a correct anatomic plane, but also enables small flexural gastric vessels to be completely clamped for amputation (Fig. 5.42).

When separating near the cardia, attention should be paid to recognizing esophageal tissue and avoiding excessive dissection, which could damage the lower esophagus (Fig. 5.43).

At the same time, the camera operator should adjust the direction of the lens direction from the lower right to the upper left, using the horizontal pancreas as the baseline (Fig. 5.44).

The dissection of LNs in the cardia is performed in a small space under the xiphoid, and good exposure by the assistant can reduce tissue

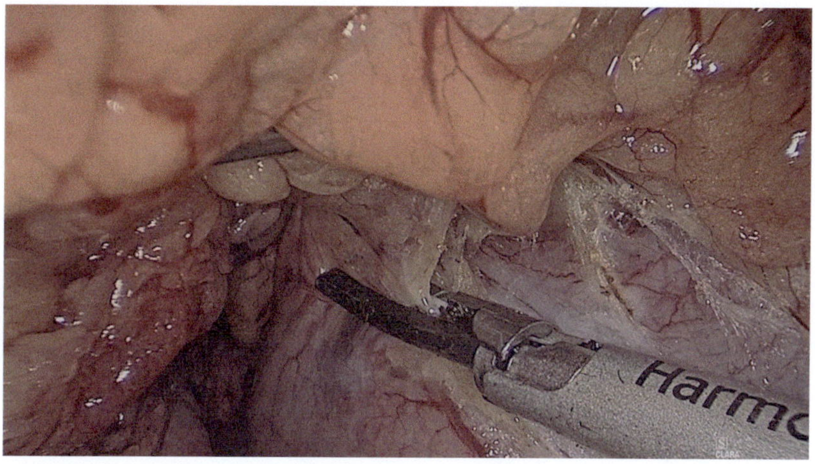

Fig. 5.42 Ultrasonic scalpel completely clamps the blood vessel

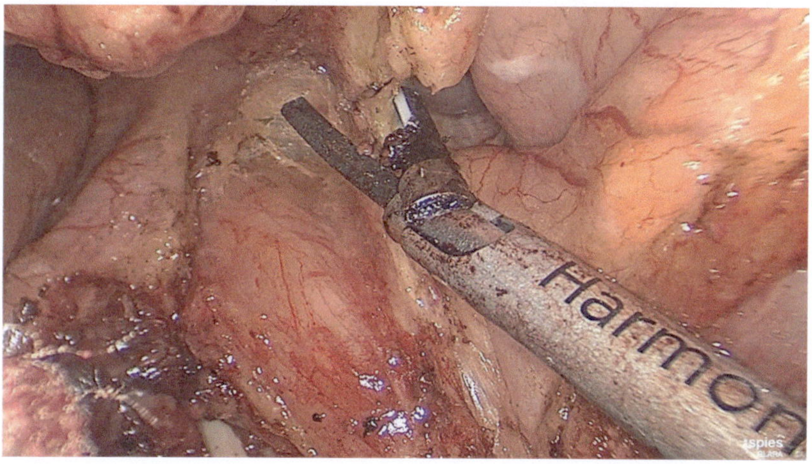

Fig. 5.43 Attention should be paid to identify esophageal tissue

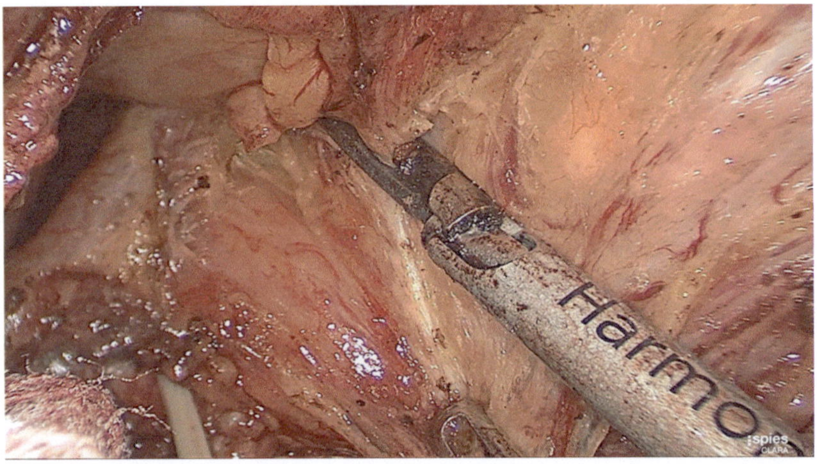

Fig. 5.44 The lens direction is from bottom right to top left

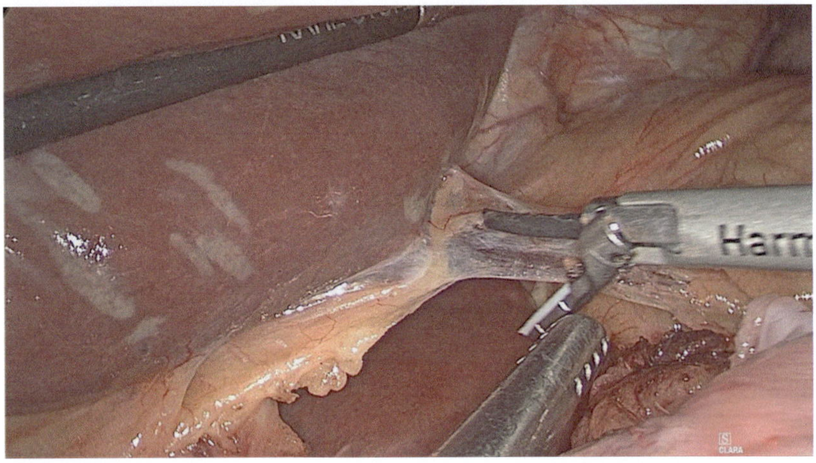

Fig. 5.45 The assistant can expose the operating view using grasping forceps in the left hand to push the left lateral lobe of the liver upwards

damage. When separating the anterior wall of the omentum, the assistant's left hand uses grasping forceps to push the left lateral hepatic lobe upwards to expose the field of view (Fig. 5.45).

After the left hepatic lateral lobe is exposed, the assistant's right hand should hold the aspirator or gastric forceps to assist the surgeon in separating the tissues and denuding the esophagus. In the process of denuding, the vagus nerve trunk should be severed first (the left trunk is generally on the front wall, and the right trunk is generally on the back wall). The fascia should then be divided between the esophagus and the esophageal hiatus to enable the mobilized esophagus to reach up to about 6 cm (Figs. 5.46 and 5.47).

Va: Vagus nerve.

The vagus nerves are mostly of high tension and brightly white stripe but their quality and elasticity are poor. The assistant should separate loose tissue between the vagus nerve and the esophagus along the longitudinal axis of the esophagus with an aspirator or gastric forceps. Then, the left and right vagus nerves should be removed along the anterior and posterior walls of the esophagus to make them easier to sever (Fig. 5.48).

According to the distribution of the terminal LGA in the gastric wall, the omentum of the lesser curvature can be regarded as an anterior layer, middle layer, and posterior layer. The surgeon should first open the omentum from the posterior layer in a region without blood vessels,

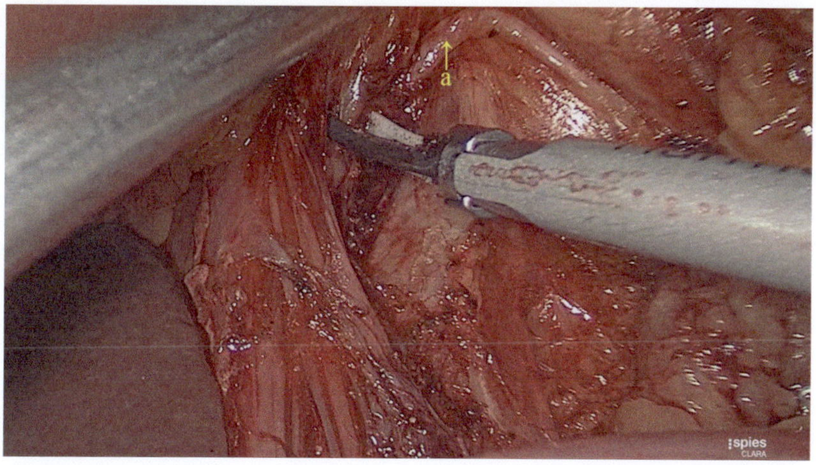

Fig. 5.46 The right trunk of the vagus nerve (**a**) is severed

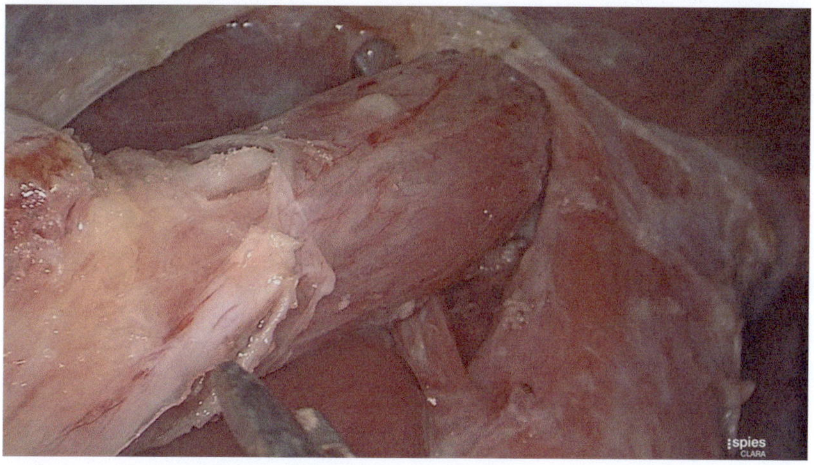

Fig. 5.47 Entirely mobilized abdominal segment of the esophagus

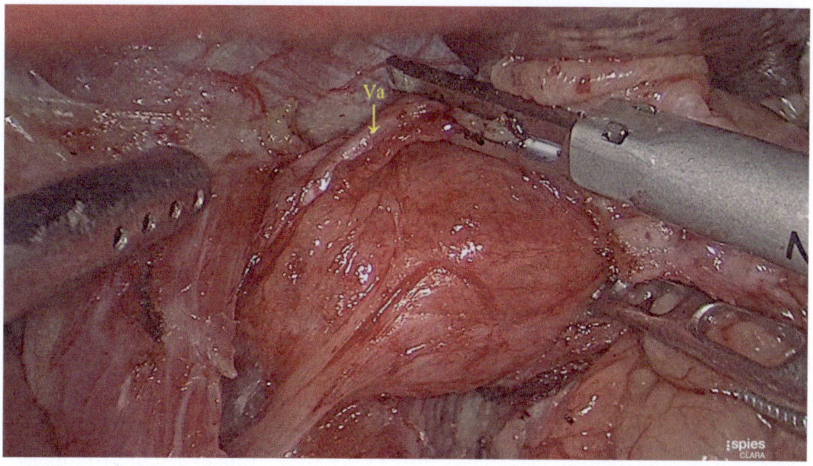

Fig. 5.48 The assistant separates the left vagus nerve with an aspirator or gastric forceps and picks apart the free vagus nerves from the esophagus

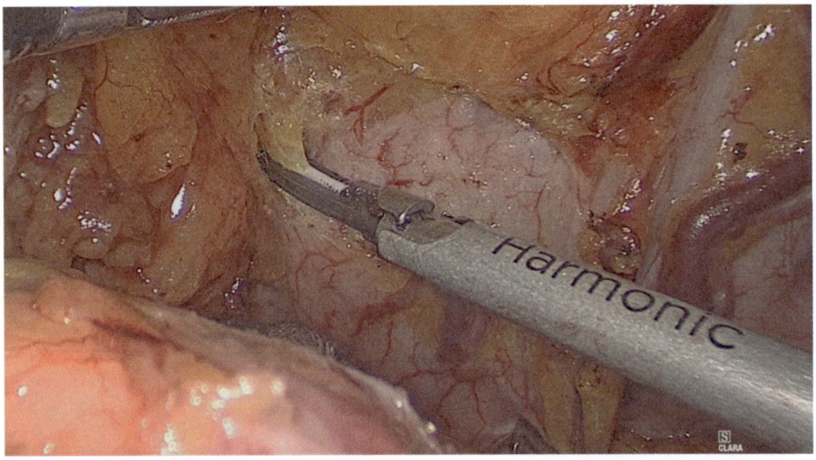

Fig. 5.49 Division of the middle layer of the lesser omentum

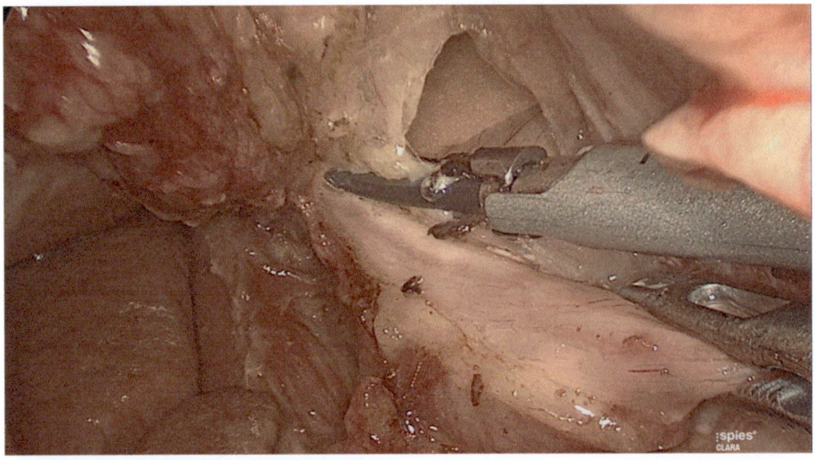

Fig. 5.50 Division of the anterior layer of the lesser omentum

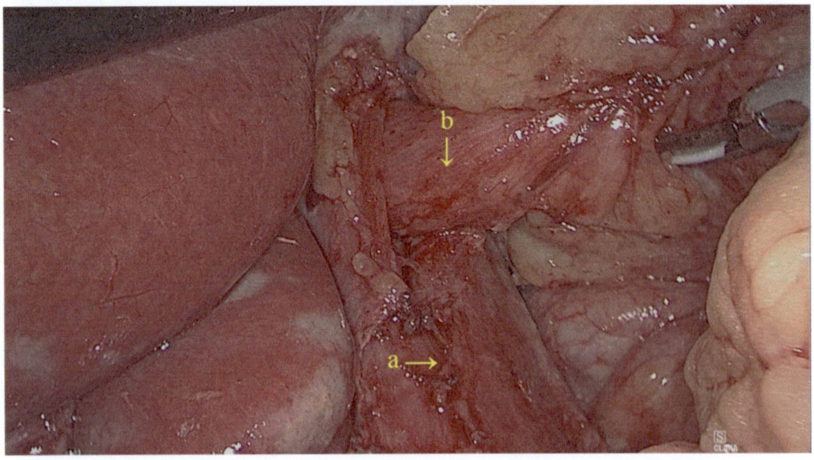

Fig. 5.51 LGA has branches (**a**) to supply to the diaphragm; the esophagus (**b**)

and continue to separate this layer and its blood vessels when performing the dissection. Next, the medial omentum should be separates, followed by the anterior omentum (Figs. 5.49 and 5.50).

Sometimes the LGA has blood vessels that innervate the diaphragm; these should be cut off to avoid causing hemorrhage when the lesser curvature is denuded (Fig. 5.51).

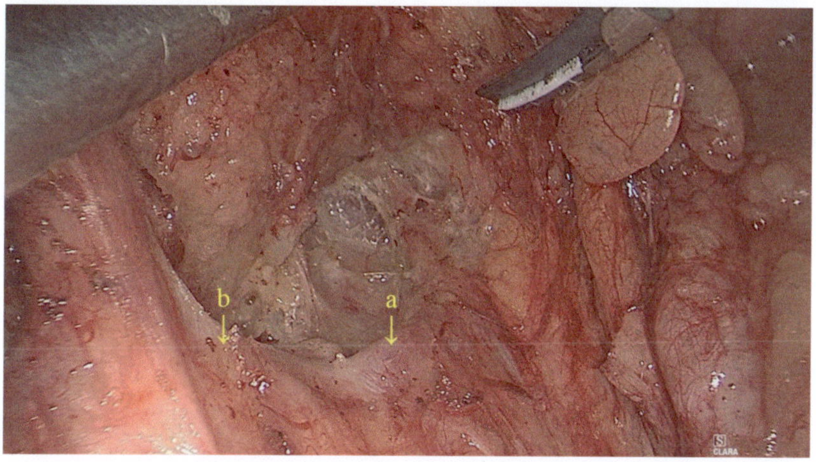

Fig. 5.52 The LIPA (**a**) originates from the celiac trunk (**b**), and may be susceptible to injury because of its superficial location

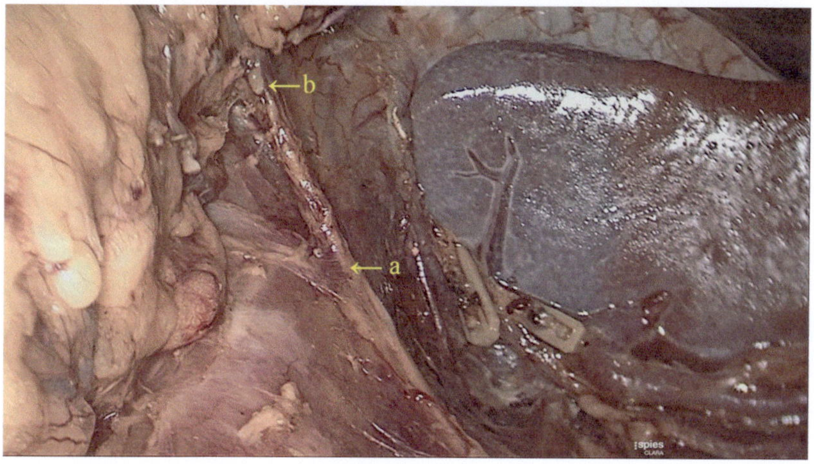

Fig. 5.53 Severing the fundic branch (**b**) arising from the LIPA (**a**)

When separating the gastrophrenic ligament along the left diaphragmatic angle, attention should be paid to the LIPA and its fundus. This is especially true when the LIPA originates from the celiac trunk because its superficial location may cause injury (Fig. 5.52).

When meeting the fundic branch arising from the LIPA, it should be severed by the surgeon at its root, taking care not to damage the left infrapatellar artery (Fig. 5.53).

Clarification

All images of the chapter come from FuJian Medical University gastric surgery database and video database.

Reference

1. Huang C-M, Zheng C-H, editors. Laparoscopic gastrectomy for gastric cancer: Springer; 2015.

6 Total Laparoscopic Reconstruction of the Digestive Tract After Radical Gastrectomy for Gastric Cancer

With the wide application of laparoscopic technology and accumulated experience in laparoscopic surgery, the reconstruction of digestive tract after laparoscopic gastrectomy has become a hot topic in surgical field. Currently, there are various methods for the total laparoscopic reconstruction of the digestive tract after radical gastrectomy of gastric cancer, including Billroth I anastomosis, Billroth II anastomosis, Roux-en-Y anastomosis after total laparoscopic gastrectomy of distal gastric cancer, functional esophageal-jejunal lateral-lateral anastomosis, Orvil anastomosis and overlapping techniques.

In this chapter, we introduce triangle anastomosis (Billroth I), Billroth II after distal gastrectomy, and functional esophageal jejunostomy after total gastrectomy. During the reconstruction of the digestive tract, the trocar site, the patient's location, and the surgeon's location are the same as those during the LN dissection (see Chap. 1 of this book).

The procedure was approved by the institutional review board of Fujian Medical University Union Hospital. All patients received written informed consent prior to surgery.

6.1 Modified Delta-Shaped Billroth I Anastomosis After TLDG

6.1.1 Anastomosis Method

The DSG is a functional anastomosis end-to-end of the posterior gastric wall and the posterior duodenal bulb wall, using endoscopic linear staplers. DSG is named after the internal triangular anastomosis line.

6.1.2 Technical Tips

After completing laparoscopic LN dissection, a linear stapler is inserted through the left upper major trocar, positioned across the duodenum vertical to the long axis in the predetermined position, and fired to transect the duodenum by rotating 90° from back to front (Fig. 6.1).

Two staplers were used to resect the stomach from the greater to the lesser curvature (Fig. 6.2).

The specimen is placed in a plastic bag. A small incision is created on the posterior duodenum wall and another incision is created on the remnant stomach greater curvature (Figs. 6.3 and 6.4).

C.-M. Huang et al., *Atlas of Laparoscopic Gastrectomy for Gastric Cancer*,
https://doi.org/10.1007/978-981-13-2862-6_6

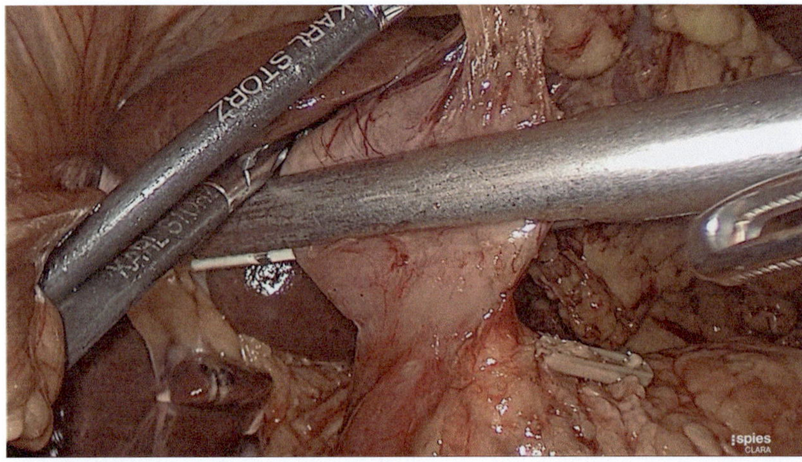

Fig. 6.1 Transecting the duodenum using linear stapler

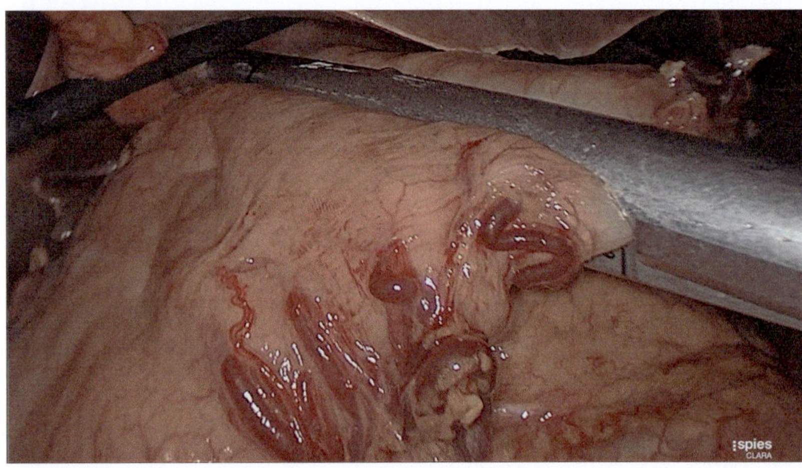

Fig. 6.2 Resecting the stomach using linear stapler

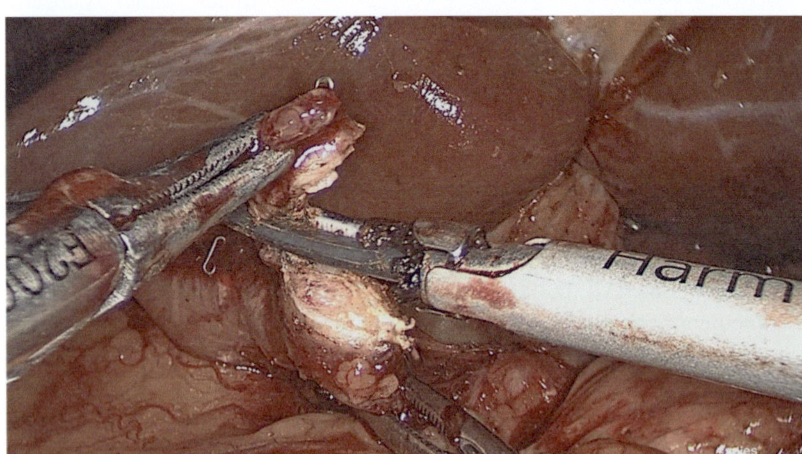

Fig. 6.3 A small incision is created on the posterior duodenum wall

Due to the greater mobility of the stomach, one limb of the stapler is first inserted into the incision on the greater curvature side of the remnant stomach, and the predetermined anastomotic site on the posterior wall should be 2 cm away from the cutting edge. Another limb of the stapler is insected on the duodenum posterior side, and the cutting edge of the duodenum is rotated 90° in a counterclockwise direction. The duodenum posterior side is anastomosed to the remnant stomach (Fig. 6.5).

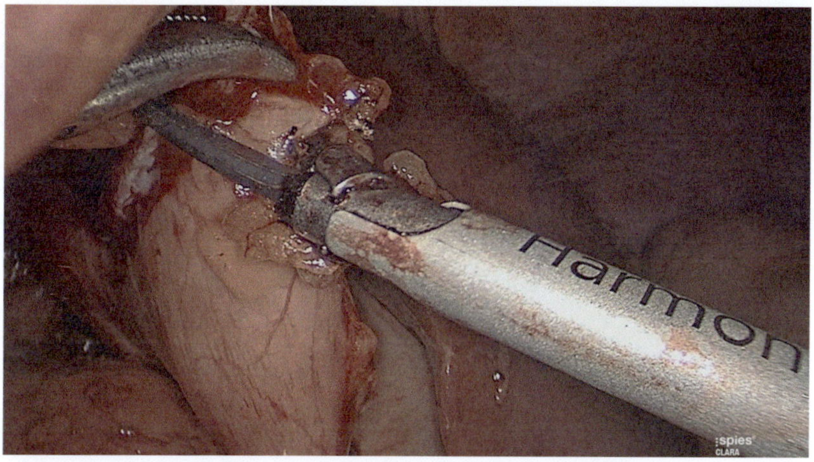

Fig. 6.4 A small incision is created on the remnant stomach greater curvature

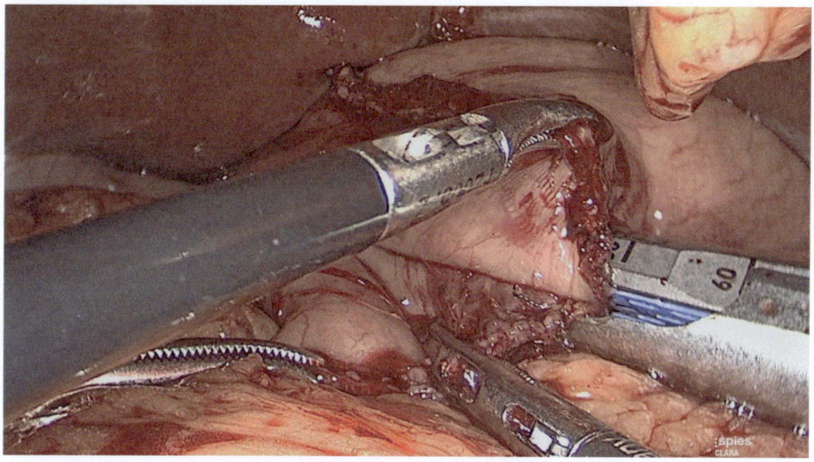

Fig. 6.5 The posterior duodenum was anastomosed with the residual stomach using a linear stapler

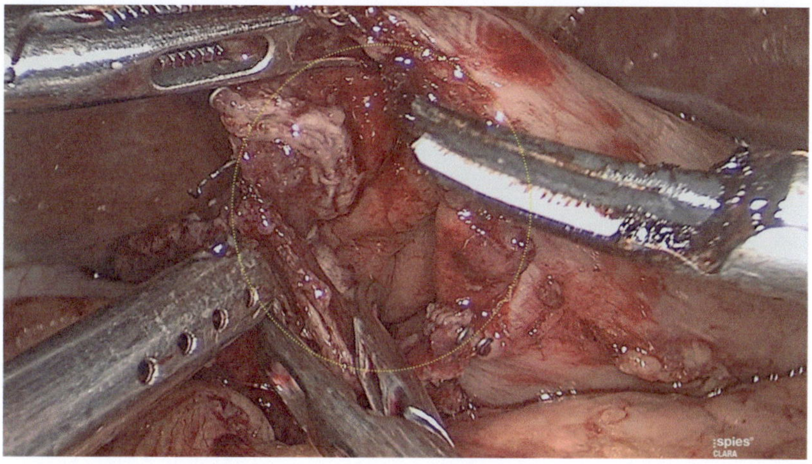

Fig. 6.6 The common stapler incision is checked

After the anastomosis quality was confirmed through the common incision (Fig. 6.6), three sutures were created at each end of the common incision and at the cutting edge of the stomach and duodenum for better involution and pull (Fig. 6.7). Finally, the common incision is closed using the linear stapler (Fig. 6.8), resulting in the modified DSG (Figs. 6.9 and 6.10). The trocar incision below the umbilicus was prolonged to 3 cm to withdraw the specimen.

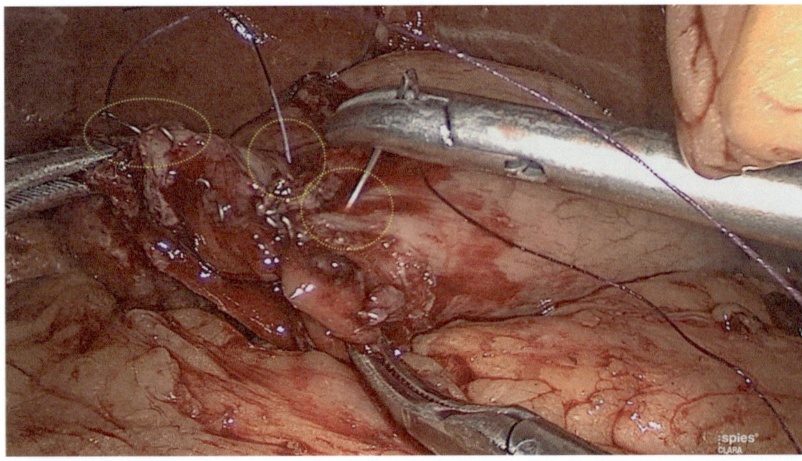

Fig. 6.7 Three sutures are created to each end and the middle position of the common incision

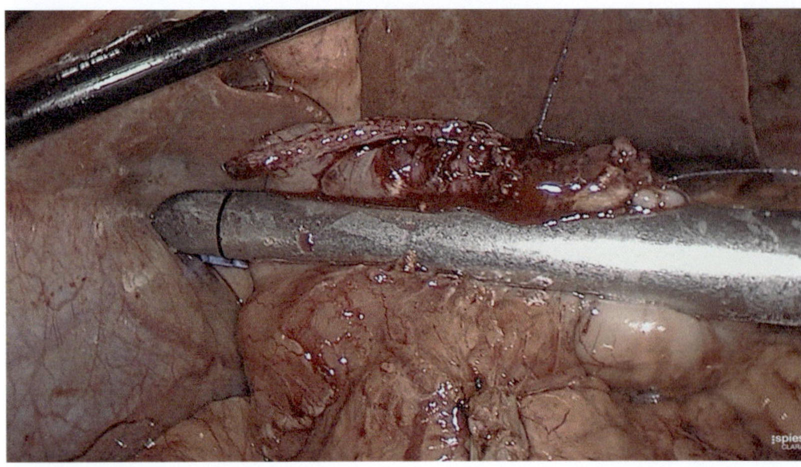

Fig. 6.8 The common incision is closed using the linear stapler

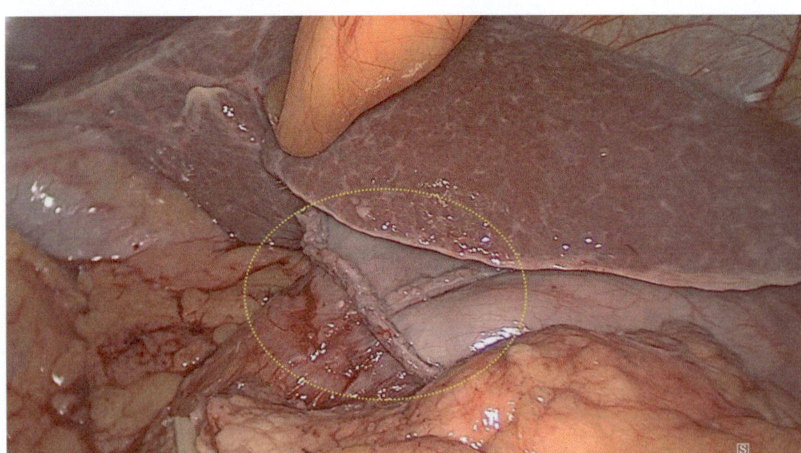

Fig. 6.9 The appearance of the modified DSG anastomosis

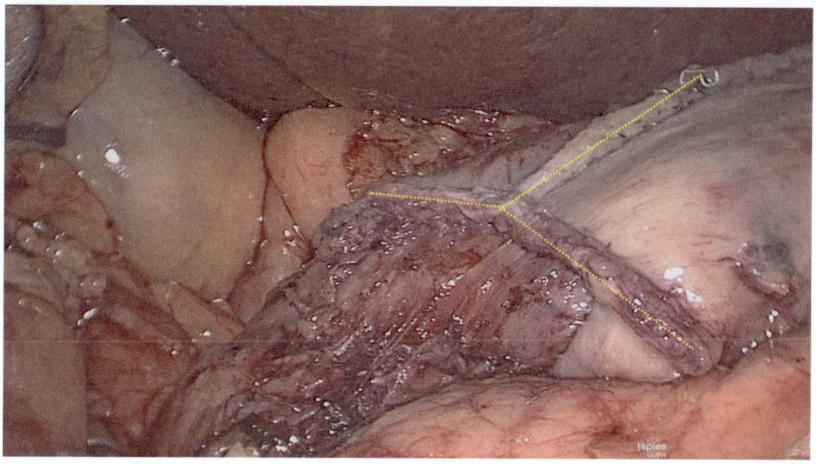

Fig. 6.10 The inverted "T" shaped appearance of the modified DSG anastomosis

6.2 Billroth II Anastomosis After TLDG

6.2.1 Anastomosis Method

The linear stapler under total laparoscopy is used to create functional lateral-lateral gastrojejunostomy. Billroth II anastomosis can also be safely performed to achieve R0 resection, even if the tumor invades the pylorus or duodenum.

6.2.2 Technical Tips

The digestive tract is reconstructed using a linear stapler after laparoscopic LN dissection. Linear endoscopic stapler is used to transect duodenum at a predetermined position after complete dissociation, and two staplers were used to resect the stomach from the greater curvature to the lesser curvature. Then, the specimen is placed into a plastic specimen bag. Small incisions are created on the greater curvature of the remnant stomach and the anti-mesenteric side of the jejunum located 12–15 cm distal to the Treitz ligament (Fig. 6.11).

After the 60-mm endoscopic linear stapler is opened, one stapler limb is first inserted into the jejunum incision towards the direction of the jejunal proximal end, and the stapler is closed temporarily. The jejunum is pulled out forward, and the other limb of stapler is inserted into the incision on the remnant stomach greater curvature. The stapler is fired to complete a side-to-side gastrojejunostomy with a common stab incision (Fig. 6.12).

During anastomosis, the afferent loop of the proximal jejunum should not be long, as it may cause internal herniation or ischemic necrosis by tortuosity or torsion of the intestine. After checking the anastomosis through the common incision (Fig. 6.13), using atraumatic grasping device to stretch both ends of common stab incision to align both ends of the common stab incision are pulled to be aligned, using atraumatic graspers. Three sutures are added at each end of the common stab incision to achieve better involution and tension. The common stab incision is closed using the 60-mm linear stapler (Fig. 6.14), performing the reconstruction (Fig. 6.15). The trocar incision below the umbilicus is prolonged to 3 cm to withdraw the specimen.

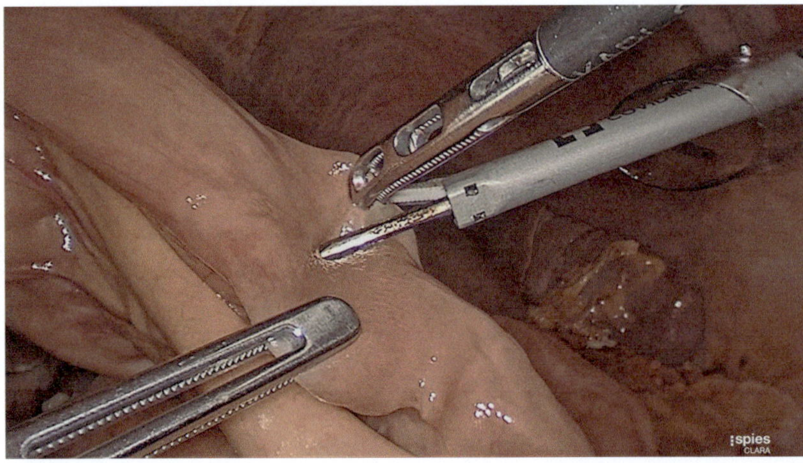

Fig. 6.11 A small incision is created on the antemesenteric side of jejunum 12–15 cm from the distal end of the Treitz ligament

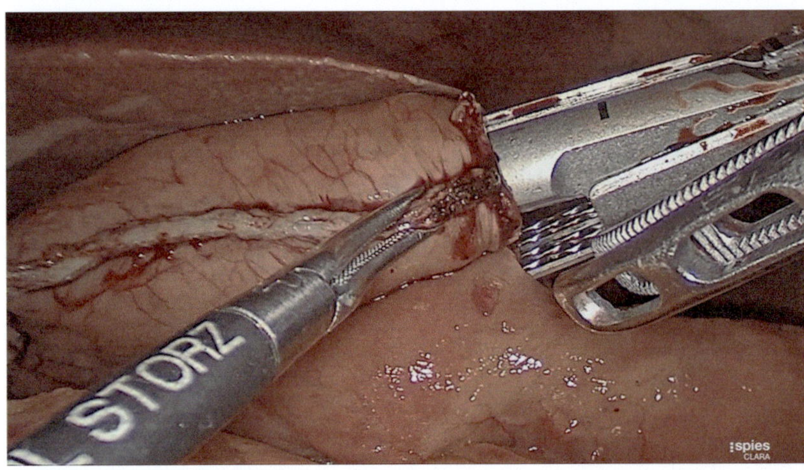

Fig. 6.12 The linear stapler is fired to complete the side-to-side gastrojejunostomy

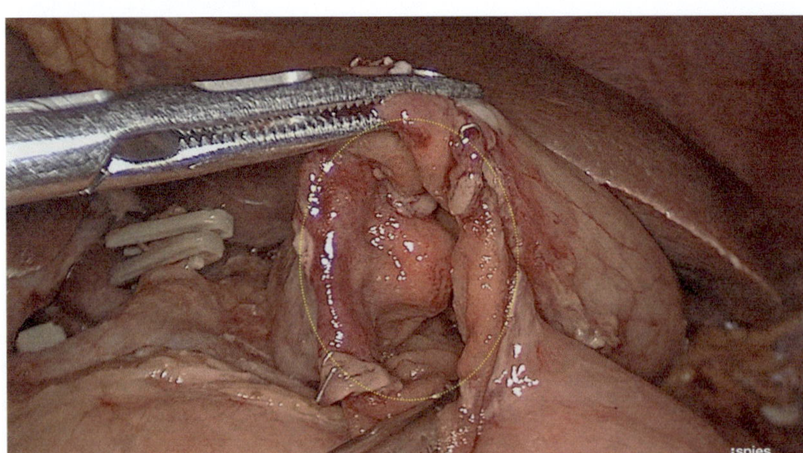

Fig. 6.13 Anastomosis quality is confirmed via the common incision

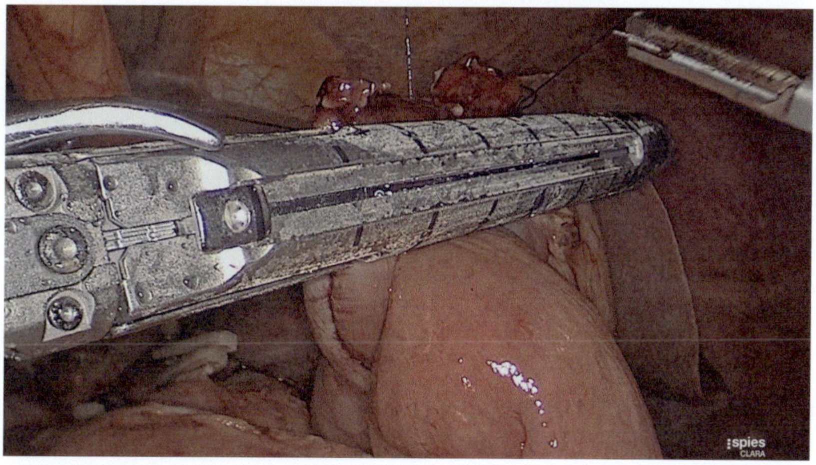

Fig. 6.14 The common incision is closed with the linear stapler

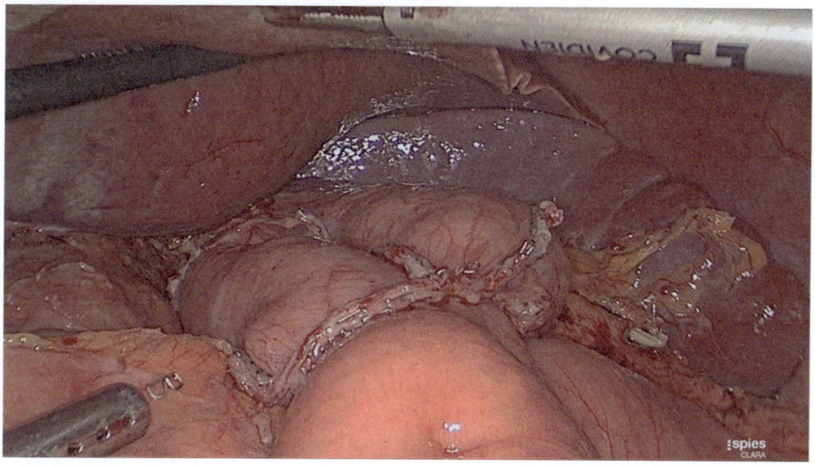

Fig. 6.15 The appearance of the anastomosis after reconstruction

6.3 Isoperistaltic Jejunum-Later-Cut Overlap for Esophagojejunostomy Anastomosis After Total Laparoscopic Total Gastrectomy

6.3.1 Anastomosis Method

After laparoscopic LN dissection and mobilization of the esophagus and duodenum, they were transected in a predetermined position employing a linear stapler. After isoperistaltic side-to-side esophagojejunostomy anastomosis, the jejunum is transected and side-to-side jejunojejunostomy is completed.

6.3.2 Technical Tips

After laparoscopic LN dissection, the stomach is pulled to expose and dissect the vagus nerve, and the esophagus is mobilized at least 5 cm above the tumor margin to confirm negative cutting margin. The duodenum is transected in predetermined positions using a linear stapler, following adequate mobilization, (Fig. 6.16). The esophagus is transected away from the cardia appling a linear stapler (Fig. 6.17).

Small incisions are made on the left side of the esophagectomy margin and on the boundary of the mesenteric membrane of the jejunum about 20 cm from the Treitz ligament (Figs. 6.18 and 6.19).

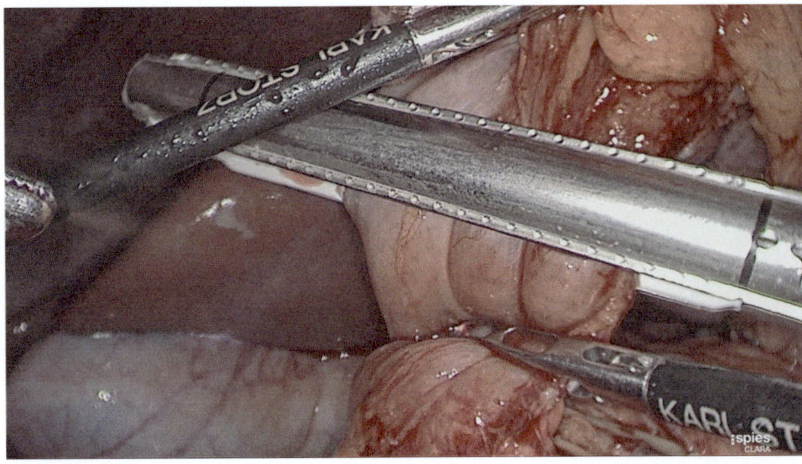

Fig. 6.16 A linear stapler is used to transect the duodenum

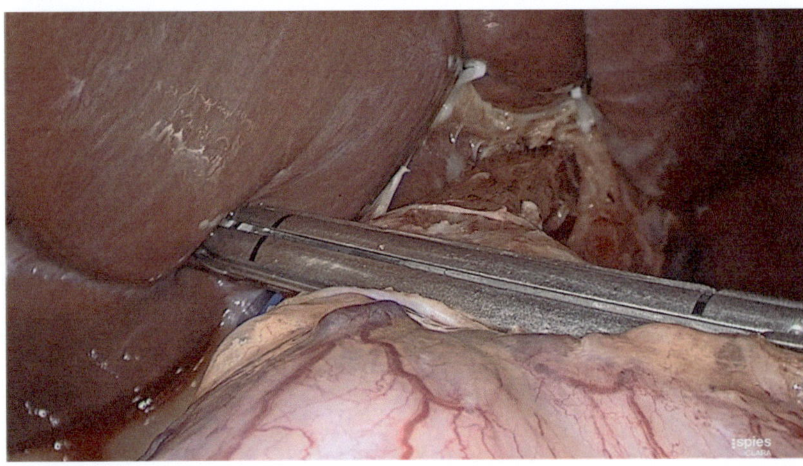

Fig. 6.17 The abdominal esophagus is transected with an endoscopic linear stapler

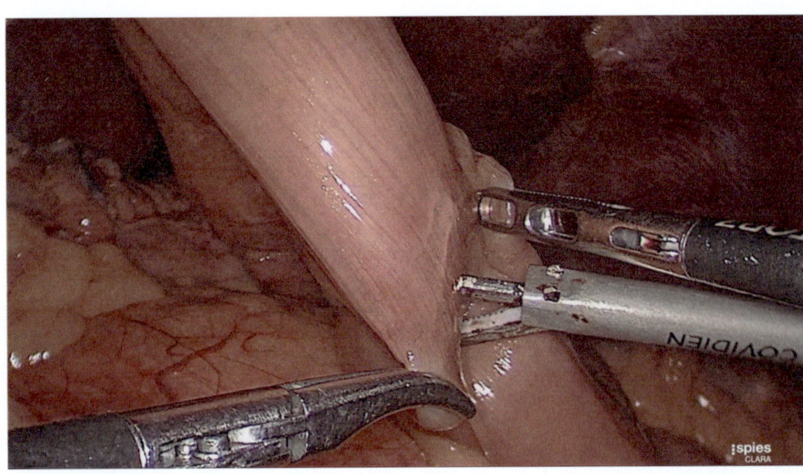

Fig. 6.18 Small incisions are created on the antimesenteric border of the jejunum

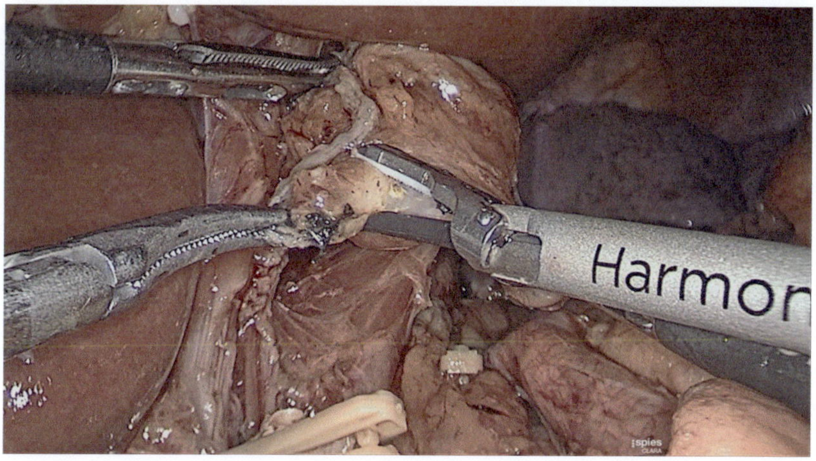

Fig. 6.19 Small incisions are created on the left side of the resection margin of the esophagus

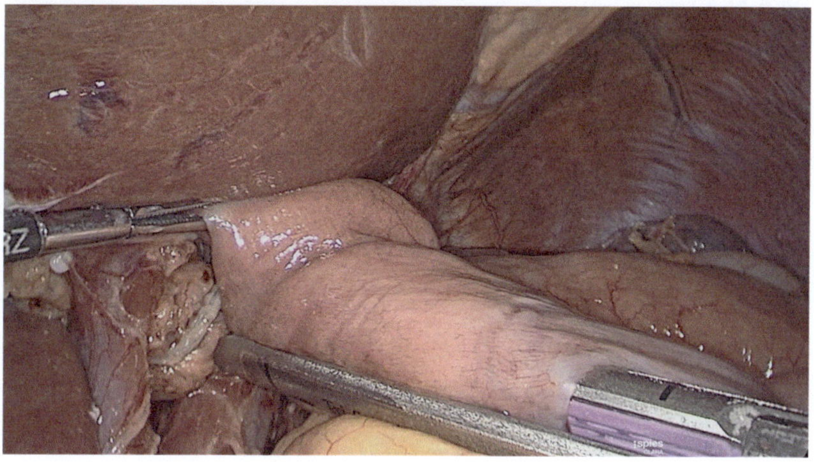

Fig. 6.20 One limb of the linear stapler is first inserted into the jejunum incision

After each incision is inserted into one of the limbs of the stapler, the fork of the stapler is closed and fired to perform a side-to-side esophagojejunostomy. Due to the larger mobility of jejunum, one limb of the 60 mm endoscopic linear stapler is first positioned on the jejunum incision and the other limb was inserted into the esophagus.

After inserting one limb of the stapler in each incision, the forks of the stapler are closed and fired, carrying out side-to-side esophagojejunostomy. Because of the greater mobility of the jejunum, one limb of the 60 mm endoscopic linear stapler is first inserted into the jejunum incision and the other limb is positioned on the esophagus. The stapler's fork is then closed and fired for a contralateral esophageal jejunostomy. Confirmation of no injury or bleeding is made via the common stab incision, which is then manually sutured (Figs. 6.20 and 6.21).

Confirmation of no injury or bleeding is made through the common incision (Fig. 6.22), which is then manually sutured (Figs. 6.23 and 6.24).

After mobilize the mesenteric border around 1 cm from the jejunum wall and around 3 cm from

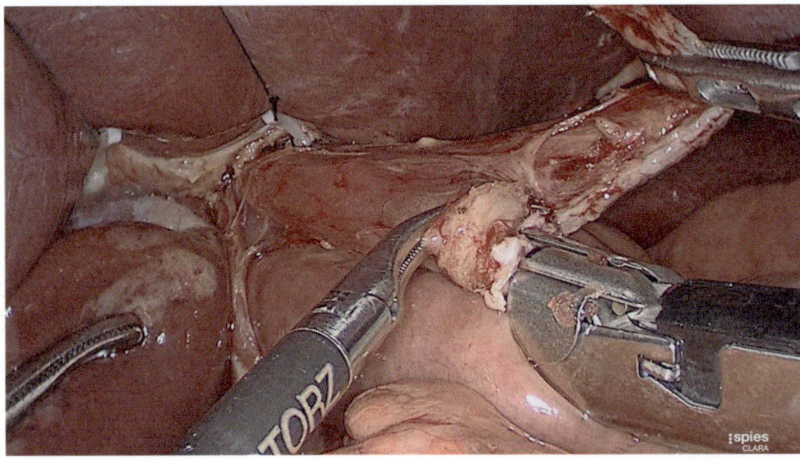

Fig. 6.21 An endoscopic linear stapler is applied to perform side-to-side esophagojejunostomy

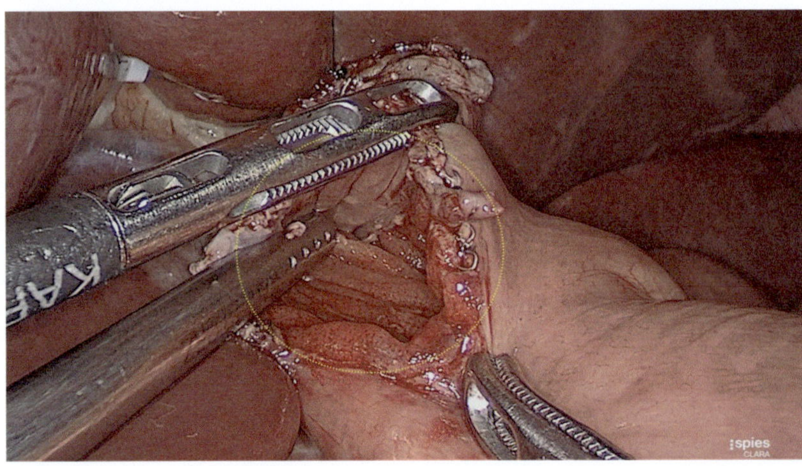

Fig. 6.22 Checking the common stab incision

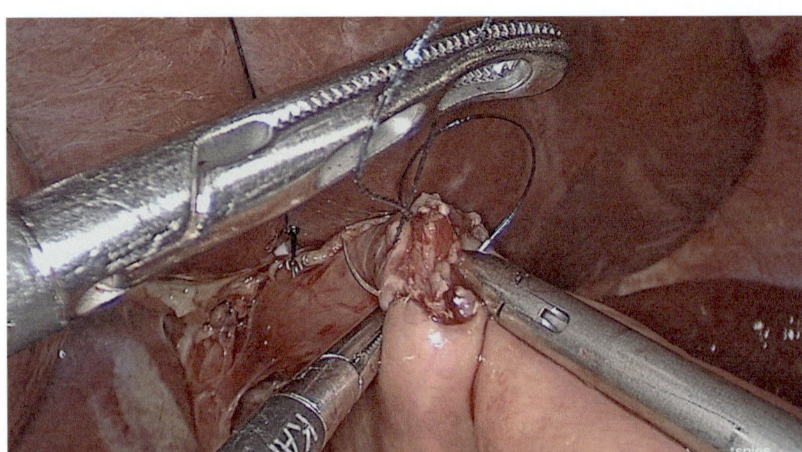

Fig. 6.23 Manually suturing the common stab incision

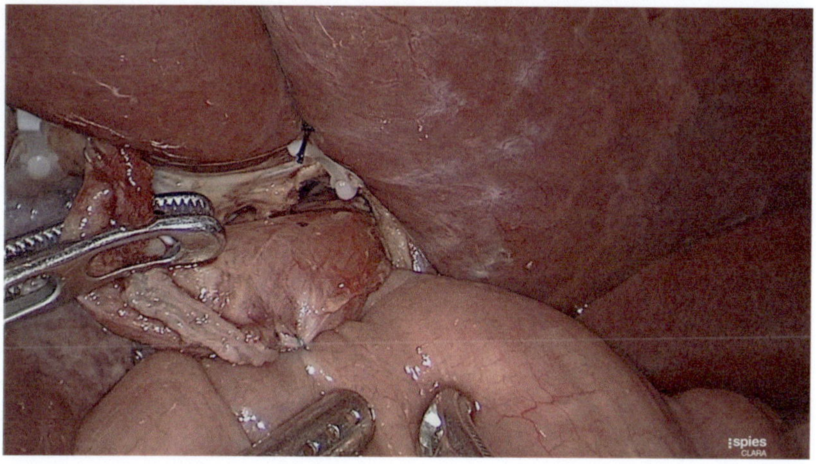

Fig. 6.24 The esophagojejunostomy is completed

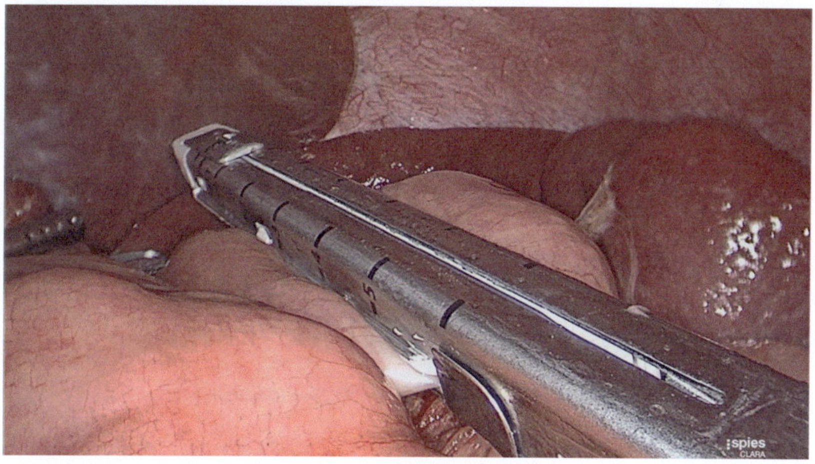

Fig. 6.25 Jejunum-later-cut method using an endoscopic linear stapler

the esophagojejunostomy, the jejunum is transected (Fig. 6.25).

Small incisions were made at the boundary of the antimesentery of the proximal jejunum and the boundary of the distal jejunum, about 40-45 cm from the esophageal-jejunum anastomosis. Then, a limb of the stapler is inserted into each incision, and the stapler fork is closed and fired to achieve lateral-lateral jejunojejunostomy (Fig. 6.26). The jejunal mucosa was confirmed free of injury or bleeding through the common stab incision, then it is laparoscopically sutured (Figs. 6.27 and 6.28).

The appearance of the incision after total laparoscopic radical gastrectomy for gastric cancer (Fig. 6.29).

Clarification

All images of the chapter come from FuJian Medical University gastric surgery database and video database.

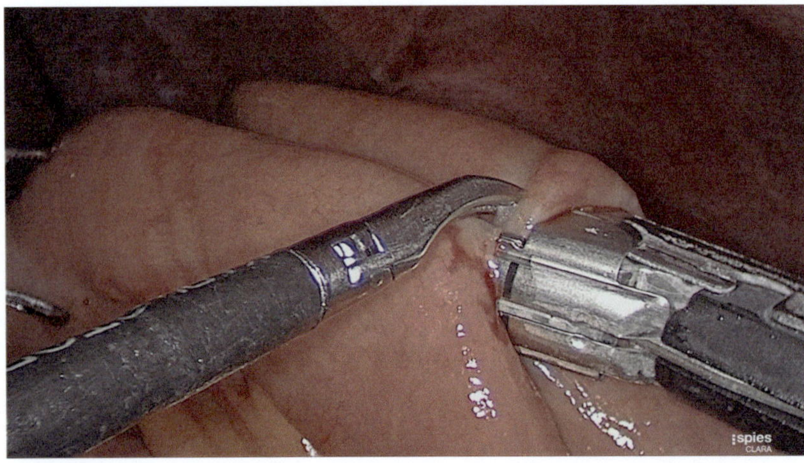

Fig. 6.26 Closing and firing the forks of the stapler to achieve side-to-side jejunojejunostomy

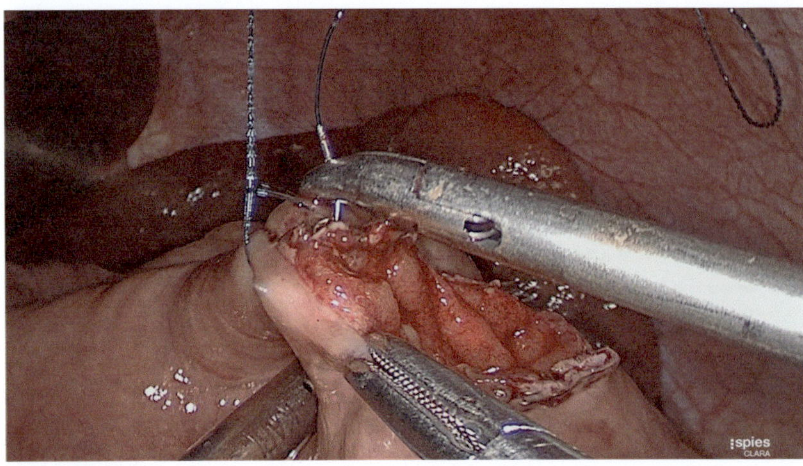

Fig. 6.27 Suturing the common stab under laparoscopy

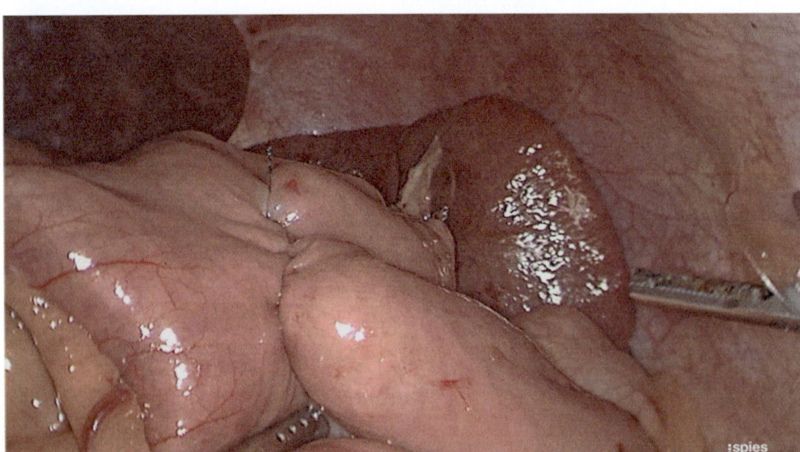

Fig. 6.28 Completing side-to-side jejunojejunostomy

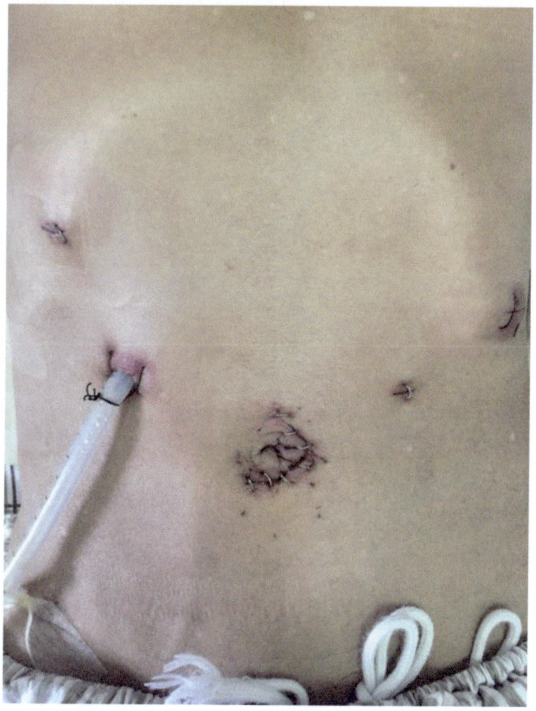

Fig. 6.29 The appearance of the incision after total laparoscopic gastrectomy

MIX
Papier aus verantwortungsvollen Quellen
Paper from responsible sources
FSC® C105338

If you have any concerns about our products,
you can contact us on
ProductSafety@springernature.com

In case Publisher is established outside the EU,
the EU authorized representative is:
Springer Nature Customer Service Center GmbH
Europaplatz 3, 69115 Heidelberg, Germany

Printed by Libri Plureos GmbH
in Hamburg, Germany